Experts' Perspectives on Medical Advances

This book series presents Chinese experts' perspectives on recent developments in clinical medicine. Written by leading Chinese experts in related fields, a wide variety of emerging and hot topics in internal medicine, surgery, oncology, neurosurgery, and ophthalmonology, etc., is covered by the series. Each title in this series covers a disease or a group of diseases, focusing on the basic knowledge, development and the latest research progress of clinical practice. This series is a practical and useful resource for researchers and practitioners in related subjects, as well as for general interest readers.

Jianqiang Cai
Editor

Chunguang Guo • Dongbing Zhao
Translators

Interpretation of Gastric Cancer Cases

科学技术文献出版社
SCIENTIFIC AND TECHNICAL DOCUMENTATION PRESS
·北京·

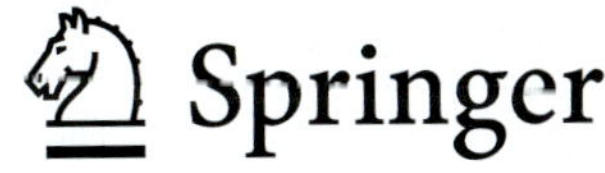

Editor
Jianqiang Cai
Department of Hepatobiliary Surgery
National Cancer Center/National Clinical Research for Cancer/Cancer Hospital
Chinese Academy of Medical Sciences and Peking Union Medical College
Beijing, China

Translators
Chunguang Guo
Department of Pancreatic and Gastric Surgical Oncology
National Cancer Center/National Clinical Research for Cancer/Cancer Hospital, Chinese Academy of Medical Sciences and Peking Union Medical College
Beijing, China

Dongbing Zhao
Department of Pancreatic and Gastric Surgical Oncology
National Cancer Center/National Clinical Research for Cancer/Cancer Hospital, Chinese Academy of Medical Sciences and Peking Union Medical College
Beijing, China

ISSN 2948-1023 ISSN 2948-1031 (electronic)
Experts' Perspectives on Medical Advances
ISBN 978-981-99-5304-2 ISBN 978-981-99-5302-8 (eBook)
https://doi.org/10.1007/978-981-99-5302-8
Jointly published with Scientific and Technical Documentation Press

This Springer imprint is published by the registered company Springer Nature Singapore Pte Ltd.
The registered company address is: 152 Beach Road, #21-01/04 Gateway East, Singapore 189721, Singapore

Preface

Gastric cancer is a common malignant tumor of digestive tract in China, with incidence rate and mortality ranking second in malignant tumors. On a global scale, China is also a major country in gastric cancer, with nearly half of the world's gastric cancer cases occurring in China. Along with the heavy burden of tumors, the overall efficacy of gastric cancer is not ideal, which is related to the late discovery of gastric cancer and poor comprehensive treatment effect. Most gastric cancer patients are diagnosed as mid to late stage at the first visit, which poses great difficulties in improving the efficacy of gastric cancer. Therefore, the focus of gastric cancer treatment in China is to promote tumor screening, early diagnosis, and treatment for high-risk populations on the one hand; on the other hand, emphasis is placed on the comprehensive treatment of mid- to late-stage cases.

After decades of exploration in basic clinical research on cancer, the comprehensive efficacy of gastric cancer has significantly improved. Especially in recent years, with the advent of a large number of new drugs and the progress of surgical technology, such as laparoscopy, perioperative chemotherapy, multidisciplinary diagnosis and treatment mode, targeted and immunotherapy, the quality of life and prognosis of gastric cancer patients have been greatly improved. In the era of evidence-based medicine, how to standardize the application of new technologies and new concepts, promote the replacement of new and old medical knowledge, and promote the progress of the overall diagnosis and treatment level of clinicians is an urgent problem facing current medical education. Especially in the face of China's vast territory and uneven regional medical development level, it is particularly important to drive the improvement of the technical level of grassroots medical units. The National Cancer Center/Cancer Hospital of the Chinese Academy of Medical Sciences is a specialized oncology medical center with a 60-year history. It undertakes a large number of clinical drug research and development and clinical research tasks every year and has rich experience in the diagnosis and treatment of gastric cancer surgery and comprehensive treatment. Therefore, this book carefully selects several representative cases, covering minimally invasive procedure, transformation research, individualized treatment, and many other aspects of gastric cancer. I hope to comprehensively introduce the latest diagnostic and treatment technologies for gastric cancer through the analysis of specific cases, from shallow to deep, and popularize the treatment methods and concepts for gastric cancer.

For the convenience of reading, this book divides the content into the following aspects based on the hot topics of gastric cancer, such as treatment options for early gastric cancer, progress and application of laparoscopic gastric cancer surgery, management of complications in gastric cancer surgery, exploration of transformation therapy for advanced gastric cancer, and treatment of special types of gastric cancer. Each case should be emphasized and fully explained. We hope that this book will not only serve as a reference book, but also help readers navigate the map and solve the confusion of specific clinical scenarios. We also hope to provide valuable insights and stimulate thinking. For the convenience of reading, a large number of images and surgical videos are also provided in the article, in order to comprehensively review the original appearance of the case.

During the compilation process of this book, thanks to the strong assistance of our brother departments and the hard work of the editorial committee, we were able to complete it as scheduled during the busy clinical work. We sincerely appreciate this! We have repeatedly checked and revised the content of the entire book, striving for accuracy. Due to limited knowledge and the rapid development of clinical knowledge, mistakes are inevitable. We sincerely request criticism and correction from colleagues.

Beijing, China Jianqiang Cai

Contents

About the Editors

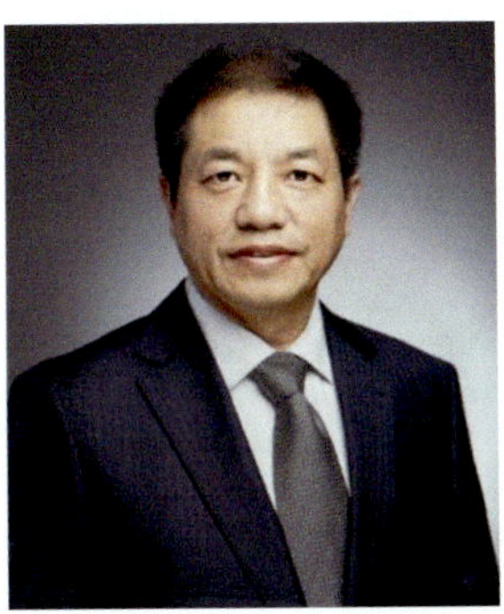

Jianqiang Cai Chief physician, professor, doctoral supervisor. He is now the deputy director of the National Cancer Center, the vice president of the Cancer Hospital of the Chinese Academy of Medical Sciences, and enjoys the special allowance of the State Council. He is a young and middle-aged expert with outstanding contributions from the National Health and Family Planning Commission. He is also a member of the Surgery Branch of the Chinese Medical Association, a standing member of the Oncology Branch of the Chinese Medical Association, a vice chairman of the Liver Cancer Committee of the Chinese Medical Association, a vice chairman of the Prevention and Control Committee of the Hepatobiliary and Pancreatic Diseases of the Chinese Preventive Medicine Association, a chairman of the Colorectal Cancer Liver Metastasis Treatment Committee of the China Association for International Exchange and Promotion of Health Care, a chairman of the Sarcoma Committee of the Chinese Anti-Cancer Association.

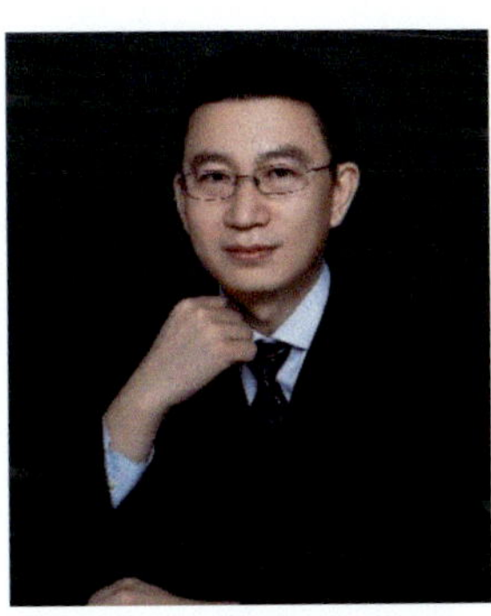

Chunguang Guo Associate Chief Physician of Pancreatogastric Surgery, PhD in Cancer Hospital Chinese Academy of Medical Sciences. I have been working in the surgery of digestive tract tumors for over 10 years, specializing in the surgical treatment of gastrointestinal and pancreatic tumors, especially laparoscopic minimally invasive treatment. Currently, research is mainly focused on predicting the risk of lymph node metastasis in early gastric cancer and the transformation therapy of gastric cancer. I have undertaken and participated in multiple national level projects and published over ten Chinese and English academic works. I served as the leader of the Upper Gastrointestinal Cancer Technical Group of the National Urban Cancer Early Diagnosis and Treatment Project of the National Cancer Center. Visiting scholar at the Dana Farber Cancer Center at Harvard Medical School in the United States. I also served as a young member of the Gastric Cancer Professional Committee of the China Anti-Cancer Association, a member of the Gastric Cancer Professional Committee of the Beijing Cancer Prevention and Treatment Association, a member of the Rehabilitation Association of the China Anti-Cancer Association, the Abdominal Tumor Professional Committee of the China Medical Education Association, a member of the Health

Science Popularization Branch, Colorectal Disease Branch, Pancreatic Gland Disease Branch of the China Medical Promotion Association, and other academic groups.

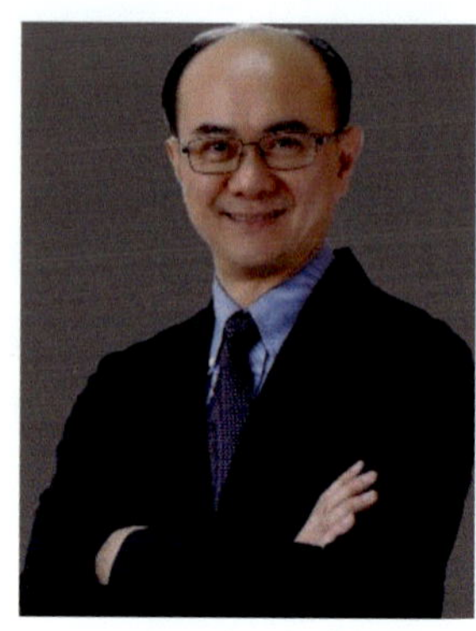

Dongbing Zhao Chief Physician, Professor, Doctoral Supervisor, PhD in Cancer Hospital Chinese Academy of Medical Sciences. Deputy Director and Secretary of the Pancreatogastric Surgery Department of the National Cancer Center/Cancer Hospital of the Chinese Academy of Medical Sciences, Chairman of the Neuroendocrine Oncology Professional Committee of the Chinese Medical Association, Chairman of the Gastric Cancer Professional Committee of the Beijing Oncology Society, Deputy Leader of the Gastrointestinal Group of the Surgical Professional Committee of the Beijing Medical Association, Deputy Chairman of the Gastrointestinal Oncology Professional Committee of the National Telemedicine and Internet Center, and Standing Committee Member of the Endoscopy Professional Committee of the Chinese Anti-Cancer Association, Member of the Standing Committee of the Oncology Branch of the Beijing Medical Association, Member of the Gastric Cancer Professional Committee of the China Anti-Cancer Association, Member of the Surgical Oncology Professional Committee of the Chinese Medical Doctor Association, Member of the International Hepatobiliary Pancreatic Association, Member of the Beijing Cancer Treatment Quality Control and Improvement Center, Member of the Beijing Medical Accident Evaluation Committee, Visiting Scholar at the Royal Cancer Institute and Hong Kong Christian Hospital.

1 The Surgical Management of the Early Gastric Cancer

Hong Zhou, Chunguang Guo, Yingtai Chen, and Dongbing Zhao

1.1 Case 1: Rescue Surgery for Early Gastric Cancer After Endoscopic Submucosal Dissection

1.1.1 Brief History

The patient, a 49-year-old female, presented with a chief complaint of persistent epigastric discomfort over a span of 4 months, with a recent exacerbation within the past month. Initially, the patient experienced intermittent epigastric discomfort of unknown etiology, which subsequently intensified following meals, accompanied by symptoms of acid reflux and heartburn. Upon upper gastrointestinal endoscopy examination, a superficial depressed lesion was observed in the gastric sinus, raising suspicion of early gastric cancer or a precancerous lesion (see Fig. 1.1). Pathological analysis of the biopsy sample revealed severe atypical hyperplasia, suggesting the potential for local infiltration. Ultrasound endoscopy unveiled thickening of the gastric wall's mucosal layer, with a maximum thickness measuring approximately 4.6 mm (see Fig. 1.2). The lesion exhibited a close association with the submucosal layer of the gastric wall at various levels, and demarcation between the two was indistinct. Conversely, the intrinsic muscular and plasma layers of the gastric wall remained transparent, continuous, and intact. The lesion primarily involved the mucosal layer, extending into the submucosal layer. Computed tomography (CT) scanning did not reveal any abnormalities. Although the patient's medical history lacked noteworthy aspects, the physical examination yielded negative findings.

1.1.2 Treatment

Following the comprehensive examination, successful endoscopic submucosal dissection (ESD) was performed in the Endoscopy Department (see Fig. 1.3). The subsequent postoperative pathology evaluation revealed the macroscopic features of a mucosal tissue specimen measuring 4.5 cm × 4.0 cm × 0.2 cm, displaying a slightly depressed area with grayish yellow mucosa located 1.1 cm from the nearest cutting edge (anal edge). Microscopically, the tumor was found to have invaded the submucosal layer, reaching a depth of 1200 μm (1325 μm in thick-

H. Zhou
Department of Breast Surgical Oncology, National Cancer Center/National Clinical Research Center for Cancer/Cancer Hospital & Shenzhen Hospital, Chinese Academy of Medical Sciences and Peking Union Medical College, Shenzhen, China

C. Guo (✉) · Y. Chen · D. Zhao
Department of Pancreatic and Gastric Surgical Oncology, National Cancer Center/National Clinical Research for Cancer/Cancer Hospital, Chinese Academy of Medical Sciences and Peking Union Medical College, Beijing, China

J. Cai (ed.), *Interpretation of Gastric Cancer Cases*, Experts' Perspectives on Medical Advances,
https://doi.org/10.1007/978-981-99-5302-8_1

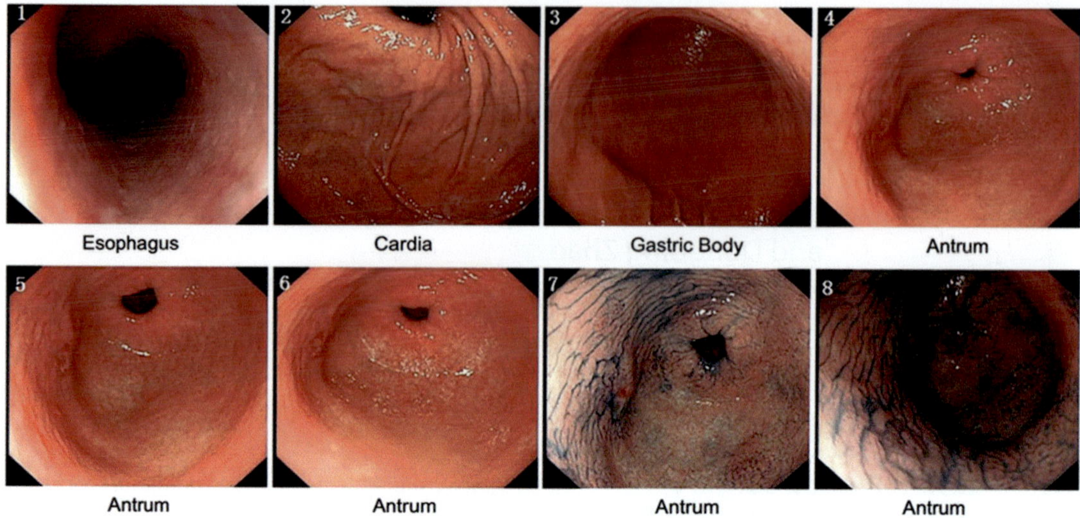

Fig. 1.1 Gastroscopy revealed the presence of a shallow concave lesion located in the gastric antrum, suggesting an early gastric cancer or a precancerous lesion

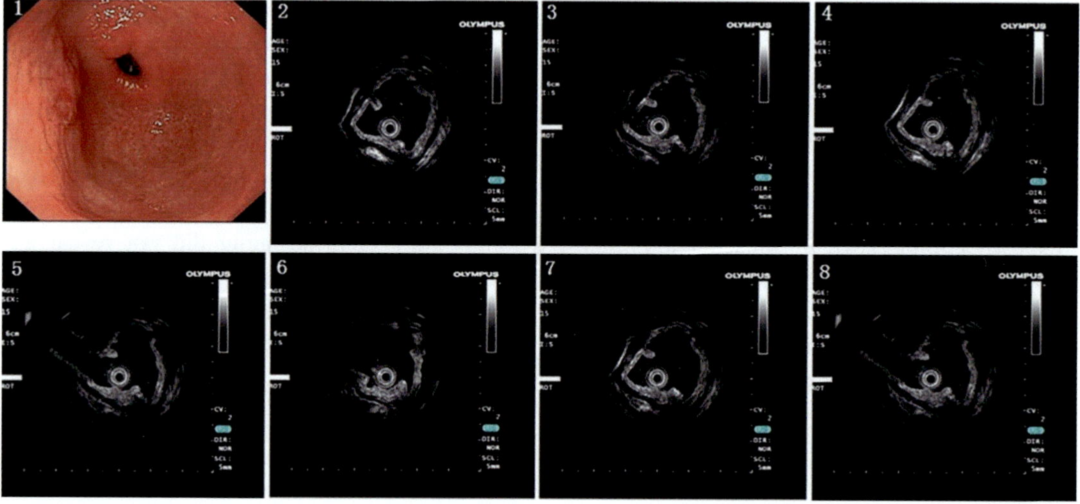

Fig. 1.2 Endoscopic ultrasonography demonstrated predominant thickening of the gastric wall's mucosal layer, with the maximum thickness measuring approximately 4.6 mm. The lesions exhibited a close association with the submucosa of the gastric wall, and the demarcation between them was not clearly discernible

ness when examined under microscopy). Immunohistochemistry results further suggested suspicious invasion of the wall of small veins by the tumor. The surrounding gastric mucosa exhibited focal chronic atrophic gastritis with focal intestinal epithelial hyperplasia and mild atypical hyperplasia in focal glands. No carcinoma or atypical hyperplasia was detected in the lateral and basal margins.

Considering the invasion depth of the submucosal layer exceeding 500 μm and the suspicion of venous invasion, an additional laparoscopic-assisted radical gastrectomy was performed, followed by Billroth I reconstruction. The patient's recovery progressed uneventfully, with a transition to a liquid diet on the third day and removal of the abdominal drainage tube on the sixth day postoperatively. Ultimately, the patient was discharged 12 days after the procedure.

Pathological evaluation of the resected specimen revealed the macroscopic features of the dis-

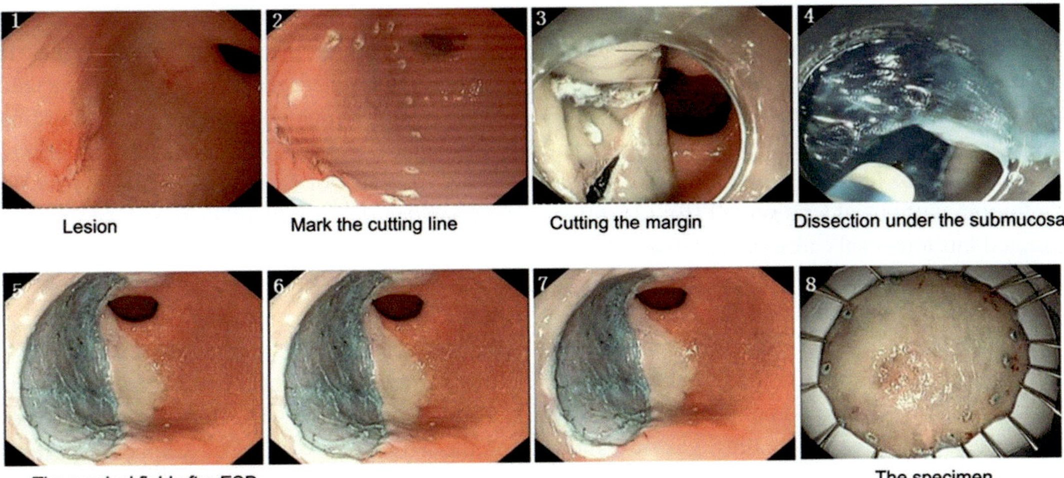

Fig. 1.3 Sequential depiction of the Endoscopic Submucosal Dissection (ESD) treatment procedure

tal partial stomach measuring 10 cm × 7 cm, with a small portion of the duodenal section measuring 5 cm in circumference and 1 cm in length. Thickening of the gastric wall near the duodenum was observed, along with a flat coarse granular area of mucosa measuring 4.5 cm × 3.0 cm located 1 cm from the upper margin. Microscopic examination, following ample sampling and immunohistochemical analysis, indicated the absence of any residual tumor in the gastric wall tissue. Various tissue alterations, including inflammatory cell infiltration, fibrous tissue proliferation, and foam cell aggregation, were consistent with histological changes following treatment. No tumor was identified at the upper margin, lower margin, or greater omentum. Furthermore, no lymph node metastasis was detected among the 18 lymph nodes examined (0/18). The final TNM staging was classified as pT1bN0M0.

1.1.3 Case Analysis

Early gastric cancer (EGC) refers to lesions that are limited to the mucosa or submucosa, regardless of lymph node metastasis. Unlike advanced gastric cancer, EGC exhibits a low rate of lymph node metastasis and generally has a favorable prognosis. Traditional gastrectomy, however, is associated with various short- and long-term drawbacks, including postoperative gastrointestinal symptoms such as weight loss, malnutrition, and anemia. These complications significantly impact long-term quality of life. With the advancement of minimally invasive surgical techniques, preserving gastric function has become a prominent focus in the management of EGC.

Endoscopic Submucosal Dissection (ESD) is a minimally invasive procedure commonly used to treat benign lesions, such as polyps and early gastrointestinal tumors. During the ESD procedure, a separator is injected into the deeper layer surrounding the lesion, and the physician carefully removes the mucosal or submucosal layers using an electric knife, effectively excising the lesion. ESD evolved from the earlier technique known as endoscopic mucosal resection (EMR). However, EMR faces limitations in the en bloc removal of lesions larger than 2 cm in diameter and determining tumor staging and margins, which can lead to residual lesions and recurrence. In order to overcome these limitations, Japanese scholars pioneered the ESD technique. Although technically more challenging than EMR and associated with longer operative times and a higher complication rate, ESD offers a higher likelihood of achieving complete resection, enables thorough histopathological evaluation, and reduces the risk of recurrence. As a result, ESD has replaced EMR as the preferred endoscopic approach for early gastrointestinal tumors.

The Expert Consensus Opinion on Standardized Endoscopic Resection of Early Gastric Cancer (2018, Beijing) outlines the indications for endoscopic treatment, categorized as absolute and relative indications. Absolute indications include: (1) differentiated intramucosal carcinoma without ulceration (cT1a); (2) differentiated intramucosal carcinoma with ulceration, provided it is less than 3 cm in diameter (cT1a); (3) high-grade intraepithelial neoplasia of gastric mucosa. Relative indications encompass undifferentiated intramucosal carcinoma (cT1a) with lesion size ≤2 cm and no ulceration [1]. The Japanese Guidelines for treating gastric cancer classify indications as absolute, expanded, and relative. Absolute indications for ESD or EMR include differentiated adenocarcinoma without ulceration, with a maximum tumor diameter of ≤2 cm and clinically diagnosed as T1a. Relative indications consist of: (1) differentiated carcinoma without ulceration confined to the mucosa, with a diameter >2 cm; (2) differentiated carcinoma with ulceration, limited to the mucosa, and a maximum diameter ≤3 cm. Expanded indications cover undifferentiated carcinoma without ulceration, located within the mucosal layer and ≤2 cm in maximum diameter, although these cases are not included in the absolute indications due to insufficient evidence. Patients who do not meet the absolute or expanded indications fall under the category of relative indications. In such cases, endoscopic resection may be suggested after thorough communication between the physician and patient, particularly for patients with severe comorbidities or a high surgical risk.

With advancements in endoscopic techniques, an increasing number of early gastric cancer patients are undergoing endoscopic treatment. However, there have been cases of excessive resection without reliable methods to evaluate lymph node metastasis. To address this issue, the Japanese Guidelines for the Treatment of Gastric Cancer have established criteria for evaluating the curative potential of endoscopic resection [2]. Studies have shown that 10.3–29.3% of early gastric cancer cases treated with ESD did not meet the criteria for curative resection [3–5].

Two factors significantly impact the curative potential of endoscopic resection for early gastric cancer: (1) complete resection of the tumor and (2) the risk of lymph node metastasis. According to the Japanese endoscopic treatment guidelines, cases with a risk of lymph node metastasis <1% are considered absolute indications for treatment and meet the criteria for curative resection.

The evaluation of resection integrity includes assessing whether the tumor is removed en bloc and whether the resection margin is negative. If either criterion is not met, the resection is deemed non-curative. The Japanese Guidelines for the Treatment of Gastric Cancer have also established criteria for the degree of endoscopic cure (Fig. 1.4). Endoscopic cure grade A (eCura A) refers to cases where the tumor is en bloc resected, confined to the mucosa, predominantly differentiated cancer, without vascular invasion, negative margins, and no ulceration, or the tumor diameter is ≤3 cm despite the presence of an ulcer. Endoscopic cure grade B (eCura B) includes cases where the tumor is en bloc resected, with negative margins, no vascular invasion, and meets one of the following conditions: (1) predominantly undifferentiated cancer without ulceration, pT1a, tumor diameter ≤2 cm; (2) pT1b, predominantly differentiated carcinoma, with SM1 (submucosal infiltration <500 μm), and tumor diameter ≤3 cm. Cases that do not meet the criteria for eCura A or eCura B are defined as eCura C. If the tumor is well differentiated, cases that do not meet the requirements of eCura A or eCura B solely due to non-en bloc resection or positive vertical margins are classified as eCura C1. Other cases that do not meet the criteria for eCura A or eCura B are classified as eCura C2. Regular and close follow-up is recommended for patients classified as eCura A and eCura B after surgery. For eCura C1 patients with only positive vertical margins or unknown margins, a second ESD, cautery, additional surgery, or close follow-up may be considered. Further surgery is recommended for other patients classified as eCura C1 and those classified as eCura C2.

In the presented case, the tumor invaded the submucosa to a depth of 1200 μm, exceeding the

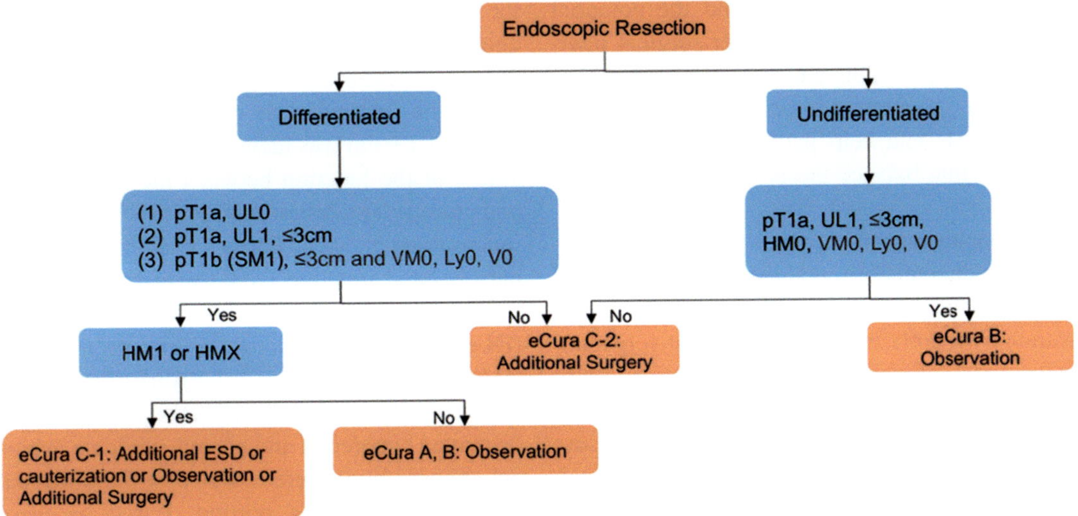

Fig. 1.4 The Cure Criteria of Endoscopic Resection in the Japanese Guidelines for the Treatment of Gastric Cancer

threshold of 500 μm, classifying it as eCura C2. Additionally, the risk of lymph node metastasis was determined to be of medium risk (2 points, based on vascular invasion and submucosal infiltration ≥500 μm). Therefore, additional surgery was recommended. However, the postoperative pathology did not reveal any residual tumor or lymph node metastasis, highlighting the challenges of accurately predicting outcomes using conventional criteria. It may be beneficial to explore alternative approaches that assess the risk of lymph node metastasis based on individual factors, as this could potentially enhance prediction accuracy [6].

It is important to note that the cure criteria provided in the Japanese Guidelines for the Treatment of Gastric Cancer are primarily based on retrospective data from Japan. Whether these criteria are entirely applicable to the Chinese population, given the differences in medical environments between the two countries, remains to be verified. Furthermore, the Japanese endoscopic non-curative criteria are regularly updated as new data accumulates.

For patients with early gastric cancer who have undergone non-curative endoscopic resection, it is crucial for healthcare professionals to fully inform them about the risk of tumor recurrence. Additionally, the medical team should develop a personalized treatment plan that takes into consideration the patient's age, physical condition, and surgical preferences.

1.1.4 Expert Comments

The increasing number of cases involving early gastric cancer after endoscopic resection has highlighted the importance of addressing non-curative resections. In order to effectively manage these cases, several key considerations should be taken into account. Firstly, a comprehensive preoperative evaluation is essential, which should include standardized endoscopy and endoscopic ultrasound. Accurate staging is fundamental to guiding appropriate treatment decisions.

Secondly, clinicians need to stay updated with the evolving guidelines for endoscopic therapy. This ensures that patients are recommended the most suitable treatment approach, avoiding both excessive and insufficient treatment. Adhering to current guidelines improves the chances of achieving curative resections and optimizing patient outcomes.

Lastly, it is vital to correctly interpret the non-curative factors described in pathology reports. This requires a thorough understanding of the implications and implications of these factors on the risk of tumor recurrence and the potential benefits and drawbacks of further surgical interventions. By providing patients with comprehensive and accurate information, healthcare professionals can help patients make informed decisions that balance the potential benefits and risks.

In conclusion, a meticulous preoperative evaluation, adherence to updated guidelines, and accurate interpretation of non-curative factors in pathology reports are critical for effectively managing cases of non-curative resections in early gastric cancer. This comprehensive approach aims to optimize patient outcomes and ensure that treatment decisions are based on a thorough understanding of the individual patient's condition.

Case provider: Hong Zhou, Yingtai Chen.

Commentary: Dongbing Zhao.

1.2 Case 2: Laparoscopic Sentinel Node Mapping in the Management of Early Gastric Cancer

1.2.1 Brief History

The patient, a 44-year-old female, presented with a chief complaint of persistent upper and middle abdominal discomfort for over a year, alongside the discovery of intragastric lesions 6 months ago. During the gastroscopic examination conducted 2 months ago (Fig. 1.5), a superficial and flat lesion (classified as type 0~IIb) measuring 1.5 cm × 1.0 cm was identified at the greater curvature of the junction between the gastric body and antrum. The lesion surface exhibited a white mucosal appearance. Further examination using narrow-band imaging (NBI) with magnification revealed positive findings for dilated lymphatics (DL+), irregular microvascular proliferation (IMVP+), and irregular microsurface structure pattern (IMSP+). Additionally, the pyloric region displayed hyperemia and edema, while no apparent abnormalities were detected in the duodenal bulb and descending portion. Based on these findings, an initial diagnosis of early gastric cancer was considered. It is noteworthy that the patient underwent surgery due to a right ankle joint fracture concurrent with the diagnosis.

Diagnosis: early gastric cancer (cT1N0M0), postoperative status of right ankle fracture

1.2.2 Treatment

After completing the preoperative evaluation, a combined approach of endoscopic submucosal dissection (ESD) and laparoscopic sentinel lymph node biopsy was carried out for the patient with early gastric cancer. Prior to surgery, the

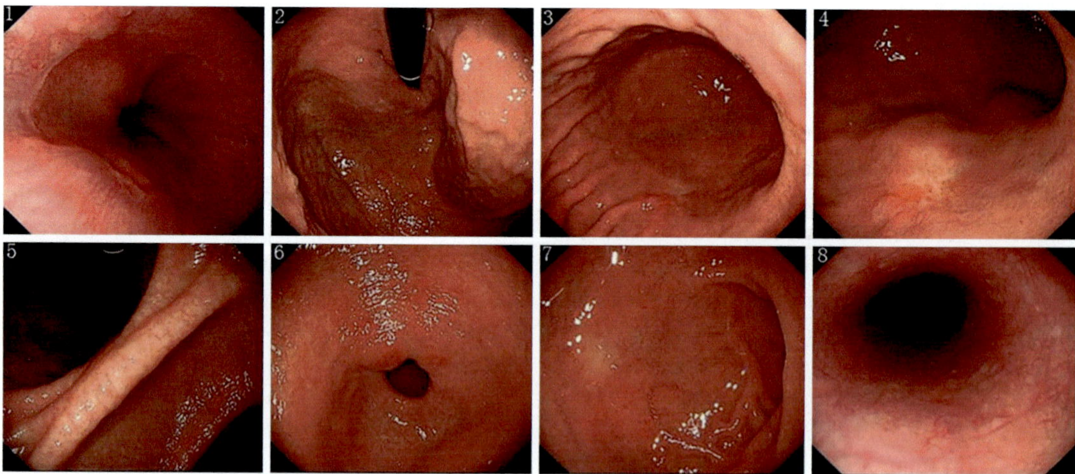

Fig. 1.5 A superficial flat lesion (0-II b type) located on the greater curvature side of the junction between the gastric body and sinus. The lesion measures approximately 1.5 cm × 1.0 cm in size

lesion was marked by the endoscopy team. A total of 2 mL of indocyanine green, with a concentration of 2.5 mg/mL, was injected into the submucosa at four points surrounding the tumor. The surgical team performed laparoscopic sentinel lymph node biopsy using the five-hole method to establish pneumoperitoneum. With the aid of fluorescent laparoscopy, the fluorescent-stained lymph nodes were identified and completely removed within the lymph node area where the staining lymph nodes were detected (Fig. 1.6). Following the procedure, the operative area was carefully re-examined to ensure that no stained lymph nodes were inadvertently left behind in the vicinity of the stomach.

The lymph nodes were carefully examined and distinguished based on their staining patterns (Fig. 1.7). Each identified lymph node was then sent for intraoperative frozen pathological examination. The results of the frozen pathology confirmed the absence of metastatic cancer in the examined lymph nodes. After a thorough examination of the surgical site, no bleeding was observed. To facilitate drainage, an abdominal drainage tube was inserted through the right abdominal wall and properly secured.

ESD was performed with the patient positioned in the left recumbent position (Fig. 1.8). Following the procedure, the patient was safely transferred back to the ward. Postoperatively, the patient was instructed to maintain fasting and refrain from water intake. On the fifth day after the surgery, both the gastric tube and abdominal drainage tube were removed, and the patient began consuming liquid food. After 6 days, the patient was discharged and instructed to continue a liquid diet for 2 weeks at home, followed by a gradual transition to a semi-liquid and soft food diet.

Pathology: Macroscopic examination revealed a superficial and flat lesion measuring 1.5 × 1.2 cm on the mucosal tissue, with an overall size of 4.5 × 4 × 0.2 cm. The lesion was located 1 cm from the nearest lateral margin. Microscopic observation showed a 0-IIB low-differentiated adenocarcinoma (Lauren typing: diffuse), with partial involvement of signet ring cell carcinoma. The cancer area measured 2.2 × 1.4 cm. Invasion into the submucosa was noted at a depth of 800 μm (submucosal depth: 840 μm). The tumor margin was 40 μm from the basal cutting margin, and no residual cancer was found at the lateral cutting edge. The surrounding gastric mucosa exhibited mild and chronic non-atrophic inflammation. None of the examined lymph nodes showed evidence of metastasis (0/3). The pathological staging was determined as pT1bN0 according to the pTNM classification.

Two months following the initial surgery, the patient expressed strong concerns about the potential risk of tumor residue and requested a distal subtotal gastrectomy. After completing the necessary evaluations, the lesion was localized

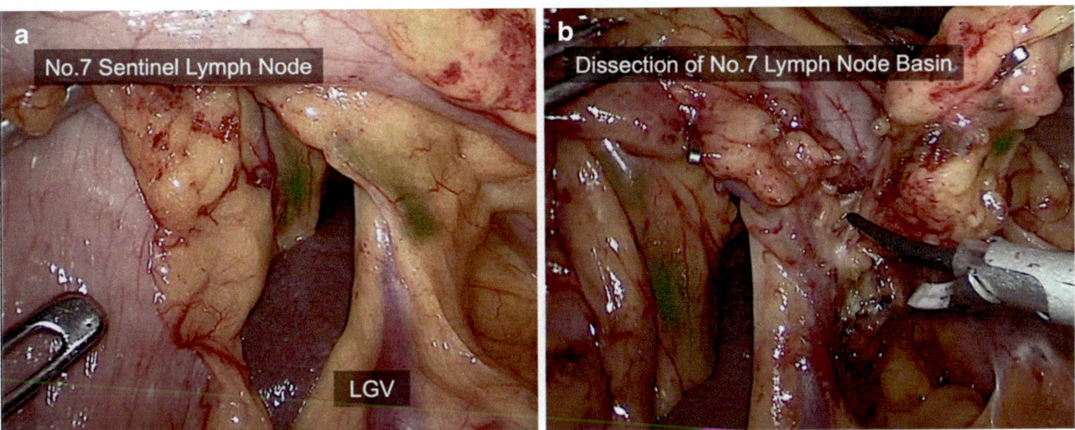

Fig. 1.6 The identification of lymph staining areas (**a**) and the selection of lymph nodes under laparoscopy (**b**)

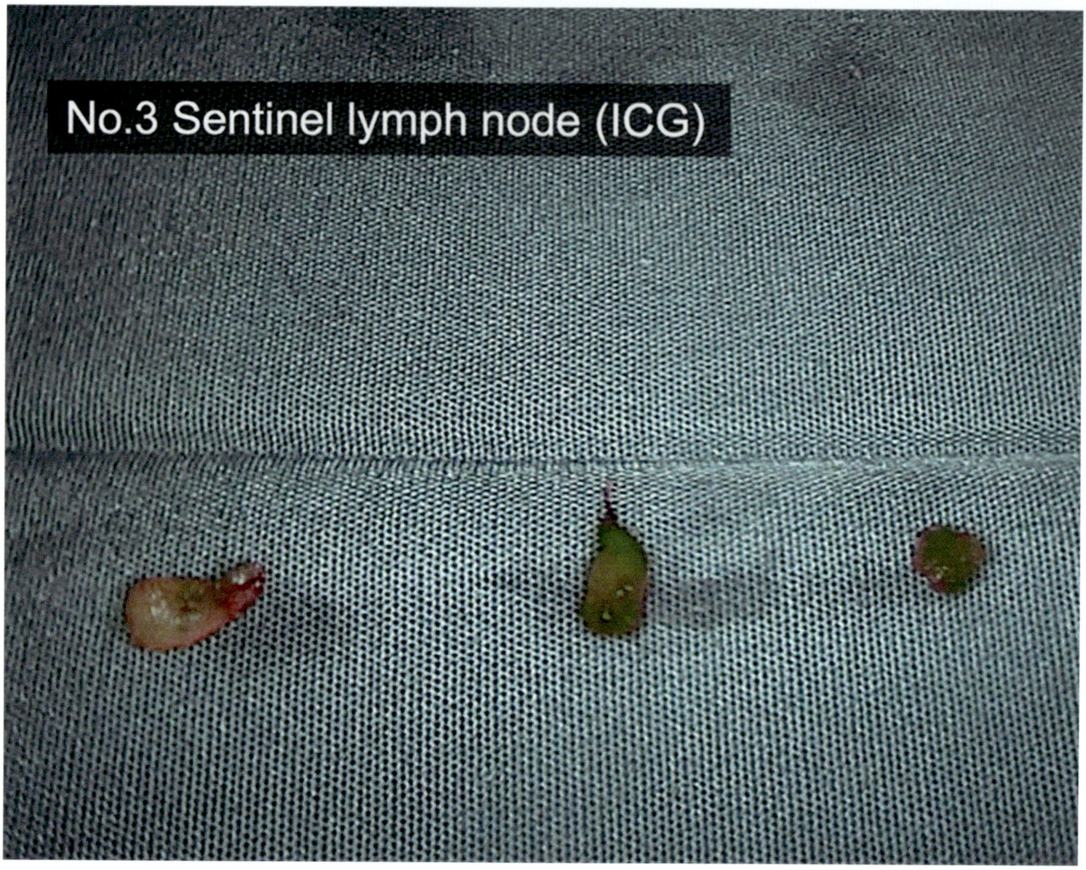

No.3 Sentinel lymph node (ICG)

Fig. 1.7 The stained lymph nodes (sentinel lymph nodes)

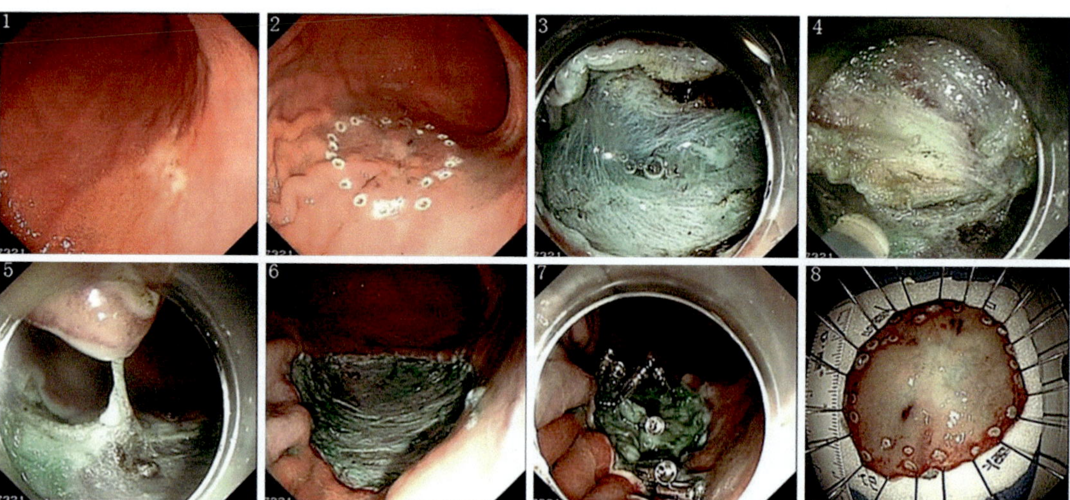

Fig. 1.8 ESD Process

using a titanium clip under endoscopic guidance (Fig. 1.9). Subsequently, laparoscopic distal subtotal gastrectomy with D2 lymph node dissection was performed. No residual cancer was identified in the surgical specimen, greater omentum, or surgical margins. Additionally, no metastatic lymph nodes were detected among the 16 lymph nodes examined.

1.2.3 Case Analysis

With advancements in endoscopic technology and its increasing utilization in diagnosis, the detection rate of early gastric cancer has been on the rise. In fact, the proportion of early gastric cancer cases has exceeded 50% in Japan [7]. Similarly, in China, the detection rate of early gastric cancer significantly improved from 2014 to 2016, reaching 19.5% [8]. As per the Japanese treatment protocol for gastric cancer, endoscopic submucosal dissection (ESD) is recommended for the treatment of cT1a lesions of early gastric cancer. For undifferentiated adenocarcinoma or cT1b tumors, D1 or D1+ lymph node dissection is advised. However, it has been reported in the literature that the lymph node metastasis rate in early gastric cancer ranges from 5% to 15% [9, 10]. Consequently, many patients without lymph node metastasis undergo unnecessary gastrectomy and lymph node dissection, significantly impacting their long-term quality of life [11]. Thus, accurately assessing the lymph node status before surgery is crucial in the management of early gastric cancer.

Various preoperative assessments are available for lymph node evaluation, including ultrasonic endoscopy, CT scan, PET-CT, and others. However, these modalities have limitations and may yield results with restricted accuracy. To preserve organ function and reduce the false-negative rate of imaging, the technique of sentinel lymph node (SLN) biopsy has been developed [12]. SLN refers to the first or several lymph nodes to which the primary tumor may potentially metastasize. A negative SLN indicates a minimal probability of tumor metastasis to other lymph nodes, allowing for the avoidance of extensive lymph node dissection. Initially employed in the treatment of melanoma and breast cancer [13, 14], SLN biopsy has subsequently been applied to other tumor types, including gastric cancer.

In a prospective and multicenter clinical study, the endoscopic dual-demonstration method using dye and nuclear imaging was employed to visualize and identify the sentinel lymph node (SLN) for biopsy in patients with cT1/T2 gastric cancer. The study demonstrated a high detection rate of SLN, with 97.5% (387/397) of cases successfully identifying the SLN, and a precision rate of 99% (383/387) [15]. In 2001, Hiratsuka et al. [12]

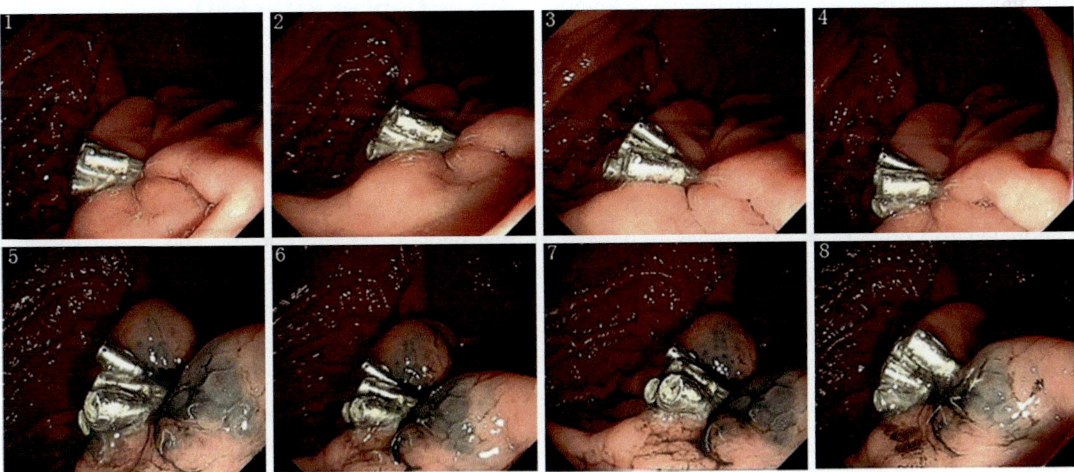

Fig. 1.9 Localization of titanium clips under endoscopy

reported the use of a single tracer, indocyanine green (ICG), in fluorescent imaging to detect the SLN, achieving a 100% detection rate (44/44). Meta-analysis has indicated that several factors influence the efficacy of ICG, including low concentration (0.5 or 0.05 mg/mL), a 20-min interval after ICG injection, and mucosal injection, which yield better results compared to instantaneous and serosal injection. Additionally, obtaining a minimum of five biopsied SLNs has shown improved sensitivity [16].

With advancements in SLN tracing technology, sentinel node navigation surgery (SNNS) for early gastric cancer has rapidly evolved. In a phase II clinical trial conducted in South Korea, patients who did not meet the absolute indications for endoscopic resection but were diagnosed as stage CT1N0M0 with a tumor diameter <4 cm were included. If quick frozen pathology during the operation yielded negative results, local resection of the stomach was performed. Otherwise, standard gastrectomy with D2 lymph node dissection was conducted. Among 100 patients, SLNs were successfully detected in 99 cases, with an average of 6.1 ± 3.9 SLNs obtained. Out of the SLNs, 11 were found to be metastatic. During follow-up, three cases of recurrence were observed, all of which occurred in the remnant stomach, while SLN biopsy results were negative. The 3-year recurrence-free survival rate and overall survival rate for patients with negative SLNs were 96.0% and 98.0%, respectively. These findings indicate the safety of laparoscopic SNNS for early gastric cancer [17]. Moreover, the quality of life after laparoscopic SNNS was found to be superior to that following traditional laparoscopic distal gastrectomy [18].

In Korea, a multicenter, randomized, and phase III clinical trial known as SENORITA was conducted to compare the outcomes of laparoscopic sentinel node navigation surgery (SNNS) with traditional laparoscopic radical gastrectomy in early gastric cancer. The preliminary results of the trial demonstrated that the rates and severity of complications between laparoscopic SNNS and laparoscopic radical gastrectomy were comparable [19]. Similar clinical research is also being carried out in Japan [20]. These findings suggest that gastric function-preserving surgery combined with SNNS has the potential to become an ideal technique for the management of early gastric cancer in the future.

1.2.4 Expert Comments

As tumor screening continues to advance, we can anticipate further improvements in the detection rate of early gastric cancer. Given the favorable prognosis associated with early-stage disease, there is increasing emphasis on minimizing surgical trauma and enhancing the quality of life for patients. The existing data demonstrates that sentinel lymph node (SLN) biopsy for early gastric cancer can provide accurate information about the status of lymph node metastasis in the perigastric region, thereby setting the stage for organ-preserving surgical approaches. With the accumulation of experience in this field, we have reasons to be optimistic that sentinel node navigation surgery (SNNS) will benefit a greater number of patients with early gastric cancer, offering them improved outcomes and quality of life.

Case provider: Hong Zhou, Yingtai Chen.

Commentary: Dongbing Zhao.

1.3 Case 3: Local Gastrectomy for the Recurred Gastric Cancer After ESD

1.3.1 Brief History

The patient, a 55-year-old female, was admitted to the hospital 6 months following an endoscopic submucosal dissection (ESD) procedure for the treatment of gastric cancer. The initial surgical intervention was performed at a different medical facility. Histopathological analysis conducted after the surgery revealed the presence of highly differentiated adenocarcinoma. Approximately 1 month prior to admission, an upper gastrointestinal endoscopy identified residual lesions located in the fundus of the stomach. Notably, the surrounding mucosa exhibited concentrated folds that appeared raised, irregular, and prone to bleeding upon contact. Narrow-band imaging (NBI) examination confirmed the presence of lesions with distinctive DL (+) characteristics and scar-like changes. The mucosal surface demonstrated irregularities in microvascular (MV) patterns and microsurface (MS) features, in addition to displaying poor gastric peristalsis. Further evaluation using endoscopic ultrasonography revealed uneven thickening of the gastric wall, with the thickest segment measuring approximately 5.7 mm. The internal echo of the lesion displayed homogeneity, while the demarcation from the surrounding mucosa remained indistinct, primarily originating from the mucosal and submucosal layers of the gastric wall. The muscularis propria layer and serous layer of the bulge exhibited clear, continuous, and intact structures. Notably, no palpable lymph nodes were observed in the vicinity of the stomach fundus (Fig. 1.10). Abdominal contrast-enhanced computed tomography (CT) exhibited gastric hypodilation and revealed dense opacities within the fundus of the stomach, consistent with postoperative changes. No significant lymphadenopathy was detected in the abdominal cavity, retroperitoneum, or inguinal region (Fig. 1.11).

Diagnosis: Recurrence of gastric cancer following endoscopic submucosal dissection (ESD).

1.3.2 Treatment

The patient underwent laparoscopic partial gastrectomy and laparoscopic lymph node dissection after completing relevant examinations, which did not reveal any contraindications for surgery. The patient received general anesthesia and was intubated, placed in a supine position with legs apart. Routine disinfection and draping were carried out, and trocars were inserted in the upper and middle abdomen on both sides to establish pneumoperitoneum. The surgical team assumed

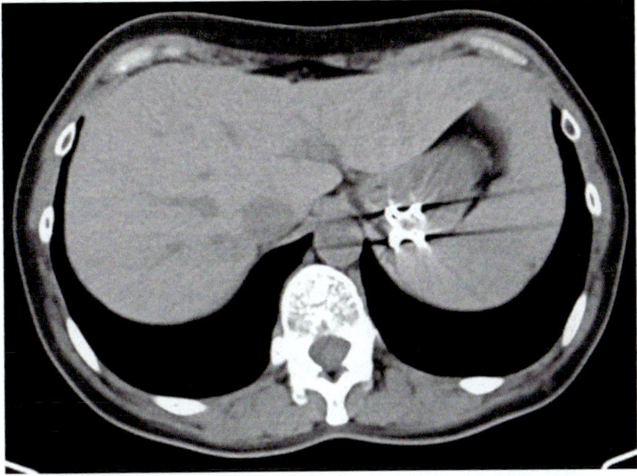

Fig. 1.11 Abdominal computed tomography (CT) demonstrated inadequate gastric dilation, with the presence of dense shadows observed at the fundus of the stomach, consistent with postoperative changes

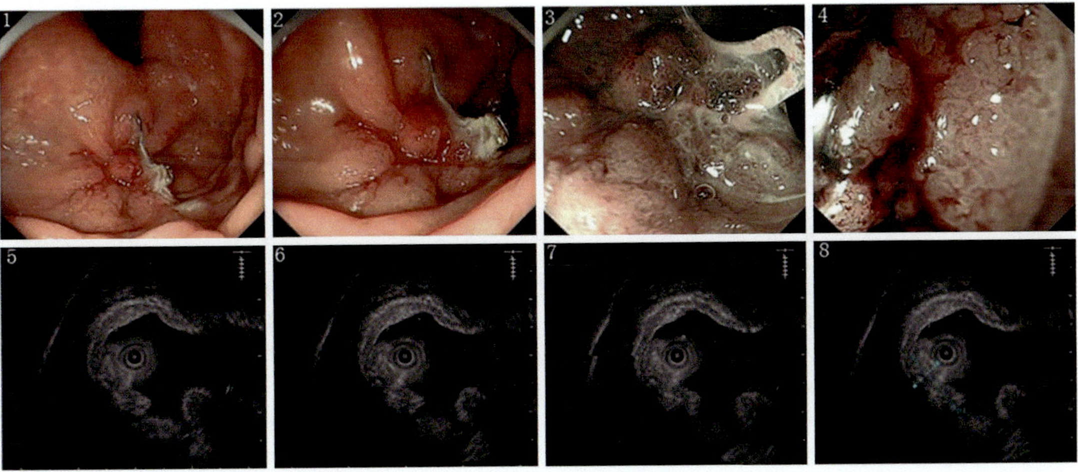

Fig. 1.10 Endoscopic ultrasonography revealed pronounced and concentrated mucosal folds surrounding the gastric fundus lesions, indicative of residual lesions

their positions, with the surgeon standing on the left side, the assistant on the right side, and the endoscopic operator positioned between the patient's legs.

A standard exploration of the abdominal cavity was performed, revealing mild adhesions in the upper abdomen but no metastatic nodules in the liver or abdominal cavity. Ligation of the left gastric vessels and short gastric vessels was performed, while the right gastric vessels and right gastroepiploic vessels were preserved. After lymph node clearance around the stomach, an auxiliary incision was made in the middle of the upper abdomen, and the abdominal cavity was accessed layer by layer. The tumor, located 2 cm away, was longitudinally closed using a cutting and closing device, along with closure of the resected lesion and the bottom of the stomach. Suturing of the entire layer was carried out, reinforced, and hemostasis was achieved. The patency of the cardia was confirmed intraoperatively. The wound was cleaned, and a drainage tube was placed for postoperative drainage at the puncture site in the right abdominal wall.

On the third day after surgery, the gastric tube was removed. A liquid diet was initiated on the fourth day, and the abdominal drainage tube was removed on the seventh day. Subsequently, the patient was discharged.

Pathology analysis revealed that the partially resected stomach specimen measured 8 cm on the greater curvature and 10 cm on the lesser curvature. There was a shrinkage area of the mucosal folds measuring 2 × 1 cm, located 1 cm from the upper margin, with the surrounding gastric mucosa appearing grayish-yellow and slightly rough. Microscopically, the diagnosis indicated early gastric adenocarcinoma of the shallow raised type (Type IIa), situated in the submucosal layer of the mucosa without involvement of the muscularis mucosae. No clear vascular tumor emboli or nerve invasion were identified. Some areas of the submucosal layer of the gastric wall exhibited fibrous scar formation, accompanied by focal multinucleated giant cell reactions and chronic inflammatory cell infiltration, indicative of postoperative changes. No tumors were detected at the upper margin, lower margin, or greater omentum. Additionally, there was no evidence of metastatic cancer in the examined lymph nodes (0/13). The TNM staging of the tumor was determined as pT1N0M0, corresponding to stage I.

1.3.3 Case Analysis

With advancements in endoscopic diagnostics and increased awareness among high-risk populations regarding regular physical examinations, the detection rate of early gastric cancer has steadily risen. Early gastric cancer is characterized by a low rate of lymph node metastasis and a prolonged postoperative survival period compared to advanced gastric cancer. Currently, due to the challenges associated with accurately assessing lymph node metastasis before surgery, approximately 80% of early gastric cancer patients, even without lymph node involvement, still undergo traditional subtotal or total gastrectomy combined with lymph node dissection. However, this approach significantly impacts the patients' postoperative quality of life due to the extensive trauma and loss of organ function caused by the surgery.

In line with the trend of minimally invasive and precise surgical management for early gastric cancer, function-preserving gastrectomy (FPG) has emerged as a research focus. FPG integrates minimally invasive techniques with the concept of preserving gastric function. Japanese scholars define FPG as a surgical approach that aims to minimize gastric resection and lymph node dissection while ensuring complete tumor removal. It emphasizes preserving pyloric and vagus nerve function [21]. FPG encompasses various procedures, including pylorus-preserving gastrectomy (PPG), segmental gastrectomy (SG), local gastrectomy (LG), and ultimately, endoscopic resection.

1. **Pylorus-preserving gastrectomy**

   Pylorus-preserving gastrectomy (PPG) originated from the pylorus-preserving gastric resection technique developed by Maki et al. [22] in 1967 for the treatment of gastric ulcers.

Over time, PPG has evolved to preserve the pylorus during the resection of early gastric cancer located in the middle third of the stomach. PPG involves preserving the upper one-third of the stomach, the pylorus, and a portion of the gastric antrum. This approach allows for food storage in the stomach and maintains normal gastric emptying, thereby reducing the incidence of postoperative dumping syndrome, gallbladder stones, and bile reflux disease, ultimately improving patients' quality of life. The first edition of the Japanese Gastric Cancer Treatment Guidelines, published in 2001, proposed PPG with vagus nerve preservation as a modified gastrectomy technique for early gastric cancer. After a decade of exploration and clinical practice, the third edition of the Japanese Gastric Cancer Treatment Guidelines, published in 2010, provided detailed recommendations regarding the indications, extent of surgical resection, and lymph node dissection for PPG. According to these guidelines, the recommended indications for PPG surgery are cT1N0M0 stage, tumors located in the middle third of the stomach, and gastric cancer patients with a tumor-to-pylorus distance of more than 4 cm [23]. Subsequently, PPG was officially included as an optional surgical treatment for early gastric cancer.

2. **Segmental gastrectomy with cardia preservation**

For early gastric cancer located in the upper portion of the stomach that does not meet the criteria for endoscopic resection, proximal gastrectomy is commonly performed. Various reconstruction methods, such as tube-like gastric anastomosis and double-channel anastomosis, have been employed. However, postoperative severe gastroesophageal reflux is often encountered regardless of the reconstruction technique. To address this issue, Japanese researchers have proposed high-segment gastrectomy for early proximal gastric cancer. This surgical approach involves resecting the upper stomach and performing local lymph node dissection while preserving the cardia, left vagus nerve liver branch, pyloric branch, and abdominal branch. Preserving the cardia is a challenging and limiting factor of this technique [24]. It is suggested that this method is suitable for early gastric cancer located in the upper third of the stomach with a minimum distance of 2 cm between the tumor edge and the gastroesophageal junction. Segmental gastrectomy with cardia preservation can reduce postoperative gastroesophageal reflux symptoms and enhance quality of life, making it advantageous for preserving gastric function. However, due to the limitations associated with the resection, this approach is currently considered a research treatment method according to the Japanese Gastric Cancer Treatment Guidelines and has not gained widespread recognition in clinical practice.

3. **Partial Gastrectomy**

Partial gastrectomy involves the partial removal of the stomach, including wedge resection and double-scope combined full-layer gastrectomy. As early as 1999, Japanese scholars began utilizing laparoscopic partial gastrectomy for the treatment of early gastric cancer and conducted preliminary investigations into its safety. However, due to the limited follow-up duration, small sample sizes, and retrospective nature of the studies, further validation of the conclusions is necessary [25]. While partial gastrectomy surgery allows for maximum preservation of gastric function and improves the patient's quality of life, the inherent limitations of the procedure restrict the extent of lymph node dissection. Therefore, careful consideration of surgical indications and patient selection is required. To ensure the completeness of these surgeries, the use of sentinel lymph node navigation technology is increasing [26]. During the operation, if no lymph node metastasis is detected, further lymph node dissection can be avoided. However, if lymph node involvement is observed, standard D2 radical surgery is necessary. Nonetheless, due to the extensive lymphatic network surrounding the stomach, complex reflux, and the propensity of gastric cancer to exhibit skip metastasis in lymph nodes, sentinel lymph node navigation surgery cannot entirely alleviate surgeons' concerns regarding the safety of achieving radical tumor cure.

4. **Double-Scope Combined Partial Gastrectomy**

   In recent years, laparoscopic endoscopic cooperative surgery (LECS), a more minimally invasive approach, has garnered attention [27]. Its primary advantage lies in the complete removal of tumors with minimal margins, allowing for maximal preservation of the gastric wall, blood vessels, and nerves, thus maintaining gastric function and enhancing postoperative quality of life. LECS has been reported as safe and feasible for undifferentiated early gastric cancer by Li et al. [28]. Moreover, minimally invasive surgery with LECS is currently covered by Japan's national health insurance program for submucosal tumors, including early gastric cancer and gastrointestinal stromal tumors [29]. Another technique, non-exposed endoscopic wall-inversion surgery (NEWS), is an improved version of LECS that is applicable to tumors in various locations, including those at the esophagogastric junction. NEWS has shown promising short-term and long-term results in the surgical treatment of submucosal tumors in Japan [30, 31]. With the advancement of minimally invasive treatment for early gastric cancer, double-scope combined lymph node regional dissection based on sentinel lymph node tracking has become an emerging research focus.

In this particular case, where residual tumors remained after endoscopic submucosal dissection (ESD) for early gastric cancer in the gastric fundus, performing proximal gastrectomy could result in severe reflux and significantly affect the patient's quality of life. Thus, after thorough communication with the patient, a partial gastrectomy was chosen to completely remove the tumor while preserving cardia function, reducing postoperative gastroesophageal reflux, improving the patient's quality of life, and simultaneously conducting regional lymph node dissection.

1.3.4 Expert Comments

The research surrounding functional preservation surgery for early gastric cancer is witnessing a surge in activity. Embracing the current inclination to merge minimally invasive approaches with organ function preservation in the management of early gastric cancer, functional preservation surgery is poised to assume the mantle as the leading trajectory for surgical interventions in this context. Nonetheless, in the practical realm, clinicians must exercise stringent vigilance in discerning the appropriate surgical indications, meticulously selecting suitable cases, and meticulously executing such functional preservation surgeries while simultaneously upholding tumor safety.

Case provider: Hong Zhou, Yingtai Chen.

Commentary: Dongbing Zhao.

References

1. 北京市科委重大项目早期胃癌治疗规范研究专家组, 柴宁莉, 翟亚奇, 等. 早期胃癌内镜下规范化切除的专家共识意见 (2018,北京). 中华胃肠内镜电子杂志, 2018,5(02):49–60.
2. Japanese Gastric Cancer A. Japanese gastric cancer treatment guidelines 2018 (5th edition). Gastric Cancer. 2021;24(1):1–21.
3. Sunagawa H, Kinoshita T, Kaito A, et al. Additional surgery for non-curative resection after endoscopic submucosal dissection for gastric cancer: a retrospective analysis of 200 cases. Surg Today. 2017;47(2):202–9.
4. Suzuki H, Oda I, Abe S, et al. Clinical outcomes of early gastric cancer patients after noncurative endoscopic submucosal dissection in a large consecutive patient series. Gastric Cancer. 2017;20(4):679–89.
5. Kim ER, Lee H, Min BH, et al. Effect of rescue surgery after non-curative endoscopic resection of early gastric cancer. Br J Surg. 2015;102(11):1394–401.
6. Guo CG, Zhao DB, Liu Q, et al. A nomogram to predict lymph node metastasis in patients with early gastric cancer. Oncotarget. 2017;8(7):12203–10.
7. Takeuchi H, Oyama T, Kamiya S, et al. Laparoscopy-assisted proximal gastrectomy with sentinel node mapping for early gastric cancer. World J Surg. 2011;35(11):2463–71.
8. Rulin M, Ziyu L. Wu Aiwen data report of China gastrointestinal oncology surgery alliance (2014–2016). Chinese J Pract Surg. 2018;38(01):90–3.
9. Lee HH, Yoo HM, Song KY, et al. Risk of limited lymph node dissection in patients with clinically early

gastric cancer: indications of extended lymph node dissection for early gastric cancer. Ann Surg Oncol. 2013;20(11):3534–40.

10. Gotoda T, Yanagisawa A, Sasako M, et al. Incidence of lymph node metastasis from early gastric cancer: estimation with a large number of cases at two large centers. Gastric Cancer. 2000;3(4):219–25.
11. Guo CG, Zhao DB, Liu Q, et al. Risk factors for lymph node metastasis in early gastric cancer with signet ring cell carcinoma. J Gastrointest Surg. 2015;19(11):1958–65.
12. Hiratsuka M, Miyashiro I, Ishikawa O, et al. Application of sentinel node biopsy to gastric cancer surgery. Surgery. 2001;129(3):335–40.
13. Giuliano AE, Kirgan DM, Guenther JM, et al. Lymphatic mapping and sentinel lymphadenectomy for breast cancer. Ann Surg. 1994;220(3):391–8, 398–401.
14. Morton DL, Wen DR, Wong JH, et al. Technical details of intraoperative lymphatic mapping for early stage melanoma. Arch Surg. 1992;127(4):392–9.
15. Kitagawa Y, Takeuchi H, Takagi Y, et al. Sentinel node mapping for gastric cancer: a prospective multicenter trial in Japan. J Clin Oncol. 2013;31(29):3704–10.
16. He M, Jiang Z, Wang C, et al. Diagnostic value of near-infrared or fluorescent indocyanine green guided sentinel lymph node mapping in gastric cancer: a systematic review and meta-analysis. J Surg Oncol. 2018;118(8):1243–56.
17. Park DJ, Park YS, Son SY, et al. Long-term oncologic outcomes of laparoscopic sentinel node navigation surgery in early gastric cancer: a single-center, single-arm, phase II trial. Ann Surg Oncol. 2018;25(8):2357–65.
18. Youn SI, Son SY, Lee K, et al. Quality of life after laparoscopic sentinel node navigation surgery in early gastric cancer: a single-center cohort study. Gastric Cancer. 2021;24:744.
19. An JY, Min JS, Hur H, et al. Laparoscopic sentinel node navigation surgery versus laparoscopic gastrectomy with lymph node dissection for early gastric cancer: short-term outcomes of a multicentre randomized controlled trial (SENORITA). Br J Surg. 2020;107(11):1429–39.
20. Kamiya S, Takeuchi H, Fukuda K, et al. A multicenter non-randomized phase III study of sentinel node navigation surgery for early gastric cancer. Jpn J Clin Oncol. 2021;51(2):305–9.
21. Nomura E, Okajima K. Function-preserving gastrectomy for gastric cancer in Japan. World J Gastroenterol. 2016;22(26):5888–95.
22. Maki T, Shiratori T, Hatafuku T, et al. Pylorus-preserving gastrectomy as an improved operation for gastric ulcer. Surgery. 1967;61(6):838–45.
23. Japanese gastric cancer treatment guidelines 2010 (ver. 3). Gastric Cancer. 2011;14(2):113–23.
24. Shinohara T, Ohyama S, Muto T, et al. Clinical outcome of high segmental gastrectomy for early gastric cancer in the upper third of the stomach. Br J Surg. 2006;93(8):975–80.
25. Seto Y, Nagawa H, Muto Y, et al. Preliminary report on local resection with lymphadenectomy for early gastric cancer. Br J Surg. 1999;86(4):526–8.
26. Mitsumori N, Nimura H, Takahashi N, et al. Sentinel lymph node navigation surgery for early stage gastric cancer. World J Gastroenterol. 2014;20(19):5685–93.
27. Matsuda T, Nunobe S, Ohashi M, et al. Laparoscopic endoscopic cooperative surgery (LECS) for the upper gastrointestinal tract. Transl Gastroenterol Hepatol. 2017;2:40.
28. Li H, Chen L, Huo Z, et al. Defining a subgroup treatable for laparoscopic and endoscopic cooperative surgery in undifferentiated early gastric cancer: the role of lymph node metastasis. J Gastrointest Surg. 2015;19(10):1763–8.
29. Hiki N, Nunobe S. Laparoscopic endoscopic cooperative surgery (LECS) for the gastrointestinal tract: updated indications. Ann Gastroenterol Surg. 2019;3(3):239–46.
30. Mitsui T, Yamashita H, Aikou S, et al. Non-exposed endoscopic wall-inversion surgery for gastrointestinal stromal tumor. Transl Gastroenterol Hepatol. 2018;3:17.
31. Tsukuda N, Komatsu S, Kumano T, et al. [Modified NEWS as a safe and inventive approach for gastrointestinal stromal tumor near the Esophagogastric junction]. Gan To Kagaku Ryoho. 2018;45(13):2153–5.

2 The Minimally Invasive Surgery for Gastric Cancer

Hu Ren, Tongbo Wang, Hong Zhou, Chunguang Guo, Xiaofeng Bai, and Dongbing Zhao

2.1 Case 4: Laparoscopic Radical Gastrectomy for Gastric Cancer

2.1.1 Brief History

A 57-year-old female presented with a chief complaint of upper abdominal pain persisting for 10 months, which worsened over the past month. Additionally, the patient experienced upper abdominal distension and discomfort after meals for the past 10 months, with intermittent episodes accompanied by back pain. Initially, the patient sought medical attention at a community hospital where she received treatment with "esomeprazole," resulting in symptom relief. However, the abdominal pain and distension reappeared 1 month ago, exacerbating the severity, although slightly alleviated with medication. Gastroscopy performed at a local hospital 20 days ago revealed the presence of ulcers in the stomach's corner. Subsequent pathological examination confirmed the infiltration of cancer cells. Abdominal examination did not reveal any abnormal findings, and tumor marker levels, including CEA, AFP, CA72–4, CA19–9, and CA24–2, were all within the normal range. Gastroscopy indicated the presence of gastric cancer, with a lesion measuring approximately 5 × 4 cm in the lower part of the gastric body, extending to the gastric angle and antrum, displaying ulcerative characteristics (Fig. 2.1). CT scan findings demonstrated localized thickening of the gastric wall along the lesser curvature of the stomach, with a maximum thickness of approximately 1.3 cm. The enhancement exhibited uneven distribution and noticeable variation, and the serous surface appeared irregular. Increased internal fat stranding and micronodules were observed, along with multiple small lymph nodes surrounding the left blood vessels of the stomach, with the largest measuring approximately 0.8 cm in short diameter (Fig. 2.2).

Diagnosis: Gastric cancer (cT2N0M0, stage I).

2.1.2 Treatment

Following admission, all relevant examinations were conducted, revealing no contraindications to surgery. The perioperative period employed a fast recovery surgical approach, wherein water fasting, skin preparation, bowel preparation, and gastric tube insertion were omitted prior to the operation.

H. Ren · T. Wang · C. Guo (✉) · X. Bai · D. Zhao
Department of Pancreatic and Gastric Surgical Oncology, National Cancer Center/National Clinical Research for Cancer/Cancer Hospital, Chinese Academy of Medical Sciences and Peking Union Medical College, Beijing, China

H. Zhou
Department of Breast Surgical Oncology, National Cancer Center/National Clinical Research Center for Cancer/Cancer Hospital & Shenzhen Hospital, Chinese Academy of Medical Sciences and Peking Union Medical College, Shenzhen, China

J. Cai (ed.), *Interpretation of Gastric Cancer Cases*, Experts' Perspectives on Medical Advances,
https://doi.org/10.1007/978-981-99-5302-8_2

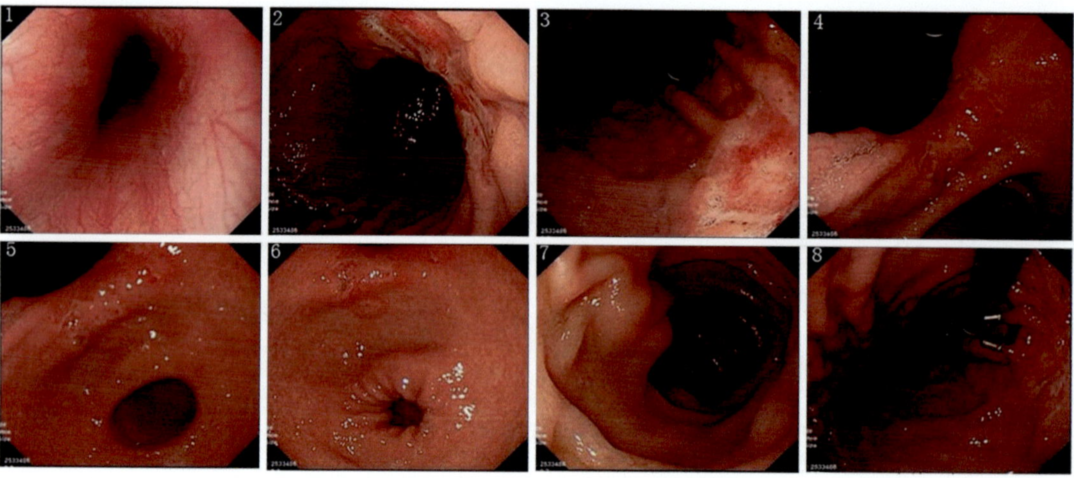

Fig. 2.1 Gastroscopy: The esophagogastric junction is located approximately 37 cm from the incisors. A distinct ulcerative lesion spanning from the lower portion of the gastric body to the gastric angle and antrum is observed, measuring approximately 5 × 4 cm in size

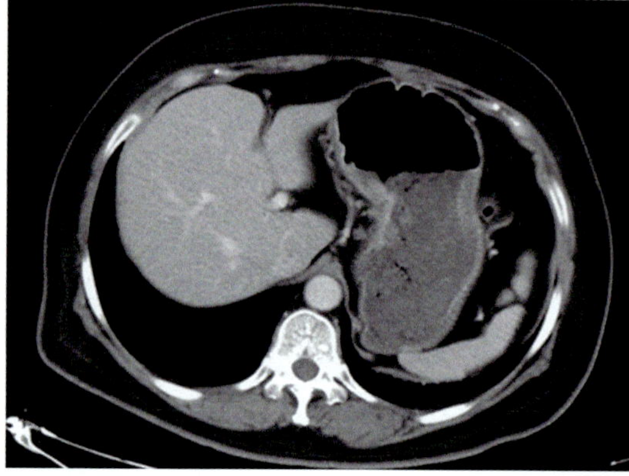

Fig. 2.2 CT: The gastric wall in the region extending from the lower portion of the gastric body to the antrum exhibits a mild thickening, accompanied by a roughened serosal surface. Scattered lymph nodes are observed in the left gastric area and mesentery, with the larger node measuring approximately 0.5 cm in short diameter

Given the early stage of the tumor, primarily located in the gastric body, laparoscopic identification of the lesion posed challenges. Therefore, on the day of the operation, the tumor was initially marked using titanium clips under gastroscopy guidance, followed by surgical intervention. Intraoperative exploration confirmed the tumor's location on the lesser curvature of the lower gastric body, without involvement of the serosa. A completely laparoscopic distal gastrectomy (Billroth II + Brown anastomosis, D2) was performed.

Postoperatively, on the first day, the gastric tube was removed, allowing for water intake. Clear fluids were initiated on the third day, followed by a liquid diet on the fifth day. The abdominal drainage tube was removed on the sixth day, and the patient was discharged from the hospital on the seventh day.

Pathological examination results are as follows: The resected specimen from the distal gastrectomy consisted of a stomach segment, with the greater curvature measuring 26 cm and the lesser curvature measuring 12 cm. A small portion of the duodenum, measuring 0.8 cm in length and 3 cm in width, was attached at the incisal margin. A shallow depression area of 4 × 2.2 cm was observed 6 cm from the pyloric ring and 4 cm from the upper incisal edge, while the surrounding gastric mucosa appeared intact. Microscopic analysis revealed a poorly differentiated superficial depressed gastric adenocarcinoma, predominantly composed of signet ring cell carcinoma (approximately 80% composition). According to the Lauren classification, the tumor was classified as diffuse type. The tumor exhibited invasion into the muscularis mucosa, without involvement of the submucosa or muscularis propria. No evidence of vascular tumor thrombus or nerve invasion was observed. Furthermore, the tumor did not infiltrate the pyloric ring or duodenum. The upper and lower incision margins, as well as the omentum, showed no evidence of cancer. The surrounding gastric mucosal tissue displayed signs of chronic atrophic gastritis. Lymph node examination revealed no metastatic cancer among the sampled 47 lymph nodes (0/47). The TNM staging was determined as pT1aN0M0, corresponding to stage I.

2.1.3 Case Analysis

In 1994, Kitano et al. [1] reported the first laparoscopic radical resection of early gastric cancer, establishing a milestone in the field of laparoscopic treatment for gastric cancer. Subsequently, in 1995, Watson et al. [2] performed the world's first total laparoscopic radical gastrectomy for early gastric cancer, highlighting the minimally invasive advantages of laparoscopy. In 2001, Goh et al. [3] successfully applied laparoscopy to advanced gastric cancer, demonstrating favorable outcomes and further validating the feasibility of laparoscopic approaches in gastric cancer treatment. In 2002, Hashizume et al. [4] in Japan introduced the da Vinci robot for radical gastric cancer surgery, ushering in a new era of intelligent laparoscopic techniques. Compared to open surgery, laparoscopic procedures offer advantages such as reduced surgical trauma, accelerated recovery of gastrointestinal function, and shorter hospital stays [5]. As laparoscopic technology became more widespread, the concept of minimally invasive gastric cancer surgery gained acceptance among gastrointestinal surgeons. Presently, laparoscopy-assisted subtotal gastrectomy has emerged as a classic surgical approach for treating gastric cancer, particularly in cases of early-stage disease.

Laparoscopic radical gastrectomy can be categorized into three types based on the surgical techniques employed: mini-incision assisted, total laparoscopic, and hand-assisted laparoscopic radical gastrectomy. First, mini-incision-assisted radical gastrectomy, also known as laparoscopy-assisted radical gastrectomy, involves laparoscopic dissection of the stomach, isolation of blood vessels surrounding the stomach, and lymph node dissection. Subsequently, a small incision is made in the upper abdomen to facilitate specimen resection and digestive tract reconstruction. This method is relatively straightforward to perform, with a short learning curve, and it is widely employed in laparoscopic gastric cancer surgery. Second, total laparoscopic radical gastrectomy has emerged in recent years due to significant advancements in laparoscopic equipment and techniques. This approach entails performing gastrectomy, lymph node dissection, and digestive tract reconstruction entirely under laparoscopic visualization. The substantially reduced incision length results in decreased surgical trauma, postoperative pain, and improved cosmetic outcomes. Third, hand-assisted laparoscopic surgery builds upon conventional laparoscopic techniques. With this method, the surgeon's hand is inserted into the patient's abdominal cavity through a small incision in the abdominal wall using a hand-assistant device (blue disc). The operation is performed with the assistance of ultrasonic scalpel and other instruments. This surgical approach represents a transition from laparotomy to laparoscopic-assisted surgery. Currently, the utilization of hand-assisted laparoscopic surgery in China is limited.

Laparoscopic radical gastrectomy encompasses different surgical approaches based on the location of the tumor, including laparoscopic proximal gastrectomy, distal gastrectomy, and total gastrectomy. The reconstruction methods following laparoscopic distal radical gastrectomy include Billroth I, Billroth II, and Roux-en-Y gastrojejunostomy. Billroth I anastomosis involves a direct connection between the proximal stomach and duodenum. This type of anastomosis closely aligns with the physiological state of the human body and is relatively straightforward to perform. It is a classic choice for anastomosis after distal gastric cancer surgery. With advancements in total endoscopic technology, an improved version of Billroth I anastomosis, known as triangular anastomosis, has been developed. Triangular anastomosis utilizes linear cutting closure for the remnant gastroduodenal anastomosis. This approach can be performed entirely under laparoscopic visualization, further minimizing the abdominal incision. Clinical studies have demonstrated the safety and reliability of triangular anastomosis [6]. Billroth II anastomosis involves an anastomosis between the remnant stomach and the proximal jejunum. The advantage of this method is that it allows for the resection of more distal gastric tissue during the operation, resulting in reduced tension at the anastomosis and relative simplicity of the procedure. However, it is associated with a higher incidence of postoperative reflux gastritis. To address this issue, Brown anastomosis is often added as a preventive measure. Billroth II anastomosis with Brown anastomosis is the most commonly used method for digestive tract reconstruction in laparoscopic distal gastrectomy. Roux-en-Y anastomosis involves dividing the jejunum at the distal end of Trez's ligament, anastomosing the distal jejunum with the remnant stomach, and performing an end-to-side anastomosis of the proximal jejunum with the distal small intestine at the gastrointestinal anastomosis. Roux-en-Y aims to align the flow direction of digestive juices with human physiology and overcome the disadvantages associated with the Billroth II formula, such as reflux. However, the incidence of Roux-en-Y retention syndrome is relatively high in practice. To address this issue, the uncut Roux-en-Y anastomosis technique has been developed [7]. This technique is based on Billroth II + Brown anastomosis, with ligation of the input loop of the small intestine. This approach preserves the normal flow of the digestive tract while avoiding the need for jejunum division.

For laparoscopic proximal gastrectomy, the available digestive tract reconstruction methods include esophagogastrostomy, jejunal interposition, and double-tract remnant gastrojejunal anastomosis. Esophagogastrostomy is a common approach for digestive tract reconstruction after proximal gastric cancer surgery. It involves directly anastomosing the remnant stomach with the esophagus, which aligns with human physiology and is relatively straightforward. However, it is associated with a high incidence of postoperative reflux esophagitis and a significant reduction in the quality of life for some patients. It is currently believed that reflux may be related to cardia resection. To address this issue, jejunal interposition and double-tract remnant gastrojejunal anastomosis have been developed. Jejunal interposition involves cutting a segment of the jejunum with a vascular pedicle from the distal end of Trez's ligament. The proximal end is anastomosed with the esophagus, the distal end is anastomosed with the greater curvature of the remnant stomach, and an end-to-end anastomosis of the jejunum is performed. Double-tract remnant gastrojejunal anastomosis entails dissecting the jejunum distally from Trez's ligament, anastomosing the distal jejunum with the esophagus, performing remnant gastrojejunostomy, and anastomosing the proximal jejunum at the distal end of the esophagojejunostomy. These two anastomotic methods effectively prevent reflux esophagitis and improve the quality of life for patients.

Commonly used digestive tract reconstruction methods after laparoscopic total gastrectomy include Roux-en-Y esophagus-jejunum anastomosis, jejunal interposition, and loop stomach replacement. Roux-en-Y esophagus-jejunum anastomosis is the most commonly used method in clinical practice. It involves creating an anastomosis between the esophagus and jejunum in a Roux-en-Y configuration. This method is simple to perform and has relatively low complications. However, in cases where transabdominal esophagojejunostomy is challenging, such as with high tumor location or obesity, the OrVil method can be considered. The OrVil technique, introduced in 2009, overcomes the difficulties associated with transabdominal placement of the esophageal nail and allows for anastomosis at a higher position to ensure an adequate margin of safety. Total laparoscopic Roux-en-Y esophagojejunostomy can be performed using two techniques: esophagojejunum functional end-to-end anastomosis (FETE) and esophagojejunum peristaltic side-to-side anastomosis (Overlap). Both approaches are relatively simple and safe but require a highly skilled surgical team. Laparoscopic radical gastrectomy has been shown to be safe and reliable in studies. The KLASS-01 trial, a multi-center prospective phase III clinical trial conducted in Korea, compared the outcomes of open surgery and laparoscopic surgery for early gastric cancer.

The results demonstrated that laparoscopic surgery for early gastric cancer is safe and reliable, with short-term and long-term curative effects comparable to laparotomy [8, 9].

As laparoscopic technology advances, laparoscopic gastric cancer surgery is being utilized in the treatment of advanced gastric cancer. Studies, such as the Japanese JLSSG 0901 study and the Korean KLASS-02 study, have shown the safety and feasibility of laparoscopic D2 lymph node dissection for locally advanced gastric cancer [10, 11]. China's CLASS-01 study, the first to complete enrollment among laparoscopic clinical studies on advanced gastric cancer, also demonstrated that laparoscopic D2 radical gastrectomy for locally advanced gastric cancer, when performed by experienced surgeons, is safe and feasible. It offers faster short-term recovery and comparable long-term survival to traditional open surgery [12]. In conclusion, laparoscopic techniques for gastric cancer surgery have shown promising results in terms of safety, feasibility, and comparable outcomes to open surgery. Laparoscopic approaches are increasingly being recommended and utilized for early and advanced gastric cancer cases [12, 13].

2.1.4 Expert Comments

Indeed, laparoscopic gastric cancer surgery has witnessed significant progress and development since its introduction in 1994 by Kitano, marking a milestone in the field. Over the course of just 30 years, laparoscopic techniques have advanced rapidly, leading to standardized dissection of lymph nodes and expanding the scope of surgeries performed. Initially, laparoscopic gastric cancer surgery focused on early gastric cancer, but with advancements in technology and surgical techniques, it has expanded to include advanced gastric cancer as well. The range of procedures has also broadened, from laparoscopic distal gastric cancer surgery to laparoscopic total gastric surgery, and from laparoscopic assisted to complete laparoscopic alimentary tract reconstruction. This progress has been driven by the incremental technical improvements made over time. The advantages of minimally invasive techniques, such as less trauma, faster recovery of gastrointestinal function, and shorter hospital stays, have been widely recognized. Evidence-based medicine has demonstrated that laparoscopic radical gastrectomy, when performed by experienced surgeons, is a safe and effective treatment option. Looking ahead, the continued promotion and adoption of laparoscopic surgery will undoubtedly benefit more gastric cancer patients. Minimally invasive techniques are expected to further improve treatment outcomes and contribute to the well-being of individuals undergoing gastric cancer surgery.

Case provider: Hu Ren, Xiaofeng Bai.

Commentary: Chunguang Guo.

2.2 Case 5: The Modified Delta-Shaped Anastomosis in Totally Laparoscopic Distal Gastrectomy

2.2.1 Brief History

The patient, a 58-year-old female, was admitted to the hospital primarily due to a persistent upper abdominal discomfort spanning a duration of 3 years, with recent aggravation over the past month. Initially, the patient experienced intermittent epigastric discomfort and dull pain without apparent triggers, which appeared 3 years ago and showed no discernible correlation with meals. Notably, the patient did not present with accompanying symptoms such as nausea, vomiting, abdominal distention, or diarrhea. Approximately 1 month prior to admission, the patient reported a worsening of abdominal discomfort, prompting her visit to a local hospital for gastroscopy, which revealed the presence of gastric cancer. Upon abdominal physical examination, no positive signs were detected. Tumor markers including CEA, AFP, CA72–4, CA19–9, and CA24–2 fell within the normal range. Gastroscopy findings indicated a superficial concave-type gastric cancer measuring approximately 3.5 cm × 2.5 cm, located at the junction of the larger curved side of the gastric body-antrum (0-IIc) (see Fig. 2.3). Biopsy pathology revealed poorly differentiated adenocarcinoma. Further evaluation through abdominal enhanced CT demonstrated mild thickening of the stomach wall extending from the lower segment of the gastric body to the antrum region, with roughening of the serous membrane. Additionally, scattered lymph nodes were observed in the left gastric region and mesentery, with the larger lymph node measuring approximately 0.5 cm in short diameter (see Fig. 2.4).

Diagnosis: Gastric cancer (cT2N0M0, stage I).

2.2.2 Treatment

Following admission, comprehensive examinations were conducted, and no contraindications were identified. During the perioperative period, a strategy of rapid rehabilitation surgery was employed, which involved forgoing water fasting, skin preparation, intestinal preparation, and preoperative tube placement.

Preoperative preparation was carried out considering the early stage of the tumor, posing challenges in laparoscopic localization. Under general anesthesia, the tumor was located using an endoscope inserted through the gastroscope. For cases with small lesions and early stages, it is customary to employ techniques such as dye or titanium clip labeling (e.g., carbon nanoparticles, methylene blue, and indocyanine green) under the gastroscope either 1 day prior to surgery or on the day of surgery.

Tracheal intubation general anesthesia was administered to the patient, who was positioned supine with legs extended. The Trocar placement followed the "five-hole method," with subumbilical puncture establishing pneumoperitoneum at a pressure of 12–15 mmHg. A 12 mm Trocar was

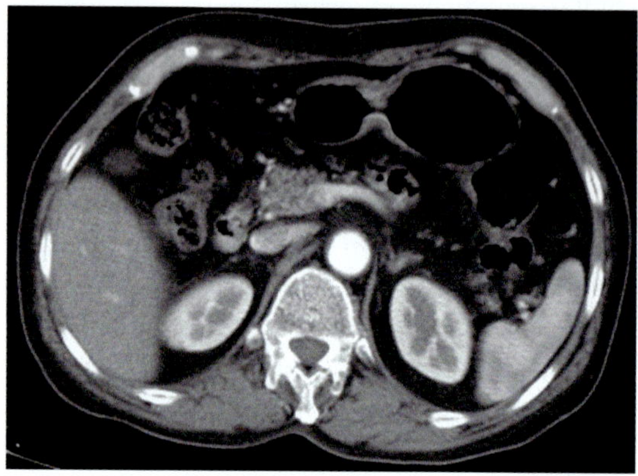

Fig. 2.4 The abdominal CT scan revealed a slight thickening of the stomach wall extending from the lower segment of the stomach body to the antrum region. Additionally, the serous surface appeared rough

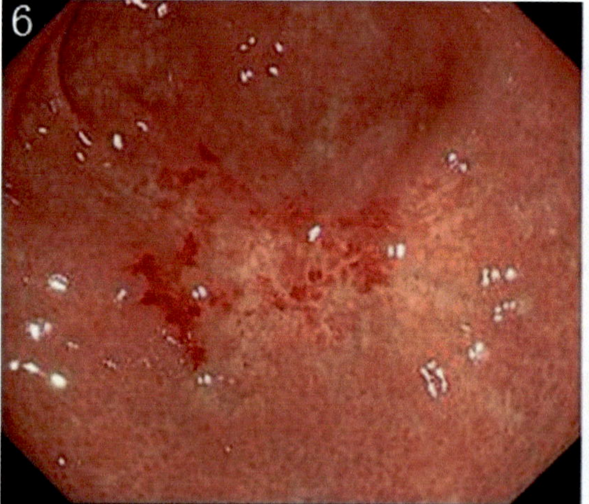

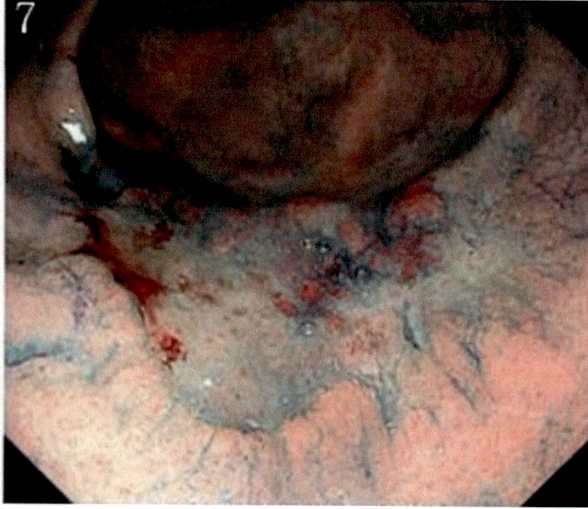

Fig. 2.3 The gastroscopic examination revealed the esophagogastric boundary positioned approximately 40 cm from the incisor. Notably, a superficial concave lesion (0-IIc) measuring approximately 3.5 cm × 2.5 cm was observed at the junction of the gastric body-antrum's larger bend

inserted as the observation hole, while the main operating holes were positioned 2 cm below the costal margin of the left anterior axillary line and 2 cm below the costal margin of the right anterior axillary line, both utilizing 12 mm Trocars. As auxiliary operation holes, 5 mm Trocars were inserted 2 cm above the umbilical cord along the left and right midclavicular lines. The surgeon stood on the patient's left side, the assistant on the right side, and the mirror holder between the patient's legs.

Intraoperatively, a routine abdominal exploration was conducted, which revealed the absence of metastasis in the liver, gallbladder, spleen, and abdominal and pelvic regions. The serous layer of the stomach wall appeared intact. By means of intraoperative gastroscopy, the tumor was localized in the greater bend of the junction between the gastric body and antrum, positioned 1 cm away from both the upper and lower boundaries of the tumor. For marking purposes, 0.5 mL of indocyanine green was injected under the mucosa (see Fig. 2.5a).

Following the Japanese protocol for gastric cancer, distal radical gastrectomy was performed, accompanied by laparoscopic D2 lymph node dissection. A linear incision closure was implemented through the main operating hole in the left upper abdomen. The duodenum was rotated clockwise by 90°, ensuring an adequate

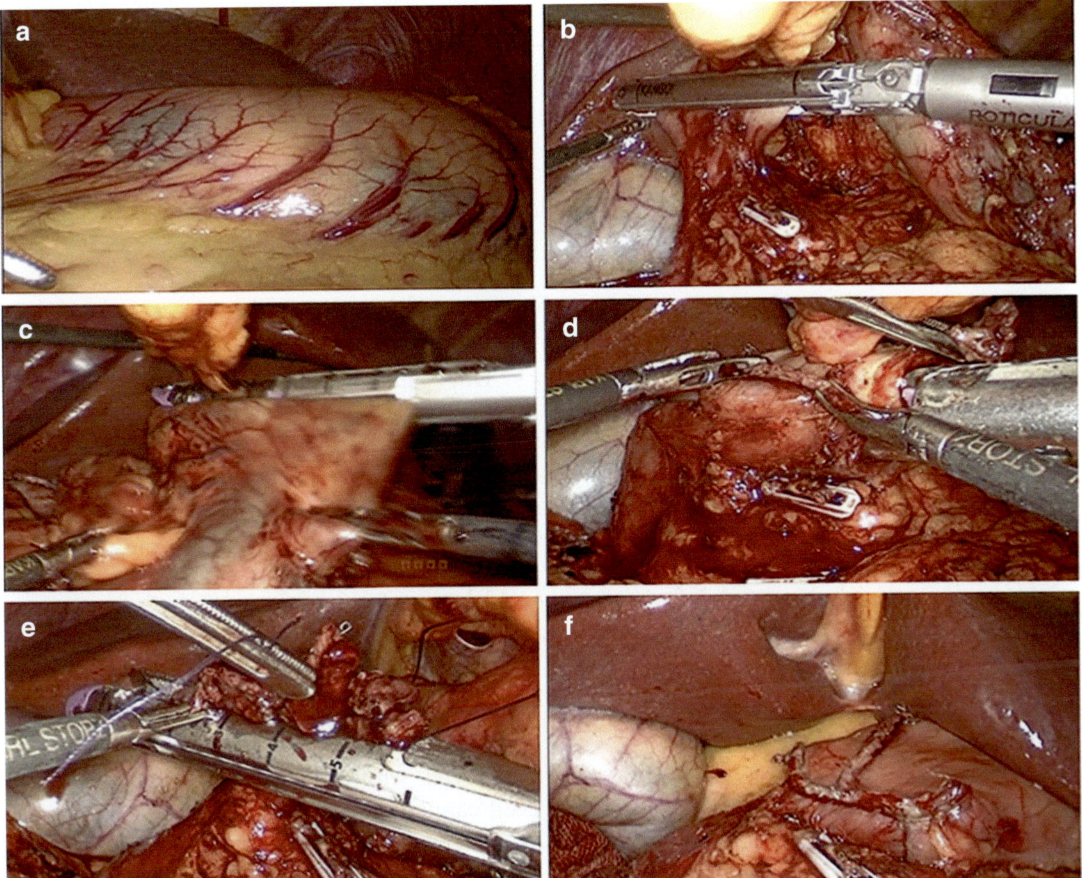

Fig. 2.5 The steps of totally laparoscopic improved triangular procedure: (**a**) Indocyanine green was utilized to locate the tumor. (**b**) The duodenum was rotated clockwise by 90° and transected from back to front. (**c**) The stomach body was surgically resected. (**d**) A linear cutting closure device was employed to perform a "V"-shaped anastomosis, matching the residual back wall of the stomach with the duodenal wall. (**e**) The joint opening was closed, and the duodenal stump was removed. (**f**) The appearance of the surgical site after the completion of the triangular anastomosis showed improvement

incisal margin, and then severed from back to front, generally leaving a stump of 2–4 cm in length. The resected stomach body was preserved 5 cm away from the upper margin of the tumor, and one-third of the proximal stomach stump was retained. The specimen was placed in a specimen bag and removed after the operation. In cases where the tumor location is uncertain or suspicion arises regarding the distance of the tumor incisal margin, the specimen can be initially removed through a small abdominal incision and examined directly or subjected to a quick intraoperative frozen pathological examination to confirm complete R0 resection. Pneumoperitoneum was reestablished following examination.

Digestive tract reconstruction was performed by creating small 1 cm openings in the greater curvature of the remaining stomach and the posterior wall of the duodenum. Both ends of the linear cutter were extended into these openings, enabling a "V"-shaped anastomosis between the posterior wall of the remnant stomach and the upper edge of the duodenum. Once the anastomosis line was inspected to ensure no bleeding and satisfactory anastomosis, the common opening was closed using the linear cutting closure device. During the anastomosis process, the assistant held the duodenal stump, placing it together with the common opening into the mouth of the cutting closure device, and closed them simultaneously. To prevent anastomotic stenosis, the closure direction of the common opening should be perpendicular to the gastric incisal margin, and careful verification of anastomotic patency should be conducted post-closure. After confirming no errors in the operative area, two peritoneal drainage tubes were placed, extracted, and secured externally (see Fig. 2.5b–f).

On the first postoperative day, the gastric tube was removed, and the patient was encouraged to drink water and mobilize. On the third day, the surgical site was cleaned, and a 5-day liquid diet was initiated. Upper gastrointestinal angiography conducted during this period did not reveal any abnormalities (see Fig. 2.6). The abdominal drainage tube was removed on the sixth day, and the patient was discharged from the hospital on the ninth day.

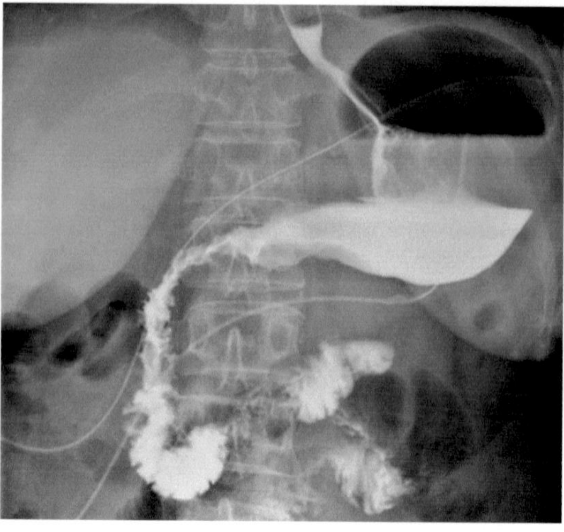

Fig. 2.6 On the fifth day after surgery, iohexol angiography showed good anastomotic passage, and no contrast extravasation was observed

Pathological examination of the distal gastrectomy specimens revealed the following details:

Gross specimen measurements:

- Minor curvature of the stomach: 11 cm long.
- Major curvature of the stomach: 13 cm long.
- Duodenum: 0.7 cm long and 3.5 cm wide.

The tumor located in the stomach body measured 2.5 × 1.5 cm in size. It was situated 4.5 cm from the superior incisal margin and 7 cm from the inferior incisal margin. Importantly, there was no involvement of the pylorus or duodenum.

According to the endoscopic diagnosis, the tumor was identified as a superficial concave poorly differentiated adenocarcinoma of the stomach (Type IIc) based on Lauren's classification. The majority of the tumor exhibited the diffuse type, with a portion displaying signet ring cell carcinoma characteristics. In terms of invasion depth, the tumor invaded the submucosa and was associated with nerve invasion. Notably, no vascular tumor embolus was observed, and there was no involvement of the pylorus or duodenum. Additionally, no carcinoma was detected in the omentum or the superior and inferior incisional margins. Importantly, no lymph node metastatic carcinoma was identified among the 25 examined lymph nodes. The overall TNM stage of the tumor was classified as pT1bN0M0, corresponding to stage I.

2.2.3 Case Analysis

1. Triangular anastomosis

   In 2002, Kanaya, a Japanese scholar, first reported the technique of total laparoscopic triangular anastomosis (Delta-anastomosis) using a straight-line cutting stapler for laparoscopic gastroduodenal anastomosis [14]. Unlike the tubular stapler technique, this method offers simplicity in operation, excellent visualization under the microscope, minimal abdominal incision, and favorable cosmetic outcomes. It represents a true total laparoscopic approach to digestive tract reconstruction. With its widespread adoption in Japan and South Korea, it has become the standard method for digestive tract reconstruction following laparoscopic gastric cancer surgery in most diagnostic and treatment centers.

   Several considerations should be noted during the operation. Triangular anastomosis is not suitable for locally advanced gastric cancer (T3–4) or tumors involving the stomach body or pylorus. To ensure the safety of the anastomosis, approximately 3–4 cm of the duodenal stump is typically preserved for surgical manipulation. Proper release of the Kocher incision during the operation can reduce tension at the anastomotic site. To protect the blood supply to the duodenum, it is essential to ensure that the stapler detaches the duodenum from back to front. During the procedure, the surgeon stands on the left side and inserts the straight-line cutting closure device through the main operating hole in the left epigastric region. As simultaneous placement of the cutting stapler into both the stomach stump and duodenum can be challenging, it is generally preferred to place a thicker stapler into the stomach cavity first, followed by a thinner stapler into the duodenal stump. The stump and duodenum are appropriately rotated, and the cut end forms a 45° angle with the cutting stapler before firing to prevent stump ischemia (Fig. 2.5b–d). Close attention should be paid to potential issues such as rotation, stenosis, bleeding, and excessive tension at the anastomotic site during the operation.

   A retrospective study has demonstrated that triangular anastomosis is a safe, reliable, and easily mastered method for digestive tract reconstruction [15]. It offers a large diameter for the anastomosis, resulting in a low complication rate and no increased occurrence of postoperative reflux gastritis. However, mastering this technique requires a steep learning curve, with an average anastomotic time of 13 min.

   Sakaguchi et al. [16] conducted a comparison study on long-term complications, body weight, and nutritional status of patients undergoing triangular anastomosis, Billroth II anastomosis, and Roux-en-Y anastomosis for digestive tract reconstruction. The results indicated that triangular anastomosis had the shortest operative time, a low postoperative complication rate, and rare anastomotic inflammation (6.7% in the first postoperative year and 15.6% in the third postoperative year).
2. Improved triangular anastomosis

   Traditional triangular anastomosis has been associated with certain risks and complications due to the "T" anastomotic intersection angles and the blind angle formed by the duodenal stump [17–19]. In China, Huang Changming et al. [17] introduced an improved triangular anastomosis method. This modification involves removing the blind angle of the duodenum and the intersection angle formed by the duodenal incisal margin, leaving only the intersection angle between the gastric incisal margin and the anastomosis line of the common opening. This reduces the three weak points of the traditional triangular anastomosis into one and results in an inverted "T" shape appearance after completion. Theoretically, this modification can reduce the occurrence of anastomotic leakage (Fig. 2.5f).

A retrospective study showed that the modified triangular anastomosis method yielded similar outcomes to the traditional method in terms of intraoperative blood loss, lymph node dissection, postoperative recovery, and complication rate. However, the modified method required less time for completion (13.9 ± 2.8 min vs. 23.9 ± 5.6 min, $P = 0.000$) [20]. Harada et al. [21] reached a similar conclusion, stating that there was no significant difference in body weight change 1 year after surgery between the two methods. However, at 1 year after the modified triangular anastomosis, gastroscopy showed a lower amount of food residue and a lower incidence of residual gastritis compared to the traditional method.

3. Indications of triangular anastomosis

Indeed, triangular anastomosis is a method of reconstructing the digestive tract, specifically for functional end-to-end anastomosis (FETE) between the residual stomach and duodenum. It is primarily used in cases of lower gastric cancer with small tumor volume and early stage, where the tumor distance from the pylorus is greater than 2 cm, due to the limitations of the anastomosis and triangulation in Bi I gastrectomy. Therefore, careful evaluation of cases is necessary before surgery to ensure optimal oncological treatment outcomes.

In cases of laparoscopic surgery for early gastric cancer, where tactile feedback may be lacking, emphasis should be placed on preoperative or intraoperative tumor localization. In this particular case, intraoperative indocyanine green (ICG) staining was used to locate the tumor, which played a crucial role in accurately determining the incisal margin.

Although the technique of triangular anastomosis is relatively simple, there are various technical aspects that need to be considered. If the anastomosis is not ideal, it can be challenging to correct intraoperatively or postoperatively. Therefore, it is recommended to perform extensive simulation experiments on animal models before the actual surgery, as this can deepen the understanding of gastrointestinal anastomotic rotation and provide valuable experience, especially in laparoscopic surgery centers [22].

2.2.4 Expert Comments

With the advancements and refinement of laparoscopic techniques, an increasing number of surgeons are favoring total laparoscopic digestive tract reconstruction after gastric cancer surgery. This approach offers benefits such as improved visualization, safer procedures, reduced trauma, faster recovery, and better cosmetic outcomes. Among the various techniques, triangular anastomosis has gained popularity since its introduction in 2002, particularly in Japan and Korea, due to its simplicity and suitability for early-stage lower gastric cancer treatment. As a functional end-to-end anastomosis method, triangular anastomosis expands the application scope of laparoscopic digestive tract reconstruction.

However, when selecting the method for digestive tract reconstruction, it is important to consider the advantages and disadvantages of different anastomotic techniques. In China, compared to Japan and Korea, the number of cases suitable for triangular anastomosis is limited due to different disease characteristics. Overusing this technique beyond its appropriate indications may compromise the oncological treatment outcomes, leading to issues such as local recurrence, positive incisal margins, and anastomotic leakage. Therefore, caution should be exercised during the application process to ensure the best therapeutic effects.

Furthermore, despite its seemingly straightforward nature, triangular anastomosis should be performed by surgeons with mature laparoscopic skills, following a step-by-step approach. This ensures the proper and orderly application of this new technology, ultimately benefiting the patients.

With the emergence of precision medicine, the landscape of early gastric cancer treatment is evolving rapidly. The approach to early gastric cancer has shifted from traditional endoscopic therapy to various forms of laparoscopic gastrectomy with a focus on functional preservation. This shift has significantly improved the quality of life for patients by minimizing the extent of surgery and preserving organ function.

However, it is crucial to adhere to established treatment guidelines and strike a balance between oncological efficacy and patients' quality of life. While functional preservation is important, the primary goal of treatment remains the eradication of cancer and prevention of disease recurrence. The choice of treatment should be based on thorough evaluation, considering factors such as tumor characteristics, stage, patient's overall health, and individual preferences.

By adhering to treatment norms and guidelines, healthcare professionals can ensure that patients receive the most appropriate and effective treatment for their early gastric cancer. This approach allows for optimal oncological outcomes while also considering and maximizing patients' quality of life.

Case provider: Tongbo Wang, Chunguang Guo.

Commentary: Dongbing Zhao.

2.3 Case 6: Totally Laparoscopic Radical Total Gastrectomy

2.3.1 Brief History

The patient, a 57-year-old female, presented with a chief complaint of persistent pain and discomfort localized to the left upper abdomen for a duration exceeding 6 months. Initially, the patient reported experiencing intermittent pain and discomfort in the left upper quadrant without any discernible triggers, accompanied by neither nausea nor acid regurgitation. Seeking medical attention, the patient underwent gastroscopy at a local hospital, which revealed the presence of "gastric mucosal lesions." Subsequent pathological examination confirmed the presence of "severe dysplasia," prompting treatment with "omeprazole" and other pharmacological interventions. Three months later, a follow-up gastroscopy demonstrated persisting "gastric mucosal lesions" with "mild-moderate dysplasia" observed pathologically. Throughout the past 6 months, the patient's abdominal pain symptoms exhibited no amelioration, and no symptoms such as dysphagia, hematemesis, or melena were reported. The patient sought consultation at our hospital approximately 20 days ago, where an abdominal examination yielded negative findings. Notably, tumor markers including CEA, AFP, CA72–4, CA19–9, and CA24–2 were all within normal limits. A subsequent gastroscopic evaluation indicated the presence of gastric cancer, specifically located in the mid-gastric body to the posterior wall of the antrum junction. Additionally, lesions on the gastric fundus and anterior wall of the lower gastric body were also consistent with gastric cancer (Fig. 2.7). Biopsy results from the posterior wall of the gastric body confirmed the presence of adenocarcinoma, while the greater curvature of the gastric fundus exhibited chronic inflammation of gastric mucosal tissue with intestinal metaplasia and atypical glandular epithelial cells. CT imaging revealed irregular thickening of the gastric wall in the lower region of the gastric body, further supporting the suspicion of gastric cancer in conjunction with the findings from gastroscopy (Fig. 2.8).

Diagnosis: Gastric cancer (cT3N0M0, stage II).

2.3.2 Treatment

Following admission, comprehensive examinations were conducted, and no contraindications for surgery were identified. Given the presence of multiple gastric lesions, with the larger lesion situated in the gastric body and the smaller lesion in the stomach fundus, a total laparoscopic gastrectomy was planned as the surgical intervention. The perioperative approach adopted in this case involved employing rapid recovery surgery techniques. Consequently, no water fasting, skin preparation, or bowel preparation were administered on the day preceding the operation. Furthermore, the placement of a gastric tube was not performed prior to surgery.

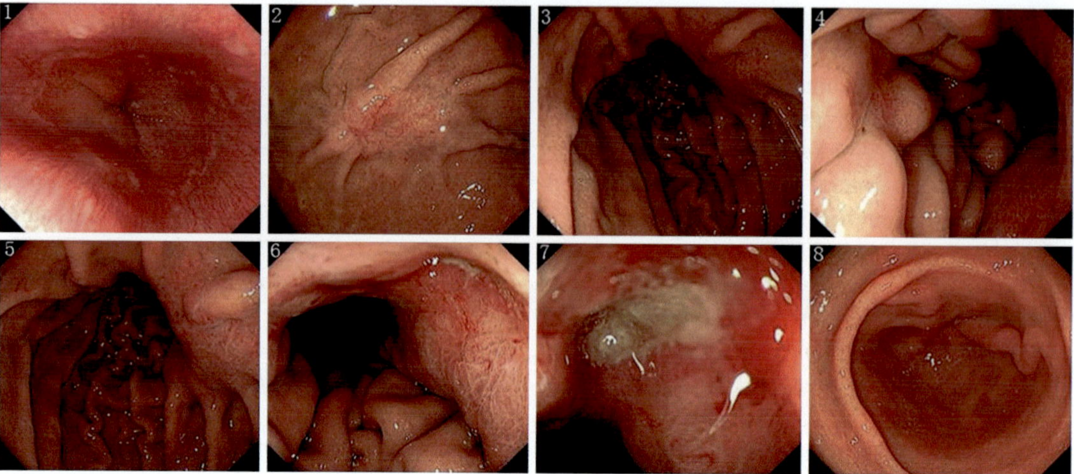

Fig. 2.7 Gastroscopy revealed that the esophagogastric junction was approximately 37 cm from the incisors. Notably, a raised lesion measuring approximately 2.0 × 1.5 cm was observed on the greater curvature of the gastric fundus. Furthermore, the lesion extended from the middle of the stomach body to the posterior wall of the junction between the body antrum and the side of the lesser curvature, located approximately 45–52 cm from the incisors

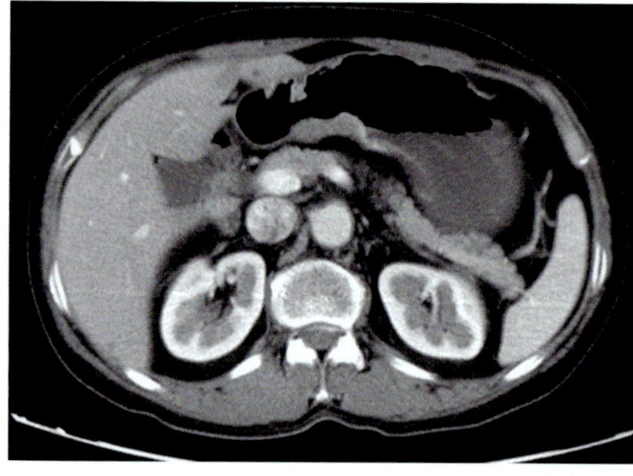

Fig. 2.8 The CT scan revealed dilation of the gastric cavity and irregular thickening of the gastric wall in the lower region of the gastric body, with the maximum thickness measuring approximately 1.0 cm. The lesion exhibited a long diameter of approximately 3.9 cm and showed enhancement upon contrast-enhanced scanning. Notably, the serosa surface appeared smooth

2.3.2.1 Surgical Steps and Technical Points

Anesthesia, Patient Positioning, and Trocar Placement

Under general anesthesia, the patient was intubated and positioned in the supine split-leg posture. Trocar insertion followed the "five-hole method," with the establishment of pneumoperitoneum achieved through subumbilical puncture at a pressure of 12–15 mmHg. An observation hole was created by inserting a 12 mm trocar. A second 12 mm trocar was placed 2 cm below the left anterior axillary margin. Auxiliary operation holes were established using 5 mm trocars positioned 2 cm below the right costal margin along the anterior axillary line and 2 cm above the umbilical level along the midclavicular line on both the left and right sides. During the procedure, the surgeon stood on the left side of the patient, the assistant on the right side, and the mirror holder in between the patient's legs.

Intraoperative Findings and Surgical Steps

Abdominal exploration revealed no metastases in the liver, gallbladder, spleen, abdomen, or pelvis. The tumor located in the posterior wall of the gastric body exhibited invasion into the serosa layer while sparing the surrounding tissues. The entire stomach and duodenum were meticulously dissected, and laparoscopic lymph node dissection was performed. The duodenum was transected using a linear cutting stapler, and the duodenal stump was closed with continuous sutures using 3–0 barbed thread, ensuring embedding in the seromuscular layer. For esophagojejunostomy, the Overlap method was employed, starting 15 cm from the Treiz ligament. A 6 cm linear cutting stapler was used to divide the jejunum, and a small opening was made on the right side of the esophagus, above the tumor. Similarly, a small opening was created on the mesenteric side, below the distal end of the jejunum, corresponding to the disrupted esophageal end. An Overlap anastomosis was performed using the linear cutting stapler, followed by closure of the common opening with a linear cutter. A midline incision of approximately 5 cm in length was made on the upper abdomen, allowing layer-by-layer access to retrieve the specimen and assess the incision margin. Side-to-side anastomosis between the distal and proximal jejunum was performed 40 cm below the esophagojejunostomy site. Continuous sutures were used to close the common opening, ensuring embedding of the seromuscular layer. The procedure concluded.

Postoperative Course and Discharge

The patient was encouraged to mobilize and leave the bed on the third day after the surgery. On the fifth day, iohexol angiography revealed no abnormalities, leading to the removal of the stomach tube, followed by the initiation of water intake. By the seventh day, the patient progressed to a liquid diet. Subsequently, on the eighth day, the abdominal drainage tube was removed, and the patient was discharged on the ninth day.

Pathology Findings

Gross specimen examination of the total gastrectomy specimen revealed specific measurements, including a length of 16 cm for the lesser curvature and 23 cm for the greater curvature. The upper esophagus measured 0.5 cm in length, while the lower duodenum ranged from 0.5 to 1 cm in length. The margins had widths of 3 cm and 4.5 cm for the lesser curvature and greater curvature, respectively. The distance between the esophagogastric junction and the lesser curvature was 5 cm. The observed mass had dimensions of 3 cm × 3.2 cm × 1 cm, featuring a gray-white solid surface with an indistinct hard boundary. The distance between the mass and the surgical margin was 6 cm. A suture mark and a 1.2 cm × 0.7 cm area of mucosal shrinkage were noted at the suture site.

Microscopic diagnosis revealed infiltrating ulcerative moderately differentiated adenocarcinoma of the stomach (Lauren classification: intestinal type). The tumor exhibited two foci with similar morphological features. The larger focus invaded the muscle layer, reaching the serosa, and demonstrated vascular tumor thrombus, nerve invasion, and extramural venous invasion. The smaller foci invaded the superficial muscle layer. Notably, there was no involvement of the esophagogastric junction, pylorus, duodenum, or omentum. Moreover, no cancer cells were detected at the upper and lower resection margins. Lymph node analysis indicated the absence of metastatic carcinoma among the examined lymph nodes (0/62). The TNM staging for the tumor was determined as pT4a (m) N0M0, corresponding to stage II.

2.3.2.2 CT Findings One Year After Operation (Fig. 2.9)

The CT scan conducted 1 year after total gastrectomy revealed poor dilation of the esophagojejunal anastomosis. The local wall exhibited slight thickening, and multiple metal density rod shadows were observed within the abdominal cavity.

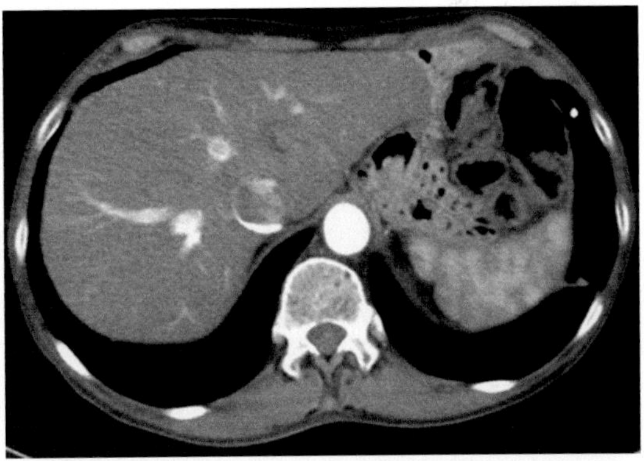

Fig. 2.9 The CT scan revealed a poorly dilated esophagojejunal anastomosis. Furthermore, there was slight thickening of the local wall, and multiple metal density rod shadows were observed within the abdominal cavity. These findings are indicative of expected postoperative changes

These findings are consistent with expected postoperative changes and are considered normal.

2.3.2.3 Gastroscopic Findings One Year After Operation (Fig. 2.10)

Gastroscopy performed 1 year after the operation did not reveal any apparent abnormalities at the anastomosis site. However, close follow-up and regular reviews are recommended to monitor the patient's condition closely.

2.3.3 Case Analysis

Total gastrectomy is the primary surgical approach employed for the treatment of esophagogastric junction tumors, gastric body tumors, leather-bottle stomach tumors, and other related malignancies. With advancements in laparoscopic technology, total laparoscopic total gastrectomy has gained popularity as a minimally invasive surgical technique in clinical practice. This approach offers reduced invasiveness and quicker recovery times. Notably, the reconstruction of the digestive tract under laparoscopy poses a significant technical challenge and has become a recent area of research interest. Esophagojejunostomy serves as a crucial aspect of digestive tract reconstruction following total laparoscopic total gastrectomy. Various anastomosis methods can be categorized into three main types: manual anastomosis, circular anastomosis, and linear anastomosis. Each of these techniques plays a significant role in achieving successful restoration of digestive continuity after surgery.

1. Manual sewing method

   Following the division of the esophagus during the procedure, the esophagojejunal anastomosis was manually sutured under laparoscopy, utilizing either an end-to-end or end-to-side anastomotic technique. This method, although cost-effective and not reliant on staplers, requires a longer operative time and demands a high level of laparoscopic proficiency from the surgical team. Not only does the surgeon need to be skilled in laparoscopic suturing techniques, but the entire surgical team must ensure optimal exposure of the surgical field and execute their tasks with precision and expertise [23].

2. Circular stapler anastomosis

   In traditional open surgery for digestive tract reconstruction, circular staplers have been widely utilized. Surgeons are accustomed to the technical aspects and operating methods associated with these devices. During the initial exploration and research of total laparoscopic digestive tract reconstruction, significant attention was given to various reconstruction techniques employing circular

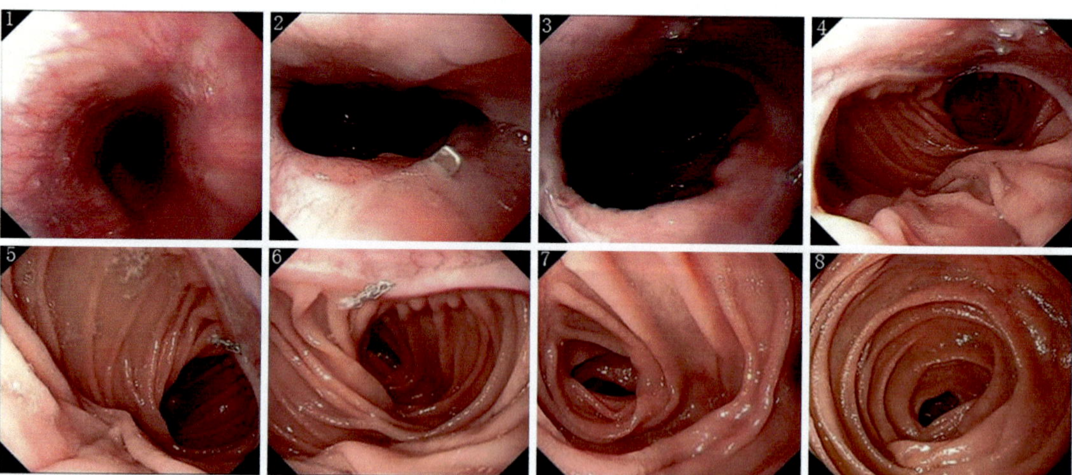

Fig. 2.10 Gastroscopy: No obvious abnormalities were found in the endoscopy 1 year after total gastrectomy

staplers. The challenge in this approach lies in the accurate placement of the distal end of the esophageal nail under direct laparoscopic visualization and its secure fixation using a purse-string suture.

(a) Purse: Bag Suture

In total laparoscopic surgery, the use of traditional purse-string forceps, commonly employed in open surgery or laparoscopic-assisted procedures, is not suitable due to their limitations such as a large head volume and short handle. To address this issue, Usui et al. [24] introduced an improved purse-string stapler specifically designed for total laparoscopic surgery. This modified purse-string suture device features a smaller head and a longer handle, allowing it to be inserted into the abdominal cavity through a 12 mm Trocar or a 4 cm auxiliary small incision in the upper middle abdomen. Once pneumoperitoneum is established, the head of the device is clamped to the predetermined resection line of the esophagus. Subsequently, under laparoscopic guidance, the purse string is inserted through the guide pin hole groove of the head, enabling the completion of the esophageal purse-string suture. For the subsequent endoscopic esophagojejunal anastomosis, an endoluminal stapler is employed. This approach allows for the completion of both the esophageal nail anvil placement and the digestive tract reconstruction within the abdominal cavity. However, some experts express concern that if the esophagus is initially severed during the operation, the esophageal stump may retract to a higher position, potentially reaching or even extending inside the diaphragm. This can make it challenging to accurately place the anvil and increase the difficulty of laparoscopic anastomosis.

(b) Anti-puncture method

The anti-puncture method, initially proposed by Omori et al. [25] in 2009, is an anastomotic technique that has undergone subsequent improvements. This technique makes use of the plastic center rod of a stapler pin holder for puncture purposes. The procedure involves the mobilization of the stomach and esophagus under laparoscopy. A suture with a needle is passed through a small hole located at the end of the central rod, tied, and fixed at the end. The nail holder with the needle is then inserted into the abdominal cavity through a small incision in the upper abdomen. The esophagus is clamped at the predetermined resection site using a clamping clamp, and a 2 cm incision is made at the upper edge of the clamp. Through this incision, the nail holder with the needle is inserted into the lower esophagus from bottom to top. The esophagus is clamped using a linear stapler close to the suture site. Subsequently, the suture is pulled firmly until the central rod of the nail seat passes completely through the esophageal wall. The stapler is then activated to close the esophageal stump and secure the nail seat in place. Finally, the laparoscopic stapler is used to perform esophagojejunostomy. The anti-puncture method eliminates the need for purse-string suturing to secure the nail seat when using a tubular stapler. Since the esophagus is not completely severed, the insertion of the nail is relatively easier, resulting in a lower incidence of esophageal injury. However, the location of the incision for this method should be carefully considered. If it is too close to the transverse incision below, it may affect the closure effect of the linear stapler. Conversely, if it is too far away, it may result in excessive esophageal resection, which can impact the subsequent esophagojejunostomy procedure.

(c) OrVil method

In 2009, Jeong et al. [26] introduced the "top-down" esophagojejunum anastomosis technique, known as the OrVil method. This technique involves the use of a guide tube to facilitate the anastomosis between the esophagus and the jejunum (or remnant stomach). The procedure begins with the dissection of the stomach and esophagus under an endoscope. The esophagus is then transected at the predetermined resection site using a linear stapler. A guide tube, with one end fixed to the stapler pin seat, is lubricated and inserted transorally into the esophageal stump with the assistance of an anesthesiologist. Under laparoscopy, a small incision is made in the esophageal stump, and the guide tube is passed through this incision. The guide tube is carefully pulled until the central rod of the stapler pin seat is fully exposed. Subsequently, endoluminal reconstruction of the digestive tract is performed. The OrVil method eliminates the challenges associated with laparoscopic purse-string suturing when using a circular stapler. It simplifies the surgical steps and reduces the overall operation time. Additionally, this technique allows for a higher surgical margin to be achieved. However, it is important to note that the implantation of the guide tube may potentially damage the esophagus and pharynx. Moreover, since the guide tube needs to be pulled out of the body through the abdominal cavity, there is an increased risk of bacterial contamination of the abdominal cavity during this process. Careful attention should be paid to minimize these risks during the procedure.

3. Linear cutting closer anastomosis

Compared to the circular stapler method, the "top-down" esophagojejunum anastomosis technique (OrVil method) offers several advantages. First, it eliminates the need to place a pin holder, simplifying the reconstruction procedure. The linear stapler can be easily inserted and removed from the abdominal cavity through a 12 mm Trocar, eliminating the need for additional small incisions. This contributes to a less invasive approach. Furthermore, this method allows for a wider anastomosis since it is not limited by the diameters of the esophagus, jejunum, and stapler pin seat. This ensures a sufficient width of the anastomosis and can significantly reduce the incidence of postoperative anastomotic stenosis, which is a common complication of digestive tract reconstruction. Overall, the OrVil method streamlines the procedure, provides more flexibility in anastomosis size, and reduces the risk of anastomotic stenosis. These advantages make it an attractive option for total laparoscopic digestive tract reconstruction.

(a) Functional end-to-end anastomosis of esophagus and jejunum (Functional end-to-end, FETE)

The laparoscopic linear cutting closure technique for digestive tract reconstruction after total gastrectomy was first reported by Uyama et al. [26] in Japan. In this method, the esophagus and jejunum were separated, and a small incision was made at the corner of the jejunal stump and the adjacent esophageal stump. A linear stapler was inserted through these incisions to perform a side-to-side esophagojejunal anastomosis. In 2009, Okabe et al. [27] further modified the technique, known as the FETE (functional end-to-end esophagojejunostomy) method, to ensure a tumor-free anastomosis. In this modified technique, the resected specimen was removed before the anastomosis. The esophagus was rotated 45° counterclockwise to allow for closure of the common opening using the "delta-shaped technique" or other methods. This type of anastomosis reduces the complexity of full-endoscopic anastomosis, ensures an adequate internal diameter of the anastomosis, and reduces the incidence of anastomotic stenosis. However, there are some drawbacks associated with these techniques. The use of closure devices increases the cost of the procedure. Additionally, the anastomosis created is not a circular passage, and there may be a small dead space present, which deviates from the normal physiological structure of the digestive tract. It is important to consider these factors and weigh the benefits and drawbacks when selecting the appropriate technique for digestive tract reconstruction after total gastrectomy.

(b) π-shaped anastomosis

The π-shaped anastomosis technique is an improvement based on the functional end-to-end anastomosis method. In this technique, after the abdominal cavity is separated, the esophagus is not cut off initially. Instead, a suture is made at the esophagogastric junction, and the esophagus is pulled downward. A small incision is then made in the right lateral wall of the esophagus and the mesenteric side of the jejunum. The common opening is closed by simultaneously cutting the esophagus and jejunum using a linear cutting stapler. The resulting shape of the anastomosis resembles the Greek letter "π," hence the name π-shaped anastomosis [28]. This method simplifies the surgical steps, reduces the time required for anastomosis, and lowers the overall cost of the operation. However, there are some considerations to keep in mind. The technique does not allow for the accurate assessment of the esophageal resection margin since the esophagus is not cut prior to anastomosis. This may pose a risk of incomplete resection margins, particularly for patients with unclear margins. Additionally, in patients with a short mesentery of the small intestine, there may be increased tension at the anastomotic site, which can lead to a higher risk of anastomotic leakage. It is important for the surgical team to carefully evaluate the individual patient's condition and consider the benefits and potential risks associated with the π-shaped anastomosis technique before selecting it as the preferred method for digestive tract reconstruction after total gastrectomy.

(c) Esophagojejunal peristaltic anastomosis (Overlap anastomosis)

In 2010, Inaba et al. [29] introduced the Overlap anastomosis technique, which involves adjusting the peristaltic direction of the small intestine after functional end-to-end (FETE) anastomosis. In this technique, the jejunal stump is placed in the proximal direction, and a small incision is made below the stump corresponding to the esophageal stump. Side-to-side anastomosis is performed using a linear stapler, and the common opening is manually sutured. This approach addresses the issue of the corner problem in side-to-side anastomosis. By allowing the small intestine to move in the direction of peristalsis after anastomosis, it facilitates better emptying of the anastomosis. When applying the Overlap anastomosis method in a case of synchronous double primary cancer, the lesions located in the fundus and the middle and lower part of the gastric body met the indication for total gastrectomy. During the surgical reconstruction, the chosen method for anastomosis was Overlap anastomosis. A small incision was made on the right lateral wall of the esophagus, and the jejunal stump was positioned in the proximal direction. Another small incision was made on the mesenteric side below the stump corresponding to the esophageal stump. This technique has the advantage of extending the esophagus first, making it easier to manipulate. After anastomosis, the small intestine moves along with peristalsis, promoting better emptying. Finally, the common opening was closed using a linear cutting stapler to prevent anastomotic stenosis. The choice of anastomosis technique depends on various factors, including the patient's condition, surgeon's expertise, and surgical team's capabilities. Each method has its advantages and considerations, and the selection should be made based on individual patient characteristics and surgical goals.

2.3.4 Expert Comments

Total laparoscopic gastrectomy offers advantages in terms of reduced trauma and faster recovery compared to open and laparoscopic-assisted surgery. However, there is currently no standard anastomosis method for digestive tract reconstruction after total laparoscopic gastrectomy. Circular anastomosis and linear anastomosis are two commonly used techniques, but their relative superiority and inferiority are still under investigation. For surgeons, it is important to be proficient in multiple anastomosis techniques, have a thorough understanding of the characteristics, advantages, and disadvantages of each method, and make individualized decisions based on factors such as tumor location and size. By selecting the most appropriate anastomosis method for each patient, surgeons can ensure the efficacy and safety of the surgical procedure. It is worth noting that advancements and ongoing research in the field of laparoscopic surgery continue to contribute to the development of new techniques and refinements of existing ones. Surgeons should stay updated with the latest literature and surgical advancements to provide the best possible care for their patients.

Case provider: Hu Ren, Chunguang Guo.

Commentary: Chunguang Guo.

2.4 Case 7: Double Tract Reconstruction in Totally Laparoscopic Proximal Gastrectomy

2.4.1 Brief History

The admission of a 64-year-old male patient was prompted by a persistent upper abdominal discomfort spanning a duration of 1 month. The patient began experiencing this discomfort without an apparent precipitating factor approximately 1 month ago. Gastroscopy performed at a previous medical facility revealed ulceration on the lesser curvature of the stomach, and subsequent biopsy results indicated the presence of high-grade intraepithelial neoplasia. Regarding the gastroscopic findings, the esophageal mucosa exhibited no evident abnormalities, with the esophagogastric junction located approximately 41 cm from the incisors. Notably, at a distance of 41–43 cm from the incisors, a superficial protrusion and shallow depression lesion (0-IIa + IIc) was observed at the cardia. The surface mucosa of this lesion appeared red, rough, eroded, and uneven, as depicted in Fig. 2.11. Furthermore, an endoscopic ultrasound examination disclosed thickening of the gastric wall at the lesion site, predominantly affecting the mucosal and submucosal layers, with the maximum thickness measuring approximately 0.68 cm. The muscularis propria and serosa of the gastric wall at the lesion site exhibited clear, continuous, and intact features. No significantly enlarged lymph nodes were detected in the vicinity of the affected gastric wall, as illustrated in Fig. 2.12. Histopathological analysis revealed moderately differentiated adenocarcinoma originating from the glandular epithelium in the mucosal layer, classified according to the Lauren classification as intestinal type. Computed tomography (CT) imaging exhibited slight thickening of the gastric wall in the cardia region, with the thickest segment measuring approximately 0.9 cm. Importantly, the outer edge of the thickened area appeared smooth, while no discernible abnormal enhancement or thickening was identified in the gastric body and antrum, as demonstrated in Fig. 2.13. The patient's medical history encompassed a 20-year duration of diabetes, managed through the administration of metformin (one tablet, three times daily) and glimepiride (one tablet, once daily). The patient self-reported a well-controlled fasting blood glucose level of 6 mmol/L. Additionally, the patient had a history of hypertension spanning over a decade, effectively regulated with pharmacological intervention. Notably, the patient had been a smoker for 40 years, consuming 20 cigarettes daily, and had a history of alcohol consumption for 20 years, consuming 150 mL of white wine per day. However, the patient has abstained from alcohol consumption for the past 3 years.

Diagnosis: Gastric malignancy (cT1N0M0), diabetes, hypertension, sinus bradycardia.

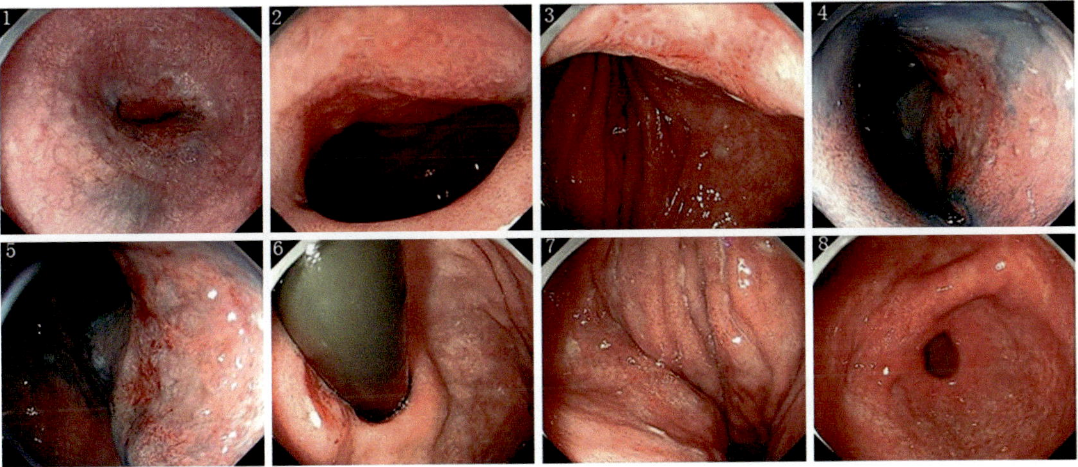

Fig. 2.11 Illustrates the presence of a superficial protrusion and shallow depression lesion located at the cardia, positioned at a distance of 41–43 cm from the incisors

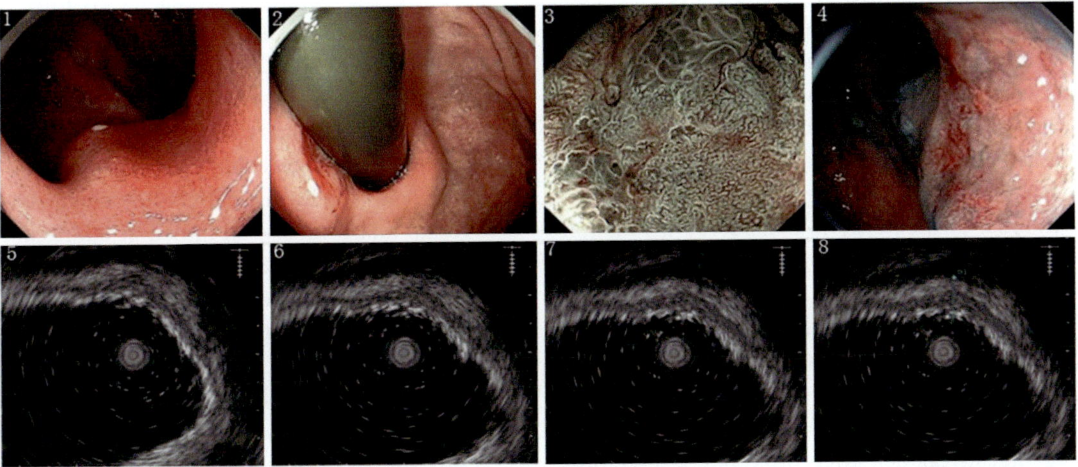

Fig. 2.12 Depicts the thickening of the gastric wall primarily affecting the mucosal layer and submucosal layer at the site of the lesion

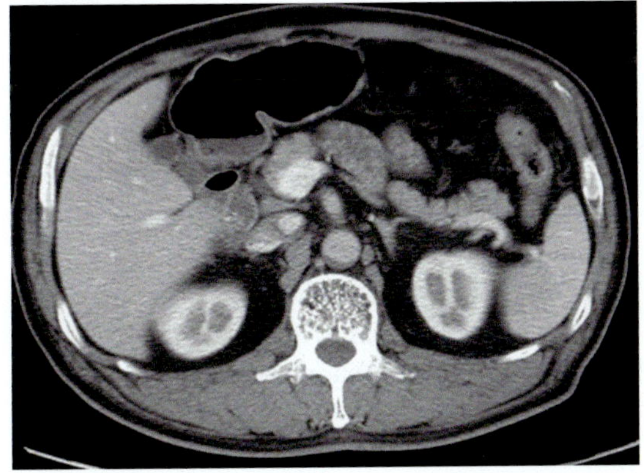

Fig. 2.13 Displays the presence of multiple small lymph nodes observed in the left gastric region and adjacent to the abdominal aorta

2.4.2 Treatment

Following the completion of preoperative evaluations, the patient underwent laparoscopic proximal gastrectomy, which included a complete D2 lymph node dissection and R0 resection. Subsequently, a double tract anastomosis procedure was performed. On the third day after surgery, the urinary catheter was removed, followed by the removal of the gastric tube on the fifth day and the abdominal drainage tube on the eighth day. The patient was discharged 12 days post-surgery.

The pathological report of the proximal stomach indicated the presence of moderately differentiated adenocarcinoma originating from the glandular epithelium. The tumor exhibited a superficial protrusion within the stomach (Lauren classification: intestinal type). Importantly, the tumor was confined to the mucosal layer and did not involve the esophagus or the greater omentum. Notably, no evident vascular tumor embolus or nerve invasion was identified. Moreover, no cancerous cells were detected at the upper and lower margins, and there was no evidence of metastatic cancer in the examined lymph nodes (0/36). The pTNM staging for the tumor was determined as pT1aN0M0.

2.4.3 Case Analysis

The global incidence of gastric cancer has been declining; however, there has been a noticeable increase in tumors occurring at the junction between the esophagus and stomach. In cases of early gastric cancer at this junction, the Japanese gastric cancer guidelines recommend proximal gastrectomy as the preferred surgical approach. Proximal gastrectomy is considered a function-preserving surgery and offers several advantages over total gastrectomy. These include the preservation of body weight, reduction in postoperative malnutrition, and decreased occurrence of vomiting and diarrhea [30].

There are different methods for reconstructing the digestive tract after proximal gastrectomy. These methods include esophagus-stomach anastomosis, jejunal interposition, and double-channel anastomosis. Among these options, direct anastomosis of the esophageal remnant and stomach can lead to severe reflux, necessitating modified procedures such as tubular stomach anastomosis and fundoplasty to address this issue.

1. **Esophagus-stomach anastomosis**

   Although the operative steps involved in esophagus-remnant stomach anastomosis are relatively straightforward, there is a high incidence of postoperative reflux. A multicenter analysis conducted in Italy demonstrated that the occurrence of reflux esophagitis and anastomotic stenosis following proximal gastrectomy with esophagus-stomach anastomosis was significantly higher compared to total gastrectomy [31]. Consequently, modified techniques for esophagus-remnant stomach anastomosis have been developed, such as tubular stomach anastomosis [32]. Tubular stomach anastomosis extends the length over which bile reflux can occur and reduces gastric acid secretion, thereby achieving a desirable anti-reflux effect. Moreover, this approach alleviates tension at the esophageal anastomosis site, thereby ensuring the safety of the anastomosis. Another method introduced by Japanese scholar Kamikawa et al. is double muscular flap reconstruction, wherein the distal end of the esophagus and the anastomotic site are embedded within the submucosa of the remnant stomach, creating a one-way valve mechanism to prevent reflux [33]. Muraoka et al. successfully performed this procedure laparoscopically and obtained satisfactory outcomes in terms of reflux prevention [34]. Other techniques include the utilization of a linear cutter for single-side overlap anastomosis, all aimed at addressing the issues of postoperative reflux of digestive fluids and anastomotic stenosis [35].

2. **Double Tract Reconstruction**

   Double tract reconstruction (DTR) is widely regarded as the most effective method of reconstruction to reduce the occurrence of reflux esophagitis. This technique offers several advantages, including an increased distance between the remnant stomach and the esophagus provided by the jejunal segment, while retaining the residual stomach-duodenal pathway for improved food storage. A retrospective analysis conducted by Jung et al. investigated the postoperative outcomes of patients with early proximal gastric cancer who underwent either DTR or total gastrectomy [36]. The findings revealed that the DTR group had a shorter operation time, reduced blood loss, and improved postoperative nutritional status compared to the total gastrectomy group. Importantly, there were no significant differences observed in terms of reflux and overall survival between the two groups. Similar conclusions were reached through a meta-analysis [37]. The ongoing Korean KLASS-05 study focuses on evaluating the short- and long-term outcomes of laparoscopic proximal gastrectomy with DTR compared to laparoscopic total gastrectomy. This study aims to provide insights into the optimal digestive tract reconstruction strategy following early proximal gastrectomy.

Laparoscopic DTR presents challenges, particularly in the esophagus-jejunum anastomosis. Prior to anastomosis, it is crucial to liberate the lower part of the esophagus to a maximum extent to avoid damage to the pleura. Ligating the gastroesophageal junction with a band can facilitate manipulation of the esophagus. A comprehensive evaluation of the tumor location and stage is necessary before surgery. The length of jejunal interposition is generally around 10 cm, as inadequate length may impede achieving an effective anti-reflux effect. After reconstruction, suturing and fixation of the distal remnant stomach and the liver-gastric ligament are performed to prevent postoperative gastric torsion [38].

3. **Intestinal Interposition Anastomosis**

   Intestinal interposition anastomosis involves the placement of a free segment of the small intestine between the esophagus and the remaining stomach, serving as an effective approach to reduce reflux esophagitis. Certain scholars argue that in comparison to double-channel reconstruction, intestinal interposition reconstruction may better preserve the patient's postoperative weight, while both methods yield similar rates of postoperative reflux esophagitis [39]. However, following intestinal interposition surgery, some patients may experience stomach discomfort due to small intestine folding, which can potentially result in delayed food emptying.

2.4.4 Expert Comments

The optimal balance between achieving a radical cure for early proximal gastric cancer and preserving postoperative quality of life is a significant and ongoing concern. The Japanese gastric cancer treatment guidelines have recognized proximal gastrectomy as a viable surgical option for early proximal gastric cancer. However, there remains a lack of consensus regarding the ideal method for digestive tract reconstruction following proximal gastrectomy. Further large-scale evidence-based studies are necessary to establish the most appropriate approach in this context.

Case provider: Hong Zhou, Yingtai Chen.

Commentary: Dongbing Zhao.

References

1. Kitano S, Iso Y, Moriyama M, Sugimachi K. Laparoscopy-assisted Billroth I gastrectomy. Surg Laparosc Endosc. 1994;4(2):146–8.
2. Watson DI, Devitt PG, Game PA. Laparoscopic Billroth II gastrectomy for early gastric cancer. Br J Surg. 1995;82(5):661–2.
3. Goh PMY, Khan AZ, So JBY, et al. Early experience with laparoscopic radical gastrectomy for advanced gastric cancer. Surg Laparosc Endosc Percutan Tech. 2001;11(2):83–7.
4. Hashizume M, Shimada M, Tomikawa M, et al. Early experiences of endoscopic procedures in general surgery assisted by a computer-enhanced surgical system. Surg Endosc. 2002;16(8):1187–91.
5. Adachi Y, Shiraishi N, Shiromizu A, Bandoh T, Aramaki M, Kitano S. Laparoscopy-assisted Billroth I gastrectomy compared with conventional open gastrectomy. Arch Surg. 2000;135(7):806–10.
6. Kim DG, Choi YY, An JY, et al. Comparing the short-term outcomes of totally intracorporeal gastroduodenostomy with extracorporeal gastroduodenostomy after laparoscopic distal gastrectomy for gastric cancer: a single surgeon's experience and a rapidly is measurable. Endoscopy. 2013;27(9):3153–61.
7. Van Stiegmann G, Goff JS. An alternative to Roux-en-Y for treatment of bile reflux gastritis. Surg Gynecol Obstet. 1988;166(1):69–70.
8. Kim HH, Han SU, Kim MC, et al. Effect of laparoscopic distal gastrectomy vs open distal gastrectomy on long-term survival among patients with stage I gastric cancer: the KLASS-01 randomized clinical trial. JAMA Oncol. 2019;5(4):506–13.
9. Kim W, Kim HH, Han SU, et al. Decreased morbidity of laparoscopic distal gastrectomy compared with open distal gastrectomy for stage I gastric cancer: short-term outcomes from a multicenter randomized controlled trial (KLASS-01). Ann Surg. 2016;263(1):28–35.
10. Inaki N, Etoh T, Ohyama T, et al. A multi-institutional, prospective, phase II feasibility study of laparoscopy-assisted distal gastrectomy with D2 lymph node

dissection for locally advanced gastric cancer (JLSSG0901). World J Surg. 2015;39(11):2734–41.
11. Hyung WJ, Yang HK, Park YK, et al. Long-term outcomes of laparoscopic distal gastrectomy for locally advanced gastric cancer: the KLASS-02-RCT randomized clinical trial. J Clin Oncol Off J Am Soc Clin Oncol. 2020;38(28):3304–13.
12. Yu J, Huang C, Sun Y, et al. Effect of laparoscopic vs open distal gastrectomy on 3-year disease-free survival in patients with locally advanced gastric cancer: the CLASS-01 randomized clinical trial. JAMA. 2019;321(20):1983–92.
13. Hu Y, Huang C, Sun Y, et al. Morbidity and mortality of laparoscopic versus open D2 distal gastrectomy for advanced gastric cancer: a randomized controlled trial. J Clin Oncol Off J Am Soc Clin Oncol. 2016;34(12):1350–7.
14. Kanaya S, Gomi T, Momoi H, et al. Delta-shaped anastomosis in totally laparoscopic Billroth I gastrectomy: new technique of intraabdominal gastroduodenostomy. J Am Coll Surg. 2002;195(2):284–7.
15. Kanaya S, Kawamura Y, Kawada H, et al. The delta-shaped anastomosis in laparoscopic distal gastrectomy: analysis of the initial 100 consecutive procedures of intracorporeal gastroduodenostomy. Gastric Cancer. 2011;14(4):365–71.
16. Sakaguchi M, Hosogi H, Tokoro Y, et al. Functional outcomes of Delta-shaped anastomosis after laparoscopic distal gastrectomy. J Gastrointest Surg. 2021;25(2):397–404.
17. Huang C, Lin M, Chen Q, et al. A modified delta-shaped gastroduodenostomy in totally laparoscopic distal gastrectomy for gastric cancer: a safe and feasible technique. PLoS One. 2014;9(7):e102736.
18. Fukunaga T, Ishibashi Y, Oka S, et al. Augmented rectangle technique for Billroth I anastomosis in totally laparoscopic distal gastrectomy for gastric cancer. Surg Endosc. 2018;32(9):4011–6.
19. Omori T, Masuzawa T, Akamatsu H, et al. A simple and safe method for Billroth I reconstruction in single-incision laparoscopic gastrectomy using a novel intracorporeal triangular anastomotic technique. J Gastrointest Surg. 2014;18(3):613–6.
20. Huang CM, Lin M, Lin JX, et al. Comparison of modified and conventional delta-shaped gastroduodenostomy in totally laparoscopic surgery. World J Gastroenterol. 2014;20(30):10478–85.
21. Harada J, Kinoshita T, Sato R, et al. Delta-shaped gastroduodenostomy after totally laparoscopic distal gastrectomy for gastric cancer: comparative study of original and modified methods. Surg Endosc. 2021;35(8):4167–74.
22. Qin X, Ji J, Zheng M, et al. Expert consensus and operational guidelines for digestive tract reconstruction in complete laparoscopic gastric cancer surgery (2018 edition). Chinese J Pract Surg. 2018;8:833–9.
23. Chen K, Wu D, Pan Y, et al. Totally laparoscopic gastrectomy using intracorporeally stapler or hand-sewn anastomosis for gastric cancer: a single-center experience of 478 consecutive cases and outcomes. World J Surg Oncol. 2016;14:115.
24. Usui S, Nagai K, Hiranuma S, et al. Laparoscopy-assisted esophagoenteral anastomosis using endoscopic purse-string suture instrument "Endo-PSI (II)" and circular stapler. Gastric Cancer. 2008;11(4):233–7.
25. Omori T, Oyama T, Mizutani S, et al. A simple and safe technique for esophagojejunostomy using the hemid-double stapling technique in laparoscopy-assisted total gastrectomy. Am J Surg. 2009;197(1):e13–7.
26. Jeong O, Park YK. Intracorporeal circular stapling esophagojejunostomy using the transorally inserted anvil (OrVil) after laparoscopic total gastrectomy. Surg Endosc. 2009;23(11):2624–30.
27. Okabe H, Obama K, Tanaka E, et al. Intracorporeal esophagojejunal anastomosis after laparoscopic total gastrectomy for patients with gastric cancer. Surg Endosc. 2009;23(9):2167–71.
28. Kwon IG, Son YG, Ryu SW. Novel Intracorporeal Esophagojejunostomy using linear staplers during laparoscopic Total gastrectomy: π-shaped Esophagojejunostomy, 3-in-1 technique. J Am Coll Surg. 2016;223:e25–9.
29. Inaba K, Satoh S, Ishida Y, et al. Overlap method: novel intracorporeal esophagojejunostomy after laparoscopic total gastrectomy. J Am Coll Surg. 2010;211(6):e25–9.
30. Takiguchi N, Takahashi M, Ikeda M, et al. Long-term quality-of-life comparison of total gastrectomy and proximal gastrectomy by postgastrectomy syndrome assessment scale (PGSAS-45): a nationwide multi-institutional study. Gastric Cancer. 2015;18(2):407–16.
31. Rosa F, Quero G, Fiorillo C, et al. Total vs proximal gastrectomy for adenocarcinoma of the upper third of the stomach: a propensity-score-matched analysis of a multicenter western experience (on behalf of the Italian Research Group for Gastric Cancer-GIRCG). Gastric Cancer. 2018;21(5):845–52.
32. Adachi Y, Inoue T, Hagino Y, et al. Surgical results of proximal gastrectomy for early-stage gastric cancer: jejunal interposition and gastric tube reconstruction. Gastric Cancer. 1999;2(1):40–5.
33. Kuroda S, Nishizaki M, Kikuchi S, et al. Double-flap technique as an antireflux procedure in Esophagogastrostomy after proximal gastrectomy. J Am Coll Surg. 2016;223(2):e7–e13.
34. Muraoka A, Kobayashi M, Kokudo Y. Laparoscopy-assisted proximal gastrectomy with the hinged double flap method. World J Surg. 2016;40(10):2419–24.
35. Yamashita Y, Yamamoto A, Tamamori Y, et al. Side overlap esophagogastrostomy to prevent reflux after proximal gastrectomy. Gastric Cancer. 2017;20(4):728–35.
36. Jung DH, Lee Y, Kim DW, et al. Laparoscopic proximal gastrectomy with double tract reconstruction is superior to laparoscopic total gastrectomy for proximal early gastric cancer. Surg Endosc. 2017;31(10):3961–9.

37. Li S, Gu L, Shen Z, et al. A meta-analysis of comparison of proximal gastrectomy with double-tract reconstruction and total gastrectomy for proximal early gastric cancer. BMC Surg. 2019;19(1):117.
38. 张永康， 廖晓锋. 全腹腔镜下近端胃切除自牵引后离断技术联合双通道吻合8例. 中国微创外科杂志. 2021;21(06):545–8.
39. Nomura E, Lee SW, Kawai M, et al. Functional outcomes by reconstruction technique following laparoscopic proximal gastrectomy for gastric cancer: double tract versus jejunal interposition. World J Surg Oncol. 2014;12:20.

3 Special Type of Surgical Resection for Gastric Cancer

Chunguang Guo, Dongbing Zhao, Yingtai Chen, Xiaofeng Bai, Yuemin Sun, Hu Ren, Chunfang Hu, Zefeng Li, Penghui Niu, Yan Song, Chongyuan Sun, Tongbo Wang, Xiaojie Zhang, Lulu Zhao, and Hong Zhou

3.1 Case 8: Laparoscopic Gastrectomy for Gastric Cancer After Neoadjuvant Chemotherapy

3.1.1 Brief History

The patient is a 70-year-old male who was admitted to the hospital after being diagnosed with gastric cancer. Three months ago, he underwent three cycles of neoadjuvant chemotherapy. The patient experienced abdominal distension 3 months ago, without any evident triggers, and did not present with additional symptoms such as abdominal pain, vomiting, hematemesis, or melena. Gastroscopy conducted at a local hospital revealed space-occupying lesions in the antrum, and subsequent pathology confirmed adenocarcinoma. Abdominal enhanced CT examination displayed irregular circumferential thickening of the gastric wall near the pylorus of the antrum, accompanied by blurred serous surface and multiple lymph nodes observed in the left gastric region, peri-antrum, and portal area of the liver (Fig. 3.1a). According to the tumor clinical stage, the cancer was categorized as cT4aN + M0. The patient received three cycles of neoadjuvant therapy using the FOLFOX regimen, which resulted in symptom relief during chemotherapy without significant toxic reactions. Subsequent enhanced CT examination conducted after chemotherapy indicated that the local gastric lesions and lymph nodes exhibited similar characteristics to the pre-treatment scan, with the treatment response being evaluated as stable disease (SD) (Fig. 3.1b). The patient has a smoking history of over 20 years, with a consumption rate of more than 20 cigarettes per day.

Diagnosis: Gastric cancer (ycT4aN + M0, received three cycles of neoadjuvant chemotherapy).

3.1.2 Treatment

Following adequate preoperative preparation, a radical distal subtotal gastrectomy

C. Guo (✉) · D. Zhao · Y. Chen · X. Bai · Y. Sun
H. Ren · Z. Li · P. Niu · C. Sun · T. Wang · X. Zhang
L. Zhao
Department of Pancreatic and Gastric Surgical Oncology, National Cancer Center/National Clinical Research for Cancer/Cancer Hospital, Chinese Academy of Medical Sciences and Peking Union Medical College, Beijing, China

C. Hu · Y. Song
Department of Pathology, National Cancer Center/National Clinical Research for Cancer/Cancer Hospital, Chinese Academy of Medical Sciences and Peking Union Medical College, Beijing, China

H. Zhou
Department of Breast Surgical Oncology, National Cancer Center/National Clinical Research Center for Cancer/Cancer Hospital & Shenzhen Hospital, Chinese Academy of Medical Sciences and Peking Union Medical College, Shenzhen, China

J. Cai (ed.), *Interpretation of Gastric Cancer Cases*, Experts' Perspectives on Medical Advances,
https://doi.org/10.1007/978-981-99-5302-8_3

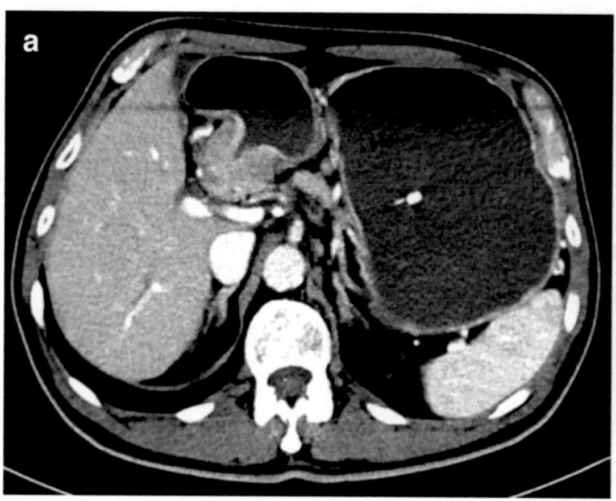
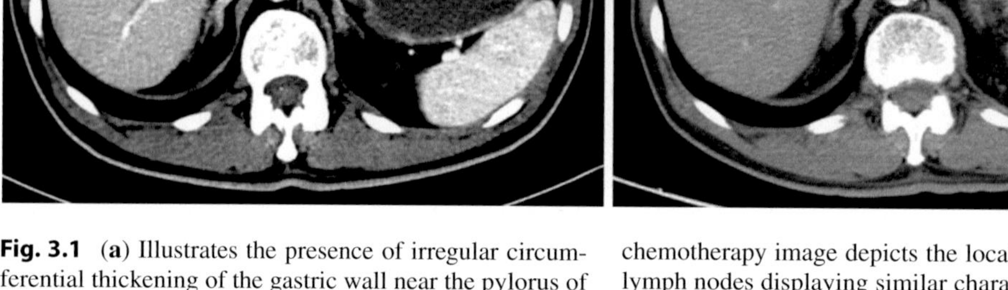

Fig. 3.1 (**a**) Illustrates the presence of irregular circumferential thickening of the gastric wall near the pylorus of the antrum before chemotherapy, with a maximum thickness of approximately 2.1 cm. In figure (**b**), the post-chemotherapy image depicts the local gastric lesions and lymph nodes displaying similar characteristics to the pre-treatment scan. The therapeutic response was evaluated as stable disease (SD)

(Billroth-II + Braun anastomosis) was performed. Intraoperative exploration revealed that the tumor was located in the gastric antrum, measuring approximately 3 cm × 4 cm, and had penetrated the serous layer of the gastric wall without infiltrating the surrounding tissues. Several enlarged lymph nodes were identified around the stomach (Fig. 3.2). The patient experienced a smooth recovery after the surgery. The gastric tube was removed on the second postoperative day, removal of gas was performed on the sixth day, drainage tube removal took place on the seventh day, and the patient was discharged on the twelfth day following the surgery.

Pathological examination revealed an antral infiltration of poorly differentiated adenocarcinoma with ulceration (Lauren type: mixed type). The tumor was observed to invade the serous membrane, and it was classified as Mandard grade TRG3. Metastatic cancer was detected in 14 out of 51 examined lymph nodes. Based on the pathological findings, the ypTNM stage was determined as ypT4aN3a.

3.1.3 Case Analysis

Studies have indicated that neoadjuvant chemotherapy for gastric cancer can lead to various pathological changes in tumor tissues, including the presence of inflammatory cells, disruption of the muscle layer structure of the gastric wall, occlusive vasculitis, tissue thrombosis, fibrosis, and changes in lymph nodes such as hyalinosis, inflammatory infiltration, and fibrosis [1, 2]. These microstructural changes have multidimensional effects on the surgical management of gastric cancer after neoadjuvant chemotherapy.

Laparoscopic radical gastrectomy was first reported by Professor Kitano et al. in Japan in 1994 [3]. Subsequent studies have confirmed the safety and feasibility of laparoscopic surgery for the treatment of advanced gastric cancer compared to open surgery [4–10]. However, the application of laparoscopy in advanced gastric cancer after neoadjuvant therapy remained uncertain due to the complex anatomy of peri-gastric tissues, long learning curve, and technical demands.

Several studies have been conducted to evaluate the use of laparoscopic surgery in gastric cancer patients after neoadjuvant chemotherapy. A small randomized controlled trial in China included 95 cases of gastric cancer after neoadjuvant chemotherapy, with 45 cases undergoing laparoscopic radical gastrectomy and 50 cases undergoing open radical gastrectomy. The study found a lower rate of postoperative complications in the laparoscopic group compared to the open surgery group (20% vs. 46%, $p = 0.007$), along with better postoperative chemotherapy tolerance in the laparoscopic group [11].

The European STOMACH trial compared laparoscopic and open surgery for total gastrec-

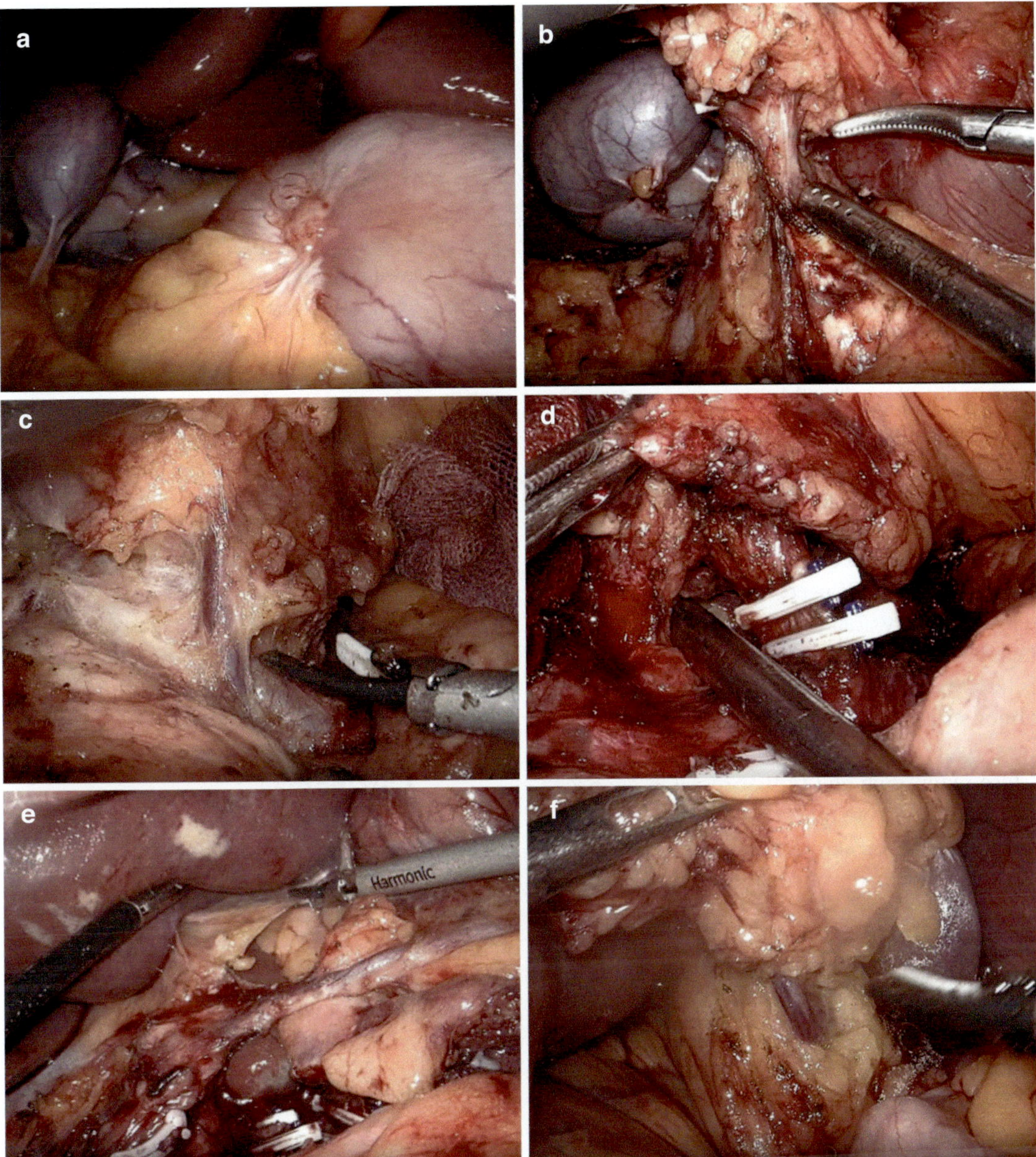

Fig. 3.2 (**a**) Showcases the laparoscopic exploration of the tumor situated in the gastric antrum, with evidence of penetration into the gastric wall. Figure (**b**) displays the ligation of the right gastro-omental vessel, while figure (**c**) depicts the dissection of lymph nodes in the superior pancreas. Additionally, figure (**d**) illustrates the dissection of the left gastric vessel, figure (**e**) demonstrates the dissection of the right gastric vessel, and figure (**f**) reveals the exposure of the left gastro-omental vessel

tomy after neoadjuvant chemotherapy in 96 patients with gastric cancer. The study found no significant difference between the two groups in terms of the number of lymph nodes dissected, negative surgical margin rates, and postoperative complications [12].

These findings suggest that laparoscopic surgery after neoadjuvant chemotherapy for gastric cancer is safe and feasible. However, it is important to consider the individual patient's condition, tumor characteristics, and the expertise of the surgical team when deciding on the appropriate surgical approach.

The survival benefit of laparoscopic surgery for gastric cancer after neoadjuvant chemotherapy remains a topic of debate. The STOMACH study, which compared laparoscopic and open surgery for total gastrectomy after neoadjuvant chemotherapy, reported similar 1-year postoperative survival rates between the laparoscopic and laparotomy groups (85.5% and 90.4%, respectively) with no statistically significant difference [12]. A meta-analysis also found no significant difference in disease-free survival time and overall survival time between the laparoscopic and open surgery groups for gastric cancer patients after neoadjuvant chemotherapy [13].

Based on the available evidence, it can be concluded that laparoscopic surgery is a safe and effective approach for gastric cancer patients after neoadjuvant chemotherapy. However, more clinical evidence is still needed to establish the long-term efficacy and survival outcomes of laparoscopic surgery in this patient population. It is important to consider individual patient factors, tumor characteristics, and the expertise of the surgical team when making treatment decisions. Close monitoring and further research are necessary to gather more robust evidence and refine the guidelines for the surgical management of gastric cancer after neoadjuvant chemotherapy.

3.1.4 Expert Comments

Indeed, laparoscopic radical gastrectomy has been demonstrated to be a safe and feasible approach for gastric cancer surgery and has gained wide acceptance. However, the impact of neoadjuvant chemotherapy on tissue inflammation and edema introduces new challenges to laparoscopic procedures.

The changes in tissue characteristics after neoadjuvant chemotherapy, such as increased inflammation and edema, may affect the surgical field visualization, anatomical landmarks, and technical aspects of the procedure. These changes can potentially increase the complexity and difficulty of laparoscopic gastric cancer surgery.

Further exploration and research are necessary to better understand the implications of neoadjuvant chemotherapy on laparoscopic procedures. This includes investigating techniques and strategies to overcome the challenges posed by tissue inflammation and edema, optimizing patient selection criteria, and refining surgical approaches to ensure optimal outcomes.

Additionally, advancements in surgical technology, such as improved imaging systems and instruments, may contribute to addressing these challenges and enhancing the safety and efficacy of laparoscopic gastric cancer surgery after neoadjuvant chemotherapy.

Overall, ongoing research and clinical experience will continue to shape the development and refinement of laparoscopic approaches for gastric cancer surgery, taking into account the unique considerations introduced by neoadjuvant chemotherapy.

Case provider: Xiaojie Zhang, Yingtai Chen.
Commentary: Yingtai Chen.

3.2 Case 9: Laparoscopic Gastrojejunostomy for Patients with Unresectable Gastric Carcinoma

3.2.1 Brief History

The patient, a 62-year-old male, presented with a chief complaint of abdominal distension and vomiting persisting for over a month. The onset of these symptoms occurred spontaneously and was not attributed to any apparent triggers. The patient also experienced a loss of appetite. Initial evaluation at an external medical facility revealed the presence of gastric masses in the body and antrum, as observed through gastroscopy. However, the procedure encountered difficulty due to luminal obstruction. Subsequent biopsy results confirmed the diagnosis of gastric adenocarcinoma. Further assessment using PET-CT demonstrated marked thickening of the gastric wall along the lesser curvature of the stomach, as well as an irregular serous surface. The analysis did not indicate involvement of the proximal duodenum or the S3 segment of the liver but suggested the likelihood of metastasis to multiple lymph nodes in the perigastric and retroperitoneal regions. The patient had a previous diagnosis of membranous nephropathy 8 years ago, for which long-term administration of hormones and tacrolimus had been discontinued. Physical examination of the abdomen did not reveal any positive signs. Tumor marker levels were as follows: CA199: 197.10 U/mL, CA242 > 150 U/mL, and CA72–4, AFP, and CEA were within normal limits. A blood routine analysis indicated a red blood cell count of 3.93×10^{12}/L and a hemoglobin level of 102 g/L. An enhanced abdominal CT scan demonstrated masses in the antrum and lesser curvature of the stomach, suggestive of gastric cancer. The tumor was found to invade the serous membrane, showing a close association with the pancreas, and exhibited a maximum thickness of 2.7 cm. Multiple lymph nodes were detected in the para-antrum, left gastric region, and retroperitoneum, with the largest lymph node measuring 1.2 cm in short diameter. Additionally, increased density of omental fat accompanied by ascites indicated the possibility of implantation metastasis (see Fig. 3.3). Pathological consultation confirmed the presence of gastric adenocarcinoma, displaying a moderate to poorly differentiated biopsy specimen, including a component of signet-ring cell carcinoma. The tumor was negative for Epstein-Barr virus-encoded small RNA (EBER) and showed human epidermal growth factor receptor 2 (HER2) immunohistochemistry 2+. Molecular pathology analysis using DNA sequencing revealed no mutations in KRAS, BRAF, NRAS, PIK3CA, CMET, or HER2 genes, no gene translocations involving ROS1, RET, or NTRK, and no amplification of the CMET gene. Moreover, no rare mutations of the epidermal growth factor receptor (EGFR) were identified. The tumor mutation load (TMB) was calculated as 8.7 mutations per megabase (Mb), and the microsatellite status was stable (MSS).

Diagnosis: (1) Gastric cancer (cT4bN3M1), (2) Pyloric obstruction, (3) Abdominal implantation metastasis, (4) Anemia, (5) Membranous nephropathy.

3.2.2 Treatment

The patient was admitted to the hospital for further examinations and management. The diagnosis indicated advanced gastric cancer with pyloric obstruction, necessitating consideration for palliative bypass surgery. Prior to the surgery, continuous gastrointestinal decompression and hypertonic saline gastric lavage were performed to address electrolyte imbalances.

Laparoscopic gastrointestinal bypass surgery was scheduled at an appropriate time. Following satisfactory anesthesia, the patient was positioned supine with the legs raised. The "four-hole method" was employed, with a trocar placed for observation in the subumbilical incision and operational access obtained through the lateral margins of the right rectus abdominis, right subcostal, and left subcostal regions. Upon exploration of the abdominal and pelvic cavities, no obvious nodules were observed in the liver. Multiple small white nodules, ranging in diameter from 0.2 to 0.5 cm, were found on the mesenteric surface. Tumors were located in the gastric antrum and pylorus, infiltrating the serous surface and closely adhering to the pancreas and retroperitoneum. Multiple cancer nodules were identified around the stomach and in the greater

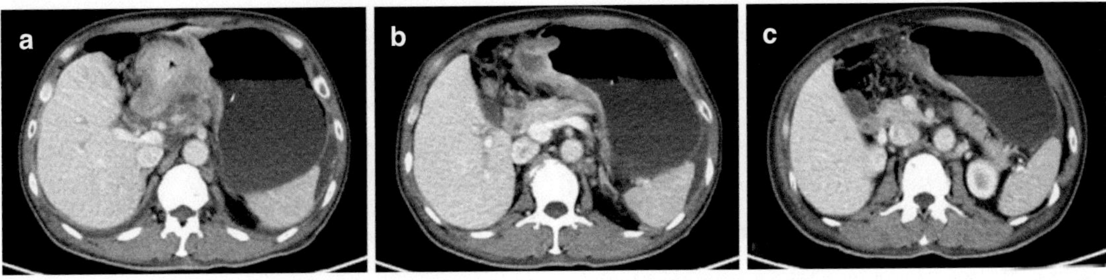

Fig. 3.3 Abdominal CT at initial examination. (**a**) Antral tumor. (**b**) Enlargement of perigastric and retroperitoneal lymph nodes. (**c**) Increased density of omental fat around the antrum, suggestive of peritoneal metastasis

omentum, with the largest measuring approximately 0.5 cm (see Fig. 3.4a). The gastrocolic ligament's middle part was incised to access the lesser omentum sac, and anastomosis was performed on the posterior walls of the stomach and intestines at a point approximately 25 cm from Qu's ligament, with closure of the common opening (see Fig. 3.4b).

The gastric tube was removed on the third day after surgery. On the fourth postoperative day, the patient experienced flatus and complained of increasing nausea and discomfort, particularly worsening at night. The abdominal drainage tube was removed on the seventh-day post-surgery. However, on the ninth day, the patient still experienced persistent abdominal distension and was unable to tolerate oral intake. Subsequent gastroscopy revealed evident mucosal congestion and edema in the output loop of the gastrointestinal anastomosis, making endoscopic passage slightly challenging. As a result, a jejunal nutrition tube was inserted (see Fig. 3.5). Symptoms gradually improved by the 17th day after surgery, and the patient was able to resume a liquid diet on the 20th day, followed by a semi-liquid diet on the 25th day. Finally, the patient was discharged on the 30th day post-surgery.

The patient received a total of 8 cycles of SOX regimen chemotherapy (oxaliplatin 200 mg intravenous infusion on day 1 + Tiggio 60 mg twice daily on days 1–14, every 3 weeks) following the surgery. Tumor marker levels were reassessed after 2 cycles of chemotherapy, revealing the following results: CA199 167.60 U/mL, CA724 7.73 U/mL, AFP 8.00 ng/mL, CEA 5.46 ng/mL, and CA242 116.295 U/mL. At the tenth-week post-surgery, a CT reexamination showed improvements in gastric wall thickening compared to the initial findings. Peritoneal density was also reduced, and there was increased absorption of abdominal fluid. The size of multiple lymph node shadows around the stomach and retroperitoneum had decreased, with the larger one measuring 0.7 cm in short diameter (see Fig. 3.6a). After 4 cycles of chemotherapy, the tumor marker levels were as follows: CA199 51.32 U/mL, CA724 6.57 U/mL, AFP 11.47 ng/mL, CEA 4.15 ng/mL, and CA242 26.719 U/mL. A CT reexamination at the 16th week after surgery showed further reduction in the size of lymph node shadows around the stomach and retroperitoneum, with the larger one measuring approximately 0.5 cm in short diameter. The remaining findings were similar to the previous examination (see Fig. 3.6b). After 6 cycles of chemotherapy, the tumor marker levels were reviewed: CA199 199.60 U/mL, CA724 6.98 U/mL, AFP 37.74 ng/mL, CEA 4.25 ng/mL, and CA242 56.014 U/mL. At the 24th week after surgery, a CT reexamination revealed smaller lymph node shadows adjacent to the antrum, left gastric region, and retroperitoneum. The larger one measured about 0.4 cm in short diameter (see Fig. 3.6c). The efficacy evaluation indicated a partial response (PR). Following the completion of 8 cycles of SOX chemotherapy, the patient transitioned to local monotherapy with S1 treatment. At 15 months post-surgery, tumor progres-

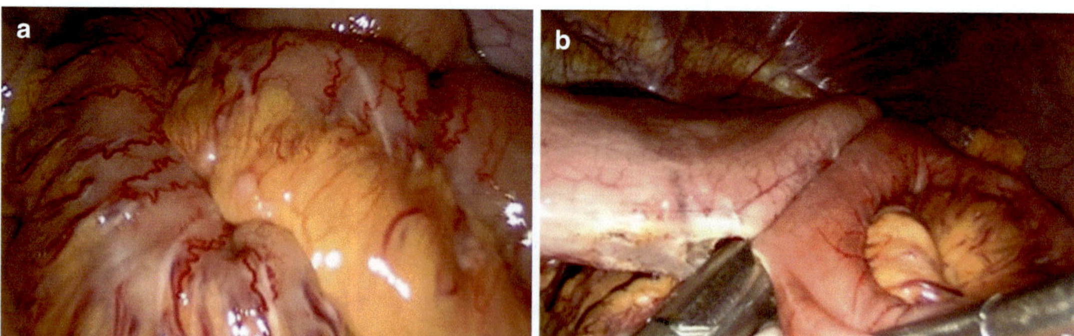

Fig. 3.4 What is seen during laparoscopy. (**a**) Multiple grayish-white implant nodules observed on the mesenteric surface. (**b**) Gastrointestinal short circuit

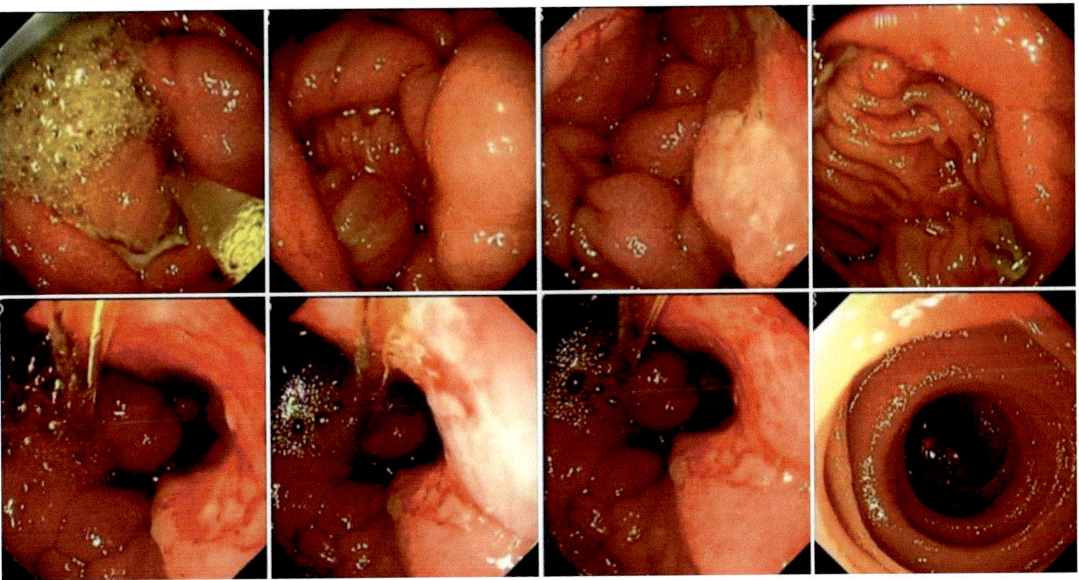

Fig. 3.5 Gastroscopy on the ninth postoperative day. The gastroscopy performed on the ninth day after surgery revealed mucosal hyperemia and edema at the anastomotic outlet

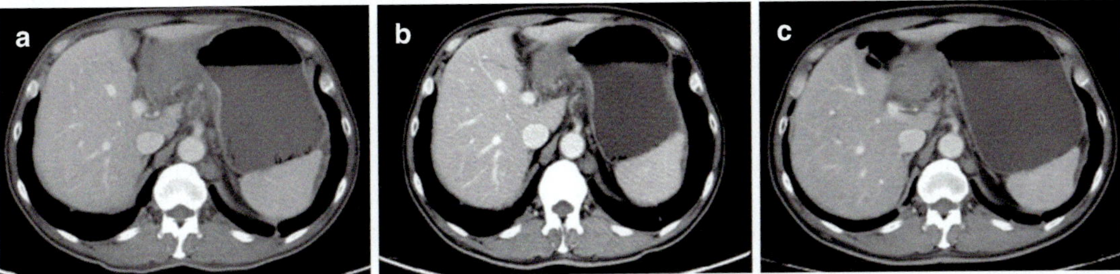

Fig. 3.6 Abdominal CT during postoperative adjuvant chemotherapy. (**a**) At the tenth week after surgery, there was improvement in gastric wall thickening, increased peritoneal density, absorption of peritoneal effusion, and reduction in multiple lymph node shadows around the stomach and retroperitoneum. (**b**) At the 16th week after surgery, there was a further decrease in the size of multiple lymph node shadows around the stomach and retroperitoneum compared to previous assessments. (**c**) At the 24th week after surgery, multiple lymph node shadows were observed in the para-antrum, left gastric region, and retroperitoneum, which were smaller than previous findings

sion was observed, leading to the initiation of local targeted therapy combined with immunotherapy. Unfortunately, 19 months after surgery, the patient succumbed to the disease.

3.2.3 Case Analysis

The primary treatment goal for advanced gastric cancer is to enhance both the quality and duration of patients' lives, primarily through systemic chemotherapy. As the disease progresses, patients with advanced gastric cancer often experience accompanying symptoms such as malnutrition (including anorexia, cachexia, and weight loss), bleeding (manifesting as hematemesis, black stools, and anemia), pain, and digestive tract obstruction (resulting in vomiting, dysphagia, and an inability to eat). Digestive tract obstruction and malnutrition are particularly significant factors that prevent patients from receiving effective drug treatments, diminish their quality of life, and shorten their survival time. Therefore, the NCCN guidelines for Gastric Cancer recommend the use of palliative gastrectomy and gastrointestinal short-circuit surgery as palliative treatments for patients with advanced gastric cancer complicated by hemorrhage and obstruction [14]. Palliative surgery can alleviate patients' symptoms, improve their nutritional status, and enhance their quality of life to a certain extent. With the advancement of endoscopic technology, the advantages of laparoscopic surgery, which entails minimal trauma and faster postoperative recovery, have become more apparent for patients in poor overall condition at an advanced stage. Laparoscopic gastrojejunostomy is a well-established surgical procedure that effectively resolves digestive tract obstruction and is widely employed in this context. Retrospective studies have demonstrated that laparoscopic gastrojejunostomy is safe and efficacious, significantly reducing the occurrence of delayed gastric emptying associated with inadequate gastric motility observed in open surgery. Moreover, it shortens the time required for postoperative oral intake and hospital stay. When compared to stent implantation, gastrojejunostomy demonstrates a marked reduction in the incidence of postoperative reobstruction [15, 16].

Palliative surgery for relieving effluent obstruction in advanced gastric cancer encompasses various surgical procedures, including laparoscopic gastroenterostomy, laparoscopic gastroenterostomy after gastric dissection, and laparoscopic jejunostomy. Gastrojejunostomy after gastric dissection is a modified technique that was first reported by Kaminishi et al. in 1997 [17]. It was employed to address gastroduodenal outflow tract obstruction in patients with advanced gastric cancer who were not suitable for radical surgery. Gastrojejunostomy offers several advantages, such as alleviating the obstruction while preserving the endoscope for tumor observation and endoscopic management of tumor-related bleeding. Additionally, it helps reduce tumor bleeding caused by food stimulation, prevents tumor spread to the gastrointestinal anastomosis, and lowers the risk of secondary obstruction. In some cases, T4b patients who have undergone chemotherapy may regain the opportunity for secondary surgical resection. Laparoscopic gastrojejunal anastomosis following gastric dissection and amputation is a minimally invasive approach that facilitates faster postoperative dietary recovery, shortens hospital stays, and enables earlier administration of antitumor therapy [18].

In 1990, O'Regan et al. first reported laparoscopic jejunostomy [19]. Since then, this procedure has been widely developed, with an increasing number of reports on single-port ostomy in recent years [20]. Laparoscopic jejunostomy can be performed using two approaches: complete intraperitoneal operation, which minimizes incision size and reduces postoperative intestinal adhesions, and laparoscopically assisted external lifting of the jejunum through a small incision. The latter technique allows direct visualization for proper placement of the nutrient tube and avoids intraluminal suturing. Various methods, such as purse-string sutures [21], Stamm inversion form [22], and Witzel tunneling [23], can be employed to secure the jejunostomy tube. Compared to open jejunostomy surgery, laparoscopic surgery is less invasive and associated with a lower incidence of incision infection and incisional hernia.

In this case, the patient presented with a poor preoperative condition and advanced tumor stage, along with multiple complications such as malnutrition, anemia, pyloric obstruction, and membranous nephropathy. Considering the patient's overall condition and the high risk of anastomotic complications, the decision was made to perform total endoscopic gastroenterostomy. Fortunately, no serious complications occurred after the surgery. The significant improvement in the patient's general condition following re-oral feeding was a crucial outcome, as it provided a foundation for subsequent systemic treatment.

It is noteworthy that the patient's overall postoperative survival was approximately 19 months, surpassing the average survival level of 12 months typically observed in advanced gastric cancer [24]. Moreover, the patient was able to maintain a good quality of life throughout the treatment period. These results highlight the positive impact of the surgical intervention and subsequent management on the patient's survival and quality of life.

3.2.4 Expert Comments

Gastric cancer in China often presents at an advanced stage, with approximately 20% of patients already having distant metastasis at the time of diagnosis. These patients face significant challenges in receiving effective treatment due to complications such as obstruction and poor nutritional status, resulting in limited survival time. Surgical intervention plays a crucial role in improving the overall condition of these patients and providing opportunities for further treatment.

The advent of laparoscopy has further revolutionized the treatment of advanced gastric cancer. Laparoscopic procedures offer advantages such as reduced trauma, faster postoperative recovery, and improved patient outcomes. The use of laparoscopy in the treatment of advanced gastric cancer is particularly advantageous due to the minimally invasive nature of the approach.

As personalized diagnosis and treatment strategies for advanced gastric cancer continue to advance, we can expect the wider utilization of laparoscopy in the management of this disease. Laparoscopic techniques, combined with individualized treatment approaches, hold great promise for improving outcomes and enhancing the quality of life for patients with advanced gastric cancer.

Case provider: Tongbo Wang, Chunguang Guo.

Expert: Chunguang Guo.

3.3 Case 10: Laparoscopic Surgery for Synchronous Double Primary Gastroenterology Neoplasm

3.3.1 Brief History

A 57-year-old male presented with a 5-month duration of sporadic abdominal discomfort, unaccompanied by nausea or acid reflux, and not notably associated with meals. However, within the past month, the symptoms have intensified, manifesting as difficulties in bowel movements. The patient reported experiencing a daily defecation pattern with meager stool output. Notably, the individual has a 10-year history of diabetes mellitus, which has been adequately managed with acceptable glycemic control.

External hospital examination:

Colonoscopy: gastric cancer and sigmoid colon cancer;

Pathological results: (Gastric) Signet-ring cell carcinoma;

(Colon) Moderately differentiated adenocarcinoma.

Our hospital examination:

Colonoscopy: Sigmoid colon cancer with incomplete bowel obstruction (Fig. 3.7).

Abdominal-pelvic enhanced CT: Irregular circumferential thickening of the bowel wall in the distal segment of the sigmoid colon, with the thickest part being about 1.5 cm and the serosa slightly blurred locally (Fig. 3.8a); irregular mass at the gastric antrum, and lymph node metastasis can be seen in the left area of gastric (Fig. 3.8b).

Diagnosis:

Sigmoid colon cancer (cT4N + M0); gastric cancer (cT1N1M0); incomplete bowel obstruction; diabetes mellitus.

An ulcerated lesion was seen at 30–35 cm from the anal verge, with a deep ulcerated base covered with white film and irregularly elevated ulcer margins and was easily bleeding when touched. Stenosis of the intestinal lumen at the lesion, making it difficult to pass the endoscope.

3.3.2 Treatment

Following the completion of preoperative preparations, the patient underwent an elective totally laparoscopic D2 radical distal gastrectomy procedure with Billroth II reconstruction and Braun anastomosis, as well as a laparoscopic-assisted radical resection of sigmoid colon cancer. The

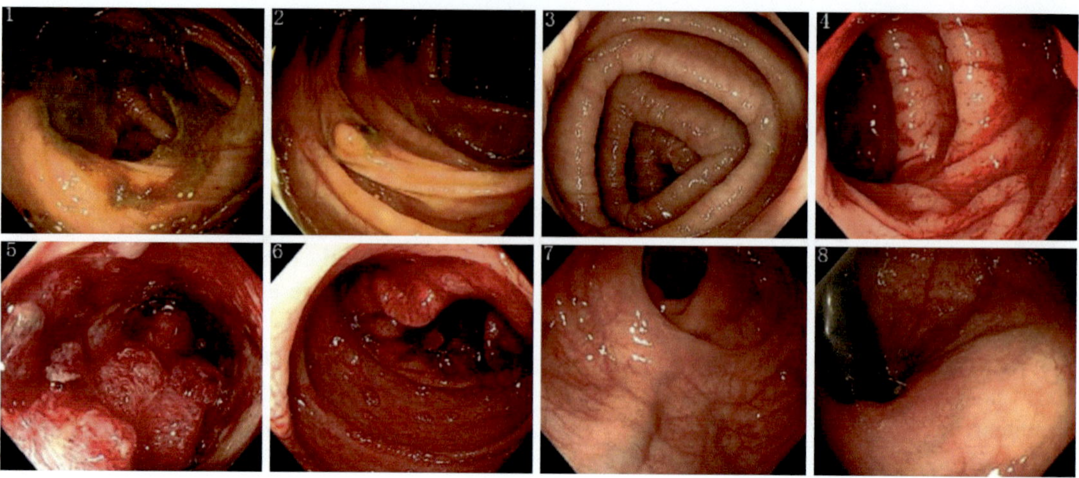

Fig. 3.7 Colonoscopy

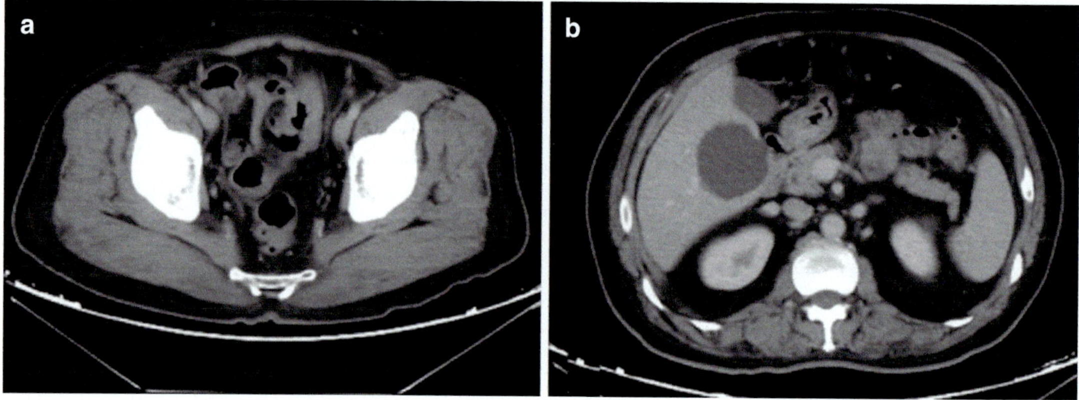

Fig. 3.8 Abdominal-pelvic enhanced CT. (**a**) Irregular circumferential thickening of the bowel wall in the distal segment of the sigmoid colon. (**b**) Irregular mass at the gastric antrum, and lymph node metastasis can be seen in the left area of gastric

patient was positioned in a lithotomy position with the head down and foot up after achieving satisfactory anesthesia.

The tumor was located in the lesser curvature of stomach and measured 3 cm × 3 cm, while the sigmoid colon tumor was 6 cm × 5 cm with circumferential growth and invasion of the serosa. An intermediate approach was employed to dissect the inferior mesenteric artery, free the sigmoid colon, and dissect the intestinal canal 5 cm from the lower edge of the tumor, subsequently setting it aside. A change in position was made, elevating the head by 15° to facilitate radical treatment of the distal gastric cancer.

The laparoscopic D2 debridement of perigastric lymph nodes was performed, followed by specimen dissection and laparoscopic gastrointestinal anastomosis. Additionally, enteroenterostomy was conducted. The patient was then repositioned with the head down and foot up. A 6 cm longitudinal incision was made in the lower abdomen, through which the gastric specimen was removed. The sigmoid colon was visually elevated and dissected, and a tubular anastomosis was placed against the staple holder. Subsequently, the pneumoperitoneum was reconstructed, and laparoscopic end-to-end reconstruction of the intestinal canal was carried out. Following the procedure, the patient was safely transferred to the ward, as depicted in Fig. 3.9. The gastric tube was removed on the second postoperative day, while the drainage tubes in the splenic fossa and duodenal stump were removed on the fifth day. On the sixth day, the pelvic drainage tube was also removed. The patient was eventually discharged on the 16th day after surgery.

Postoperative pathologic report

1. The distal subtotal gastric resection specimen was 9 cm long for the lesser curvature, 12 cm long for the greater curvature, 1.5–2 cm long for the duodenum, and 5.5 cm wide for the incisional margin. A shallow ulcer was seen on the posterior wall of the lesser curvature of the gastric sinus, measuring 4.0 cm × 2.5 cm, near the pyloric ring, 1.5 cm from the lower incisional margin and 5 cm from the upper incisional margin, with a slightly grayish margin confined to the mucosal layer, approximately 0.5 cm thick. Very little fat near the large and small curves of the stomach, no nodules were seen.

   (Microscopic diagnosis) Superficial depressed poorly differentiated adenocarcinoma of the stomach. Lauren classification: diffuse-type, mainly in the form of signet-ring cell carcinoma, with tumor invading the submucosa, involving the pylorus and duodenal mucosa, not involving the greater omentum. No definite vascular tumor thrombus and nerve invasion. No tumor at margins of excision. No metastatic carcinoma was found in lymph nodes (0/48), pTNM stage: pT1bN0.
2. Colon resection specimen, the upper resection margin of the intestinal canal was 5 cm wide and the lower resection margin was 5 cm wide. An ulcerated mass was seen at 7 cm from the upper and 7.5 cm from the lower resection margin, with a circumferential size of 5.0 cm × 6.0 cm × 1.5 cm, with a grayish, hard surface and focal involvement of the serosa.

   (Microscopic diagnosis) Sigmoid colon infiltrating ulcerated moderately differentiated adenocarcinoma. The tumor invaded the serosa membrane with clusters of poorly differentiated tumor cells and tumor outgrowth. Nerve invasion was seen, and no clear choroidal aneurysm embolus or extra-muscular vein invasion was observed. Metastatic carcinoma of lymph nodes (2/17), pTNM stage: pT4aN1b.

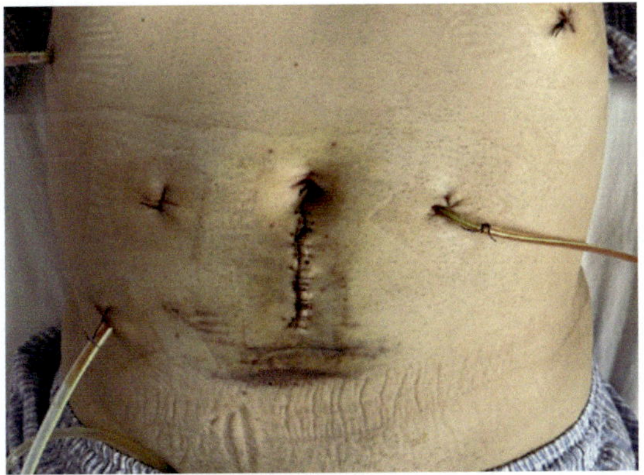

Fig. 3.9 Patient's surgical incision

3.3.3 Case Analysis

The occurrence of two or more primary malignant tumors in the same patient, either successively or simultaneously, is referred to as multiple primary carcinoma (MPC). The criteria established by Moertel for identifying MPC include the following: (1) Presence of two or more malignant tumors within the gastric cavity; (2) Each tumor exhibits its own distinct pathological pattern and does not originate from or metastasize from another tumor; (3) Cancer foci are interspersed with normal tissue and migrating bands [25].

Based on the time interval between tumor occurrences, MPC can be further categorized into synchronous carcinoma (SC), which refers to tumors that develop within 6 months of each other, and metachronous carcinoma (MC), which indicates tumors that arise more than 6 months apart.

The incidence of MPC is low at 0.3–7.3% [26, 27]. In recent years, it has been on the rise as the survival outcomes and diagnostic levels of cancer patients has been prolonged. MPC are most commonly found in the same organ, followed by the same tissue source or paired organs, with the lowest incidence in tissues and organs of different systems [28]. Moreover, MPC are most common in double primary cancers, with tumors of digestive system and respiratory system being the most common, with more males than females. The pathogenesis of MPC is unclear and may be related to the following factors: (1) family history of tumor and mutation or copy number change of tumor susceptibility gene [29]; (2) poor living and dietary habits, changes in the natural environment and microbial infections; (3) age, gender, race, hormone level, and other factors that may cause accumulation of pathogenic factors and decrease in immune function of the body; (4) tumor radiotherapy may likewise lead to the occurrence of secondary tumors.

The treatment of MPC follows that of single malignant tumors, prioritizes the treatment of tumors with high malignancy, and adopts a comprehensive treatment based on surgery. The prognosis of MPC is still inconclusive. It is generally believed that the prognosis of multiple primary cancers is worse than that of single primary cancers, which may be related to the tumor load. The prognosis of SC is worse than that of MC, and the shorter the time interval between multiple cancer foci, the worse the prognosis [30]. However, it has also been shown that the biological characteristics of MPC are similar to those of single primary carcinomas, and there is no statistical difference in the 5-year survival rate between MPC and single primary carcinomas after radical surgery [31].

For patients with double primary tumors in the stomach and intestines, various surgical approaches can be considered, including open surgery, laparoscopic surgery, and combined laparoscopic-open approaches [32]. The choice of surgical approach depends on factors such as the patient's condition, number of tumors, location of cancer foci, and histopathological grading. Historically, open surgery was the main approach for managing multiple primary gastrointestinal tumors. However, this approach is associated with long incisions, significant trauma, slow postoperative recovery, and a higher risk of complications. Laparoscopic simultaneous resection of gastric and colorectal cancers has been reported as a viable alternative [33]. Several studies have demonstrated that laparoscopic surgery offers advantages such as smaller incisions, faster postoperative recovery, and lower incidence of wound infections. Laparoscopic surgery is particularly suitable when tumors are located far apart, as it reduces the length of the incision. Importantly, long-term survival rates after laparoscopic surgery are comparable to those of open surgery [32]. However, simultaneous surgery can present challenges due to complex anatomy, extensive lymph node dissection, technical difficulties, and prolonged operation time. Clinicians must carefully select the surgical approach based on the patient's condition and their own expertise, aiming for precise and personalized minimally invasive treatment within the context of radical surgical intervention.

3.3.4 Expert Comments

MPC represent a rare category of tumors that are becoming more prevalent due to advancements in patient survival and improved diagnostic capabilities. It is crucial for clinicians to maintain vigilance in order to prevent the oversight of lesions in tumor patients. Comprehensive endoscopic and imaging evaluations play a vital role in enhancing the detection rate of MPC. Additionally, regular follow-up examinations of tumor patients are essential. The utilization of laparoscopic techniques offers significant advantages over open surgery, including reduced incision-related injuries and improved quality of life for patients.

Case provider: Chunguang Guo, Penghui Niu.
Commentary: Yuemin Sun.

3.4 Case 11: Laparoscopic and Endoscopic Cooperative Surgery for the Duodenal Lesion

3.4.1 Brief History

A 65-year-old female presented with a 6-month history of epigastric discomfort following meals, accompanied by symptoms of acid reflux and heartburn. Additionally, she had an elevated tumor marker, CA199, which was identified 1 month ago. Subsequently, a comprehensive gastrointestinal endoscopy was conducted, yielding the following findings (Figs. 3.10, 3.11, 3.12).

3.4.2 Biopsy Pathology

Neuroendocrine tumor, G1. AE1/AE3(+), CD34(−), ChrA(+), CD56(+), LCA(−), Syno(+), CDX-2(+), Villin(+) (Fig. 3.12).

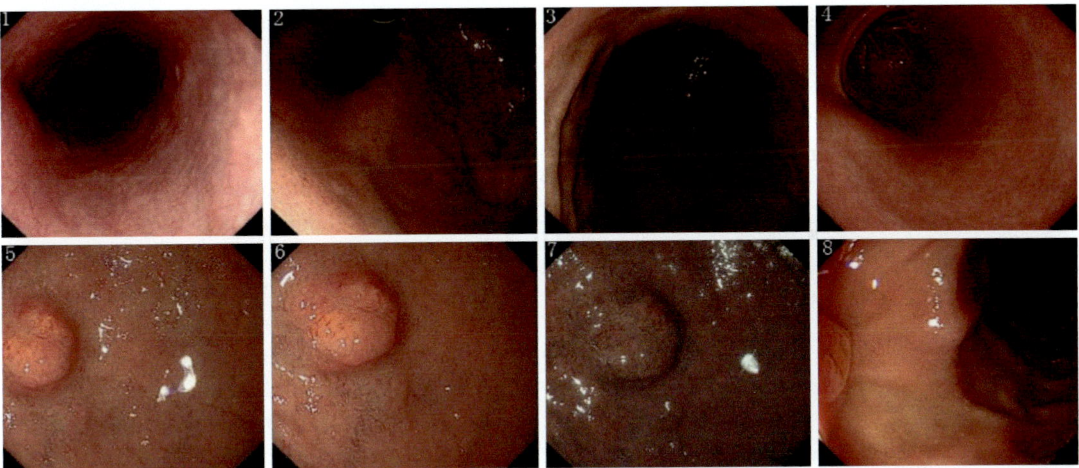

Fig. 3.10 Gastroscopy. The mucosa of the gastric sinus exhibited mild irregularities, while the pylorus appeared round and consistently patent. Within the duodenal bulb, there was a sarcoid-like lesion measuring approximately 1.0 cm × 0.8 cm. This lesion displayed a broad, non-active base and an eroded mucosal surface with rough texture

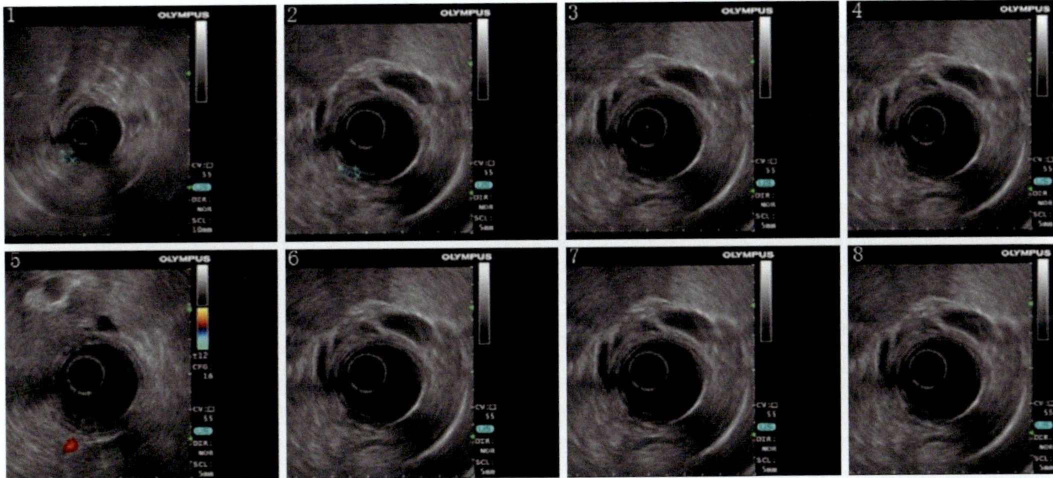

Fig. 3.11 Ultrasound endoscopy. A hypoechoic mass measuring approximately 5.5 mm × 3.5 mm was observed within the duodenal wall near the augmentation site. The mass displayed consistent internal echogenicity and well-defined borders. It primarily affected the mucosal and submucosal layers of the duodenal wall, while the intrinsic muscular layer and serosal layer at the augmentation site appeared clear, continuous, and intact. Notably, no enlarged lymph nodes were detected in the vicinity of the lesion. Given these findings, a neuroendocrine tumor was considered, predominantly localized within the mucosal and submucosal layers. Consequently, endoscopic treatment was recommended

3.4.3 Treatment

Following admission and completion of the diagnostic evaluations, a definitive diagnosis of a duodenal tumor was established. The tumor, located within the submucosal layer, exhibited no secretory activity on octreotide imaging, indicating its classification as a non-functioning neuroendocrine tumor.

Elective laparoscopic endoscopic combined duodenal mass resection was performed when preoperative examination was completed. After general anesthesia, the patient was operated in the lateral decubitus position. Endoscopic exploration revealed that the tumor was located in the anterior wall of the duodenal bulb and was about 1 cm in size, with a wide and inactive lesion base and rough and eroded mucosa on the lesion surface. The lesion was seen to be closely related to the muscularis propria layer with unclear demarcation, and endoscopic full-thickness resection was performed (Fig. 3.13). After the endoscopic resection, the patient's position was changed from lateral to lying down, and the pneumoperitoneum was established by the "five-hole method." The duodenum was closed with full-thickness sutures and the muscle sarcoplasm layer was embedded. Endoscopic examination of the duodenum revealed no strictures, and then the operation was completed. Postoperative bed activity was encouraged on the first day, the gastric tube was removed on the second day, the fluid diet was resumed on the third day, and the patient was discharged on the ninth day. Based on the pathological findings, regular review was recommended.

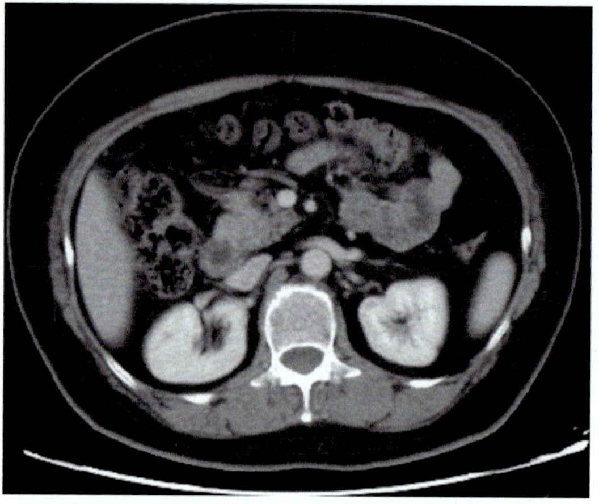

Fig. 3.12 Enhanced abdominal CT. The duodenal wall was locally thickened, with a thickening of approximately 0.7 cm, and reinforcement was seen on the enhanced scanning. No clear enlarged lymph nodes were seen in the coeliac and retroperitoneum

3.4.4 Postoperative Pathologic Report

Neuroendocrine tumor (G1). The tumor penetrated through the submucosa and invaded into

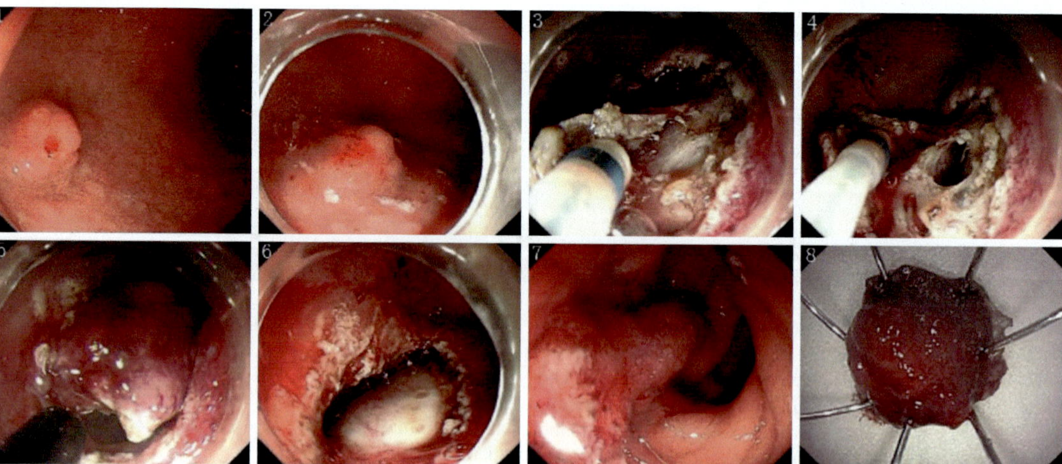

Fig. 3.13 Endoscopic surgery procedure

the superficial layer of the intrinsic muscle, nearest 300 μm from the basal surgical margin. No vascular tumor embolus or nerve invasion was seen, and no tumor was seen in the mucosal layer or basal resection margin. pTNM: pT2Nx. Immunohistochemistry: AE1/AE3(+), CD56(2+), ChrA(3+), Ki-67 (2%+), Syno(3+), Desmin (intrinsic muscles+).

3.4.5 Case Analysis

Neuroendocrine neoplasms (NENs) encompass a diverse group of tumors originating from embryonic neuroendocrine cells. These tumors possess neuroendocrine markers, have the capacity to produce peptides, and can arise in various tissues and organs throughout the body. Over recent years, the incidence of NENs has been increasing, with gastroenteropancreatic neuroendocrine tumors (GEPNENs) being the most prevalent, accounting for 65–75% of all NENs [34]. Within the GEPNEN category, duodenal neuroendocrine tumors (D-NENs) are rare, constituting less than 5% of cases [35]. Clinically, most D-NENs exhibit slow growth and primarily present with non-specific gastrointestinal symptoms, making early detection and diagnosis challenging. Symptoms such as gastrointestinal bleeding or jaundice may manifest when the tumor ruptures, bleeds, or obstructs the pancreaticobiliary duct. Carcinoid syndrome, characterized by flushing, diarrhea, abdominal pain, dyspnea, and cardiovascular abnormalities, is a distinctive feature observed in NEN patients. However, the incidence of carcinoid syndrome in D-NENs has been reported to be low, and its presence often indicates distant tumor metastasis [36].

The local diagnosis of D-NENs relies on endoscopy and imaging examination, while the qualitative diagnosis focuses on histopathological examination. Ultrasound, CT, and MRI can detect tumors larger than 1 cm in diameter, with a positive detection rate of 60–90% [37]. They are of guiding significance in assessing the relationship between tumors and adjacent organs and blood vessels, as well as the metastasis of peripheral lymph nodes, surgical feasibility, and preoperative staging. Ultrasound endoscopy has special advantages in the localization of D-NENs and can detect tumors less than 1 cm in diameter with a diagnostic sensitivity of 80–90% [38]. Preoperative ultrasound endoscopy can determine the size of the tumor, the depth of infiltration, the invasion of the surrounding adjacent organs and the presence of enlarged lymph nodes, which can provide good guidance for the preoperative staging of the tumor and the selection of clinical treatment. The final diagnosis of D-NENs needs to rely on pathological examination combined with immunohistochemical staining.

Surgery is the main treatment for D-NENs, including operative surgery and endoscopic resection. Indications of endoscopic treatment: (1) the maximum diameter of tumor is less than 1.0 cm; (2) the tumor grows outside the ampulla; (3) the lesion does not invade the muscle layer; (4) no lymph node metastasis is seen in EUS or CT examination; (5) pathological results show that the tumor cells do not have nuclear division, show inert behavior and no metastatic foci [39]. For lesions with a diameter of 1.0–2.0 cm, beyond the submucosa, laparoscopic or open resection is the best option. In cases with a diameter greater than 2.0 cm, especially those with pathology suggesting a mitotic index greater than 2 per high magnification, EUS suggesting tumor cells infiltrating the deep intestinal wall, peritumor lymph node involvement, and CT and/or MRI suggesting suspicious lymph node involvement, radical surgical resection is recommended [40].

Traditional laparotomy for gastrointestinal tumors is highly traumatic, with slow postoperative wound healing and relatively many complications. With the continuous progress of minimally invasive technology, laparoscopic resection has been applied and popularized in the treatment of NENs of the digestive tract. However, most of the NENs of the digestive tract are intraluminal in growth, and in some cases, there is no obvious change in the serosal membrane layer, so it is difficult to accurately locate the site of tumors with small diameter by simple laparoscopic surgery, and blindly cutting through the intestinal wall will cause additional damage [41]. On the other hand, the duodenal wall is thinner than the gastric wall, and there is a higher risk of perforation and bleeding in endoscopic resection of D-NENs [42]. In recent years, the clinical treatment of gastrointestinal neuroendocrine tumors by endoscopic combined with laparoscopic technology has achieved good results. The combination of two scopes can give full play to the advantages of endoscopic and laparoscopic surgery, with clearer vision and easy to accurately locate the tumor lesion. At the same time, the combination of endoscopy and laparoscopy can reduce the trauma of surgery, reduce postoperative complications, and speed up the postoperative recovery of patients. Toyonaga et al. [43] reported a patient with D-NENs who underwent successful wedge resection of duodenal bulb tumor with endoscopic guidance, and Bowers et al. [44] reported a case of laparoscopic local resection of a duodenal bulb posterior neuroendocrine tumor. In both cases, endoscopic combined with laparoscopic techniques were used to successfully perform local resection of D-NENs. However, performing laparoscopic local resection, especially when using the anastomosis, adequate surgical margins should be maintained while avoiding duodenal stricture. On the other hand, the combined technique is highly demanding and requires close cooperation between the surgeon and the endoscopist, as well as the innovation of the relevant auxiliary instruments.

3.4.6 Expert Comments

D-NENs are characterized by their rarity and slow-growing nature, often presenting with non-specific digestive symptoms. In cases that meet the appropriate indications, a combined laparoscopic endoscopic resection approach is considered feasible. This combined technique offers several advantages compared to open resection, including reduced invasiveness, decreased incidence of complications, and faster postoperative recovery. Furthermore, when compared to pure laparoscopic surgery, the combination of laparoscopy and endoscopy allows for the optimal utilization of each technique's strengths. Endoscopy enables accurate localization and precise resection of the lesion, while laparoscopy facilitates meticulous suturing, ensuring the surgical procedure's safety and achieving radical tumor removal.

Case provider: Chunguang Guo, Penghui Niu.
Commentary: Dongbing Zhao.

3.5 Case 12: Totally Laparoscopic Resection of Gastric Remnant Cancer

3.5.1 Brief History

The patient was male, 49 years old. The chief complaint was that "residual stomach cancer discovered during follow-up half a month ago." The patient underwent gastric resection 8 years ago for gastric cancer with Billroth II anastomosis. Pathological examination revealed invasion of the muscular layer and the lesser omentum by poorly differentiated adenocarcinoma. No lymph node metastasis was detected (0/27). Following surgery, the patient received six cycles of adjuvant chemotherapy. Annual regular gastroscopy was performed for surveillance. The most recent gastroscopy identified multiple white patches and granular changes at the anastomosis site, with biopsy confirming adenocarcinoma. Physical examination showed no abnormalities. Tumor markers (CA199, AFP, CEA) were within normal limits. Gastroscopy revealed scattered white patches in the residual stomach and hyperemic, rough appearance at the gastrointestinal anastomosis (Fig. 3.14). Pathology confirmed residual gastric ring-cell carcinoma and chronic active inflammation and intestinal metaplasia in the gastrointestinal anastomosis mucosal tissue. Abdominal contrast-enhanced CT scan revealed the absence of a portion of the stomach, high-density anastomosis at the stump and distal bowel anastomosis, and high-density anastomosis at the duodenal stump (Fig. 3.15).

Diagnosis: Residual gastric cancer (cT1N0M0).

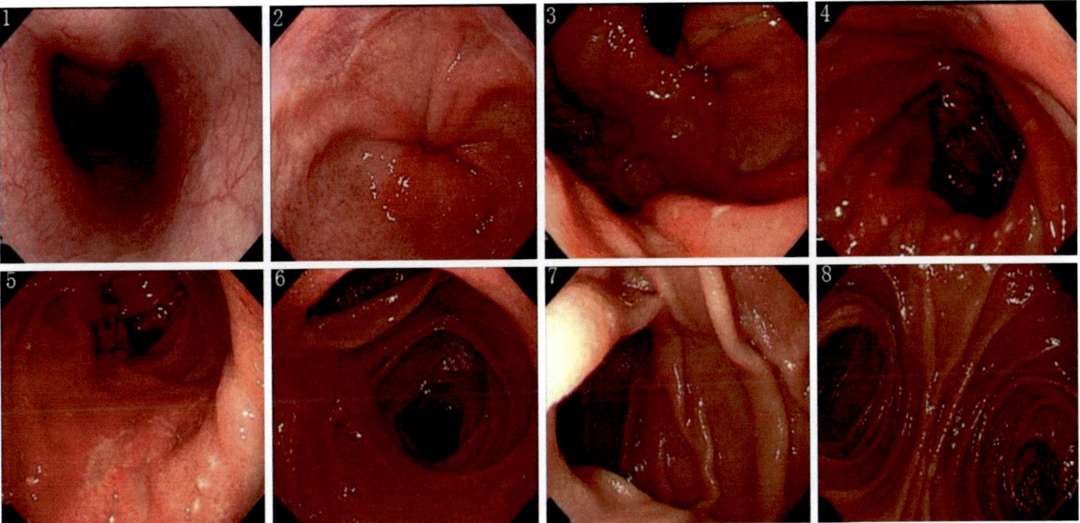

Fig. 3.14 Gastroscopic examination revealed hyperemia and edema of the remnant gastric mucosa, accompanied by scattered white patches

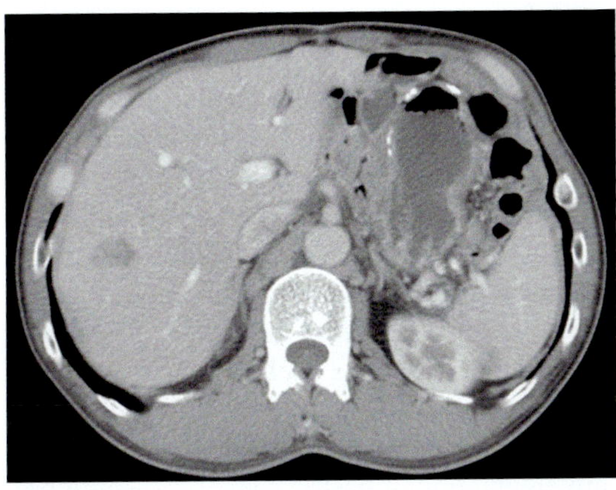

Fig. 3.15 Abdominal CT scan demonstrated the partial absence of the stomach and the presence of high-density anastomosis at the gastric stump and distal intestine

3.5.2 Treatment

Upon admission, relevant examinations before surgery and totally laparoscopic radical resection of gastric remnant carcinoma were performed. Following general anesthesia, the lithotomy position was assumed. The "five holes" technique was employed to insert trocars, and pneumoperitoneum was established using the open method of umbilicus puncture, with a pressure range of 12–15 mmHg. A 12 mm trocar was positioned as an observation port. Other 12 mm trocars were inserted 2 cm below the costal margin along the left anterior axillary line and 2 cm above umbilicus along the right midclavicular line. 5 mm trocars were placed 2 cm below the costal margin along the right anterior axillary line and 2 cm above umbilicus along the left midclavicular line. The surgeon stood on the patient's right side, the assistant on the left side, and the camera operator positioned between the patient's legs. Abdominal exploration revealed no evidence of tumor metastasis. Severe intra-abdominal adhesions were observed, with close adhesion of the remnant stomach to the original abdominal incision, proximal small intestine, and the visceral surface of the left lobe of the liver. Multiple tumor lesions were identified within the remnant stomach, ranging in size from 2 to 3 mm, without invasion of the muscular layer. No enlarged lymph nodes were found in the vicinity. Adhesions were meticulously dissected, revealing a pre-colon Billroth II + Braun anastomosis as the original reconstructive method for the digestive tract. The distance between the gastrointestinal and Braun anastomosis was approximately 20 cm.

Special attention was given to protecting the colon and disconnecting the input and output loop at the distal end of the original intestinal anastomosis. The stomach was mobilized towards the cardia, and the short gastric vessels were transected. Lymph node dissection was performed for No. 4sa and No. 2 lymph nodes, and the left crus of diaphragm was exposed. Along the lesser curvature of the stomach, the stomach was further mobilized to the left side of the cardia, vagus nerves were severed, and lower mediastinal lymph nodes were meticulously cleared. A 5 cm segment of the lower esophagus was prepared for anastomosis. The distal jejunum was elevated, and an esophagojejunal π anastomosis was performed, securing the junction with a linear cutting occluder. Lateral anastomosis between the distal and proximal jejunum was executed, 40 cm from the distal end of the esophagojejunal anastomosis. The surgical procedure progressed smoothly.

On the second day following the surgery, contrast medium flow was unobstructed, with no signs of extravasation. The patient exhibited flatus and initiated a liquid diet on the fourth day post-operation. Drainage tubes were removed on the seventh day, and the patient was discharged on the eighth day.

3.5.3 Pathology: (Gross Specimen)

The remnant gastrectomy specimen displayed an 11.5 cm long lesser curvature and a 13.5 cm long greater curvature. The small intestine with anastomosis measured 29 cm and 35 cm in length, respectively, with edges measuring 4 cm and 5 cm in width. The gastric wall mucosa exhibited a greyish-brown coloration, interspersed with greyish-yellow patches. A segment of the esophagus measuring approximately 0.8 cm in length and 2.5 cm in width was also observed.

3.5.4 Microscopic Diagnosis

Microscopic examination revealed scattered small and poorly differentiated adenocarcinoma cells within the remnant gastric wall tissue, characterized as signet ring-cell carcinoma (Lauren type: diffuse type). The tumor was confined to the lamina propria of the gastric mucosa and did not exhibit apparent vascular tumor thrombus or nerve invasion. No involvement of the small intestine or the junction between the esophagus and stomach was observed. Foam cells were sparsely distributed in the lamina propria of the peripheral gastric mucosa. Focal vascular hyperplasia and dilation of the chylous duct were noted in the intestinal mucosa. No cancer cells were identified at the surgical margins of the small intestine. Furthermore, no lymph node metastasis was detected. The TNM staging for this case is pT1aN0M0.

3.5.5 Case Analysis

In 1922, Balfour et al. [45], American scholars, first introduced the concept of gastric remnant carcinoma, which refers to primary cancer occurring in the gastric stump following subtotal gastrectomy for benign diseases. According to the ninth edition of SURGERY in China, gastric remnant carcinoma is defined as primary cancer in the gastric stump that arises more than 5 years after subtotal gastrectomy for benign diseases, with an incidence of approximately 2% [46]. In recent years, the surgical treatment of benign diseases has declined due to advancements in endoscopic therapy and the widespread use of proton pump inhibitors. Concurrently, the implementation of gastric cancer screening programs and improved standardization of surgical procedures have significantly increased the long-term survival rates of gastric cancer patients [47]. Clinically, there has been a gradual rise in the occurrence of primary cancer in the remnant stomach after gastric cancer surgery. Consequently, in the 1990s, the Japanese academic community expanded the definition of gastric remnant cancer to include primary cancer in the remnant stomach occurring more than 5 years after subtotal gastrectomy for benign lesions or more than 10 years after subtotal gastrectomy for gastric cancer [48, 49]. In 1982, Ichikawa, a Japanese scholar, argued that due to the difficulty in effectively distinguishing between new and recurrent cancers, it was more appropriate to use the term "cancer on the stump stomach" instead of "gastric remnant carcinoma" [50]. This revised definition no longer distinguishes the nature of the initial disease or the specific time interval. However, it still needs to note the nature of the initial disease, the time elapsed since surgery, and the location of the residual gastric cancer. After several rounds of discussions, the latest version of the Japanese gastric cancer management protocol adopted this concept [51] to objectively describe the clinical characteristics of gastric remnant carcinoma. Unlike the epidemiological characteristics of gastric cancer in Japan, China has a high proportion of advanced gastric cancer cases, with higher rates of local recurrence and positive resection margins. Consequently, the expert consensus in China regarding the definition of gastric remnant cancer maintains that "cancer on the gastric stump" is not equivalent to "gastric remnant carcinoma." To avoid confusion in clinical practice, it is recommended to adhere to the previous definition of "gastric remnant carcinoma," which refers to the development of new cancer in the gastric stump more than 5 years after gastrectomy for benign diseases or more than 10 years after gastrectomy for gastric cancer [52].

The scope of lymph node dissection for gastric remnant carcinoma remains a subject of debate due to changes in lymph flow direction. Studies on lymph node metastasis in gastric remnant carcinoma have reported the following rates: No. 1 30.8%, No. 2 25.0%, No. 3 44.4%, No. 4 33.3%, No. 7 33.3%, No. 8 + No. 9 23.5%, No. 10 21.4%, No. 11 14.2%, No. 12 14.2%, No. 13 6.7%, No. 14 28.6%, and 54.5% in lymph nodes along the mesojejunum, with rates ranging from 33.3 to 62.5% in No. 19, 20, 110, and 111 lymph nodes [53]. The Japanese Gastric Cancer Research Association recommends lymph node dissection for gastric remnant carcinoma, including No. 1, No. 2, No. 3, No. 4, No. 7, No. 8, No. 9, No. 10, No. 11, No. 12, and No. 13 [54]. Han et al. [55] suggested that lymph node dissection after Billroth I operation should include the No. 17 group lymph nodes, while for Billroth II operation, the mesenteric lymph nodes of the jejunum should be cleared. Liang Han [56] proposed that the scope of lymph node dissection for gastric remnant carcinoma should exceed the requirements of D2 dissection. In addition to the second station of lymph node dissection, it should also encompass No. 17, No. 13, No. 14v, the mesenteric lymph nodes of the jejunum, No. 10, No. 19, No. 20, No. 110, and No. 111 lymph nodes.

Surgery is the primary treatment method for gastric remnant carcinoma. However, the complexity of the operation is increased due to factors such as severe abdominal adhesions, unclear anatomical levels, and invasion of surrounding organs. In the past, open surgery was commonly used for these cases. However, with the introduction of laparoscopic techniques, laparoscopic surgery for gastric cancer has become the standard approach for early-stage gastric cancer due to its advantages of reduced trauma, less bleeding, and faster recovery. In 2005, the first laparoscopic surgery for gastric remnant cancer was successfully performed, following the success of laparoscopic radical gastrectomy for gastric cancer [57, 58]. Over the years, as laparoscopic surgery for gastric cancer has gained wider application and matured technology, laparoscopic surgery for gastric remnant cancer has also increased in popularity. A meta-analysis comparing open surgery and laparoscopic surgery for gastric remnant cancer between 2005 and 2014 found that although laparoscopic surgery took longer, the number of lymph node dissections and long-term survival rates were comparable [59]. One of the advantages of laparoscopic surgery is its ability to significantly reduce intraoperative bleeding [60, 61]. Studies have shown that as surgeons gain experience and cross the learning curve, the benefits of laparoscopy in treating gastric remnant cancer become apparent. The use of pneumoperitoneum in laparoscopy provides clearer visualization of the anatomical layers, and the magnifying effect of laparoscopic cameras helps reduce bleeding during the procedure.

Laparoscopic surgery for gastric remnant carcinoma has its own unique characteristics compared to open surgery. After the initial operation, the remnant stomach often retracts to the left upper abdomen, making it more convenient for the surgeon to stand on the patient's right side during the laparoscopic procedure. To minimize the risk of injury, it is recommended to place the first puncture device away from the surgical site under direct vision. During laparoscopic surgery, the tension created by pneumoperitoneum can help release abdominal adhesions. Selective removal of adhesions is performed based on the individual case, aiming to improve surgical exposure and facilitate the operation. In cases where it is challenging to differentiate between postoperative adhesions and cancerous invasion, timely conversion to open surgery or even multi-visceral resection may be necessary to ensure the completeness of the radical treatment [62].

The prognosis of gastric remnant cancer is generally considered to be worse than that of primary proximal gastric cancer. However, a meta-analysis conducted by Shimada et al. [63] involving 20 articles and 906 patients with gastric remnant cancer indicated that there was no significant difference in long-term survival between gastric remnant cancer and primary proximal gastric cancer. This finding challenges the notion that gastric remnant cancer has a worse prognosis and suggests that the long-term survival outcomes can be comparable to those of primary proximal gastric cancer when appropriate treatment is administered.

3.5.6 Expert Comments

Under the influence of evolving times and changing disease patterns, there has been a noticeable increase in the incidence of gastric remnant cancer. Consequently, the definition of this condition has also undergone alterations in both its connotation and scope. Within the realm of modern surgical practices, the pursuit of excellence has consistently driven surgeons to explore the potential of various minimally invasive techniques. Through the accumulation of technical expertise, minimally invasive surgery has undeniably yielded numerous favorable outcomes. Nonetheless, it is important to recognize that laparoscopic surgery, at its core, remains a surgical modality, and patient prognosis ultimately hinges on the implementation of standard procedures guided by sound surgical rationale.

Given the intricacies associated with gastric remnant cancer, it is imperative to strike a delicate balance between the benefits and drawbacks of novel technologies. Rather than solely pursuing the artistry of minimally invasive procedures, it is crucial to adhere to the principle of achieving a curative effect. By prioritizing the efficacy of radical treatment, we can ensure that minimally invasive surgery genuinely enhances patient outcomes.

Case provider: Chunguang Guo, Zefeng Li.
Commentary: Chunguang Guo.

3.6 Case 13: Reduced-Port Laparoscopic Gastrectomy in Gastric Cancer

3.6.1 Brief History

A 29-year-old male patient was admitted to the hospital for diagnostic evaluation following the recent diagnosis of gastric antral cancer. The patient experienced discomfort in the pharynx, prompting him to undergo gastroscopy at an external medical facility 1 week prior to admission. During the procedure, a protruding mass, measuring approximately two-third of the antrum cavity, was identified. The mass exhibited irregular characteristics, accompanied by multiple ulcerations and erosion lesions on its surface. The mucosa appeared rough, and clear demarcation from the surrounding tissues was indiscernible. The tumor extended upwards towards the gastric angle and was positioned 2 cm away from the pylorus ring in a downward direction (refer to Fig. 3.16). Pathological examination of the

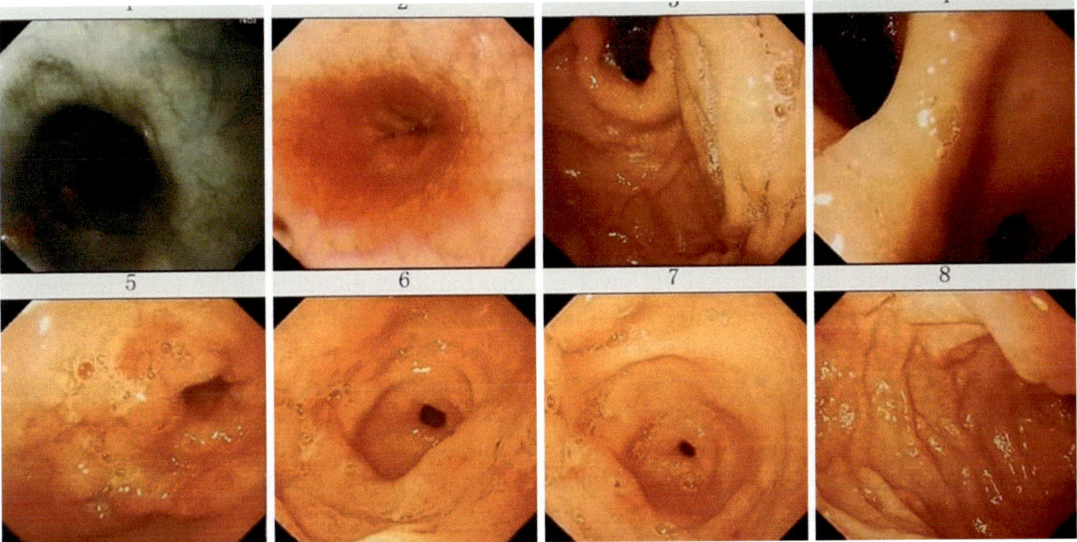

Fig. 3.16 Illustrates the findings of the gastroscopy, revealing a prominent protrusion and the presence of surface ulcers in the vicinity of the gastric antrum

biopsy specimen revealed poorly differentiated adenocarcinoma, displaying partial features of signet ring cell carcinoma. Subsequent chest, abdominal, and pelvic computed tomography (CT) scans demonstrated alterations in the gastric antrum, featuring a smooth serosal surface. Notably, no enlarged lymph nodes were detected in the abdomen or retroperitoneum following the endoscopic procedure (see Fig. 3.17).

Diagnosis: Gastric antral cancer (cT2N0M0).

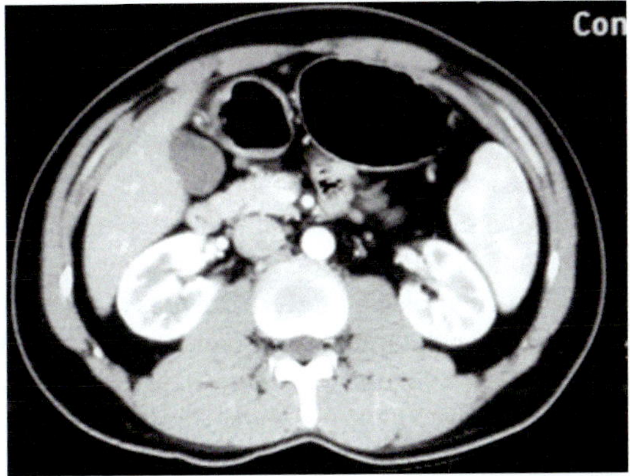

Fig. 3.17 Showcases the computed tomography (CT) findings that indicate alterations occurring in the gastric antrum

3.6.2 Treatment

Following the completion of preoperative assessments, the patient underwent laparoscopic pylorus-preserving gastrectomy with Billroth II anastomosis and Braun operation. Intraoperatively, the tumor was identified on the greater curvature of the gastric antrum, measuring approximately 2 × 3 cm in size. Visual inspection did not reveal any serosal invasion. Notably, no enlarged lymph nodes were detected in the vicinity of the pylorus, hepatic artery, or left gastric artery. The resected specimen was extracted through a 5 cm incision made around the umbilicus. The left abdominal drainage tube was removed 11 days postoperatively, while the right abdominal drainage tube was removed 13 days postoperatively. The patient was discharged from the hospital 14 days after the operation.

Pathology: A localized ulcerative lesion, measuring 2 × 2 × 0.7 cm in size, was identified at a distance of 2.5 cm from the lower resection margin. The cut surface of the lesion appeared gray-white and firm, displaying an indistinct boundary. The lesion infiltrated the muscular layer. Upon microscopic examination, the diagnosis revealed a limited ulcerative low-grade adenocarcinoma of the stomach, characterized as Lauren type: diffuse type, with partial presence of signet ring cell carcinoma. The tumor exhibited invasion into the submucosal layer, with no evident nerve invasion or vascular tumor thrombosis. Notably, the tumor did not involve the pylorus ring or greater omentum. The adjacent gastric mucosa demonstrated features of chronic atrophic gastritis with intestinal metaplasia. No tumor was detected at the proximal and distal resection margins, and lymph node examination revealed no evidence of metastatic cancer (0/30 lymph nodes examined). The final diagnosis is pT1bN0M0.

3.6.3 Case Analysis

With the advancements in the concept of minimally invasive surgery and the continuous progress of laparoscopic equipment, instruments, and techniques, reduced-port laparoscopic surgery (RPLS) has emerged as a viable approach. As the name implies, RPLS involves performing laparoscopic procedures with fewer incisions compared to conventional laparoscopic surgery, with the ultimate goal of achieving single-incision laparoscopic surgery (SILS). Reduced port/single-incision laparoscopic gastrectomy offers several advantages over traditional five-port laparoscopic gastrectomy, including reduced trauma, improved cosmetic outcomes, decreased postoperative pain, and faster recovery. The safety of single-incision laparoscopic distal gastrectomy was initially confirmed in 2011 [64], and since then, the application of single-incision laparoscopy in gastric cancer surgery has been rapidly evolving, encompassing procedures ranging from distal gastrectomy to total gastrectomy and proximal gastrectomy [65–67].

In 2016, Kunisaki et al. from Japan, reported a series of 165 cases of reduced-port laparoscopic gastrectomy. All patients were clinically diagnosed with stage I/II gastric cancer before the surgery. The surgical approach involved a combination of a navel incision and one additional port. The short-term and long-term outcomes demonstrated satisfactory results, indicating the effectiveness of this approach for stage I/II gastric cancer [68]. In 2019, researchers investigated the application of single-incision laparoscopic surgery for advanced gastric cancer and observed that the SILS group exhibited lower intraoperative bleeding and shorter postoperative hospital stays, highlighting the safety and feasibility of single-incision laparoscopic surgery for advanced gastric cancer, with favorable short-term outcomes [69].

Reduced port/single-incision laparoscopic gastrectomy is currently in the exploratory phase. Foreign literature suggests that this approach should be considered for early gastric cancer patients who are relatively slim and have less visceral fat, particularly young women [70]. To establish standardized guidelines for the development of reduced-port laparoscopic gastrectomy, domestic experts have reached a consensus regarding the indications for single-incision plus one-port laparoscopic gastrectomy, which include the following criteria [71]: (1) BMI ≤ 25 kg/m^2; (2) tumor located in the gastric antrum or body; (3) no history of upper abdominal surgery; and (4) clinical staging evaluation of cT1b-3N0-1M0 based on preoperative ultrasound gastroscopy, abdominal (pelvic) CT, or MRI.

It is important to note that reduced port/single-incision laparoscopic gastrectomy is a challenging procedure that demands high technical proficiency, particularly in the case of single-incision laparoscopic surgery. The parallel arrangement of instruments and light source can lead to a coaxial effect, and the instruments themselves can create a chopstick effect. Moreover, single-incision laparoscopic surgery is typically performed by a single surgeon without the assistance of an assistant. Therefore, pure single-incision laparoscopic gastrectomy presents greater difficulties and requires even higher technical expertise, thus limiting its widespread adoption. In some international settings, researchers have employed Da Vinci robotic surgery to mitigate the surgical complexity [72, 73]; however, the high cost associated with robotic surgery prevents its universal application.

In terms of the technical aspects of reduced port/single-incision laparoscopic gastrectomy, Su et al. [74] have highlighted the primary challenge as maintaining appropriate tissue tension throughout the procedure, which necessitates coordination between the surgeon's left and right hands. Graspers and energy instruments are utilized to apply moderate tension by pulling in different directions. Additionally, gauze strips are employed as barriers to protect surrounding tissues while providing suitable anatomical space. The patient's position may be adjusted as needed, and the gravitational pull exerted by the greater omentum and adjacent tissues can help optimize the surgical field of view by minimizing obstruction from structures such as the greater omentum, transverse colon, hepatic flexure, splenic flexure, and pancreas.

During intraoperative anastomosis, traction wires are pre-placed at the esophageal stump and jejunal opening. These wires are then moderately pulled in the opposite direction of the linear cutter insertion to facilitate the completion of the anastomosis.

In the specific case discussed, since the tumor was in the early stage, the procedure involved reduced-port laparoscopy with three ports for total laparoscopic distal gastrectomy, D2 lymph node dissection, and Billroth II reconstruction. The overall surgical procedure proceeded relatively smoothly. While the three-port approach helps mitigate instrument conflict, the absence of an assistant still presents challenges in maintaining tension. Leveraging gravity and utilizing the natural traction provided by tissue adhesions surrounding the surgical area can be advantageous in facilitating the operative steps.

3.6.4 Expert Comments

In conjunction with adhering to the principles of D2 lymph node dissection for gastric cancer, the successful execution of minimally invasive laparoscopic gastrectomy with reduced or single incision relies on maintaining optimal surgical exposure and tension. In cases where operative challenges arise, impeding the smooth progress of the procedure, it may be necessary to make additional incisions or convert to open surgery to ensure complete cancer removal and prioritize surgical safety. The development of reduced or single-incision laparoscopic techniques represents an advancement over traditional laparoscopic surgery and holds significant clinical value. However, the implementation of these new techniques must be approached with a primary focus on ensuring surgical safety.

Case providers: Hong Zhou, Chunguang Guo.

Commentary expert: Dongbing Zhao.

3.7 Case 14: Laparoscopic Surgery for Gastric Cancer in a Patient with Kyphoscoliosis

3.7.1 Brief History

The subject of interest is a 60-year-old male patient who was admitted to the hospital primarily due to persistent upper abdominal discomfort over a duration of 6 months. Initially, the patient experienced unprovoked upper abdominal discomfort, which was unresponsive to treatment with traditional Chinese medicine. Notably, 1 month ago, the patient underwent gastroscopy, revealing the presence of a gastric body ulcer. Pathological examination further confirmed poorly differentiated adenocarcinoma, with some portions displaying signet-ring cell carcinoma morphology. The patient's medical history includes a diagnosis of diabetes, hypertension, and a prolonged smoking habit. Additionally, he has endured the long-term consequences of poliomyelitis contracted over four decades ago, resulting in the development of muscular dystrophy syndrome and subsequent kyphotic deformity. Upon admission, the patient presented with a pronounced lateral curvature of the spine, rendering him unable to maintain an upright posture.

Abdominal examination did not elicit any positive findings. Serum levels of CEA, CA199, and CA242 fell within the normal range. Gastroscopic evaluation revealed the presence of an ulcer-like mass in the upper section of the stomach, approximately 40–44 cm from the incisor (see Fig. 3.18). Moreover, abdominal CT with contrast enhancement demonstrated thickening of the greater curvature of the gastric body, along with an irregular outer membrane, indicative of gastric cancer (see Fig. 3.19). Pulmonary function testing revealed severe restrictive ventilatory dysfunction.

Diagnosis: Gastric cancer (cT4N0M0), diabetes mellitus, hypertension, post poliomyelitis muscular dystrophy syndrome, kyphotic deformity, and severe restricted ventilation dysfunction.

3.7.2 Treatment

Following completion of relevant examinations, the patient underwent laparoscopic total gastrectomy at an appropriate timing. The surgical procedure and key technical points are as follows:

Under endotracheal intubation and general anesthesia, the patient was placed in a supine leg position. A "five-hole" Trocar was utilized, with the surgeon positioned on the left side and the assistant on the right side. A laparoscopic camera was positioned between the patient's legs. Conventional exploration of the abdominal cavity was performed.

During the operation, the tumor was identified as ulcerated and located in the middle of the greater curvature of the stomach, measuring larger than 2 cm from the gastroesophageal boundary, with dimensions of approximately 3 × 3 × 2 cm. No metastases were detected in the liver, gallbladder, spleen, abdomen, or pelvis. Based on the exploration findings, a decision was made to proceed with totally laparoscopic radical full stomach resection (D2, Overlap, Roux-en-Y).

The surgical procedure was executed smoothly, and post-surgery, the patient was transferred to the Intensive Care Unit (ICU) for close observation. On the first day after surgery, the patient's condition remained stable, and subsequently, he was transferred back to the ICU.

By the sixth postoperative day, the patient passed gas and began receiving liquid feeding

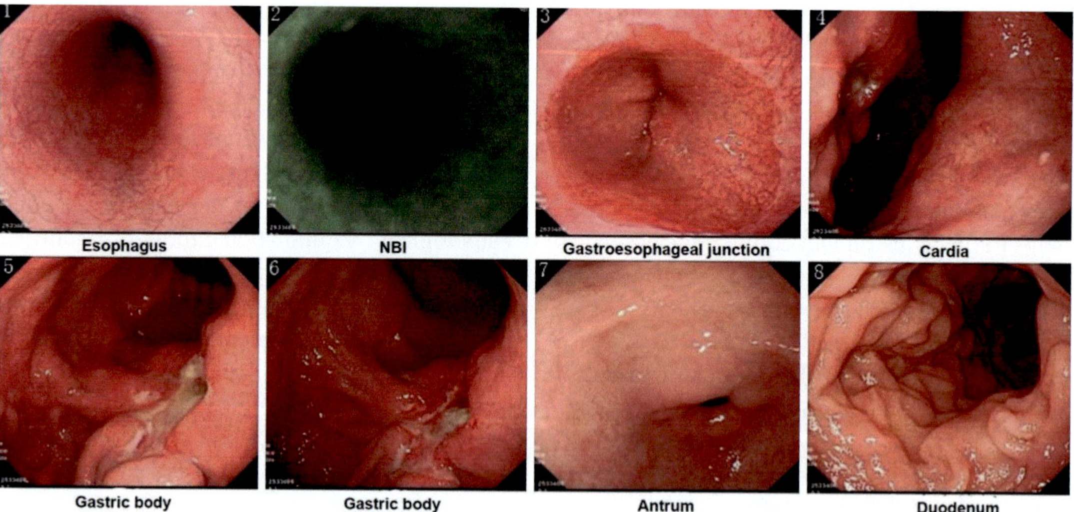

Fig. 3.18 Illustrates the gastroscope examination, revealing the presence of an ulcerous mass located in the upper region of the stomach, approximately 40–44 cm from the incisor

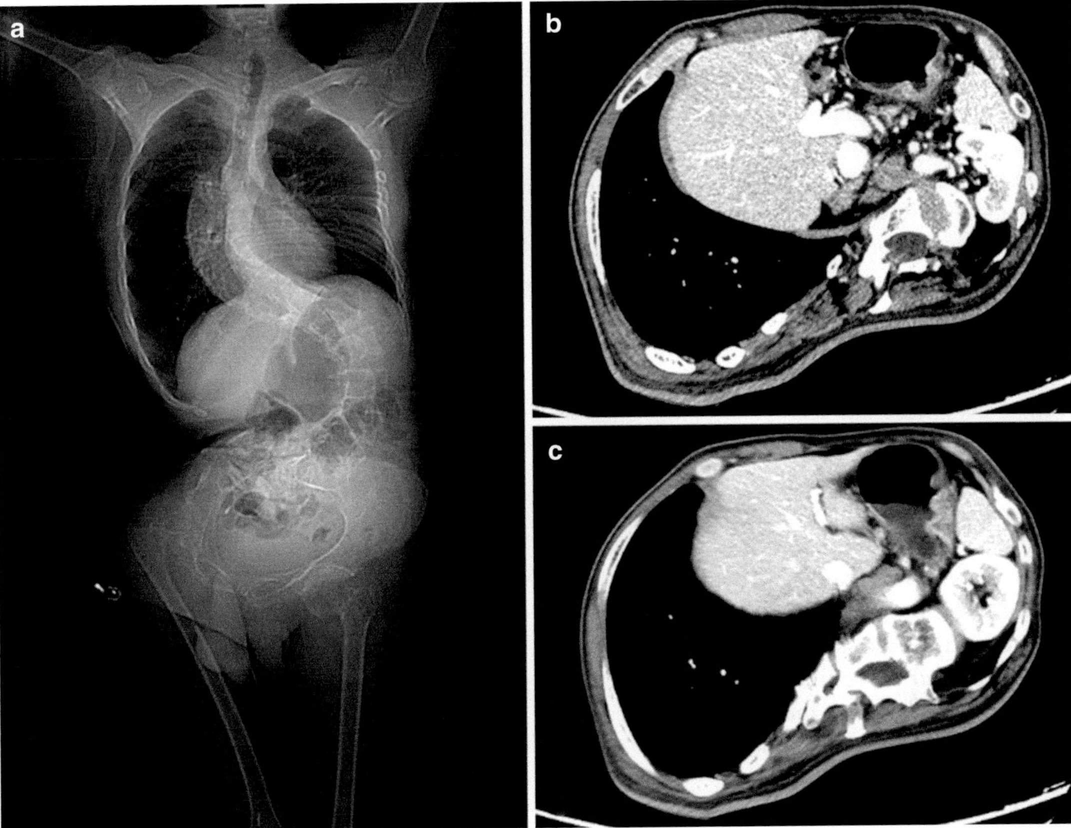

Fig. 3.19 Presents the initial abdominal CT scan, depicting the following findings: (**a**) Severe deformity of the spine. (**b**) Localized thickening of the stomach wall along the greater curvature of the gastric body, measuring approximately 1.7 cm at its thickest point. Notably, the enhancement pattern appears uneven, accompanied by a rough outer membrane. (**c**) Within the left region of the stomach, small lymph nodes with a diameter of approximately 0.5 cm can be observed

following removal of the gastric tube. The abdominal drainage tube was removed on the tenth day. Finally, on the twelfth day, the patient was discharged from the hospital.

Pathology: The histopathological analysis revealed the presence of a gastric infiltrating ulcerated moderately poorly differentiated adenocarcinoma, classified as mixed type according to the Lauren classification system. Some portions of the tumor displayed characteristics of signet-ring cell carcinoma. The tumor infiltrated the muscularis propria and extended into the subserous fibrous adipose tissue. Nerve invasion was observed, while clear evidence of vascular tumor thrombus was not identified. The tumor did not involve the pylorus, duodenum, or greater omentum. Furthermore, no carcinoma was detected in the margins of resection. Lymph node examination indicated the absence of metastatic involvement (0/25). Based on the TNM staging system, the tumor is classified as pT3N0M0, corresponding to stage IIa.

3.7.3 Case Analysis

In recent years, the advancement of laparoscopy technology has facilitated its application in minimally invasive treatment for various diseases, gaining popularity among major medical centers and patients. However, patients with anatomical malformations represent a distinct surgical group that presents unique challenges. Prolonged malformations can induce alterations in respiration, circulation, abdominal internal organs, and vascular relationships. Moreover, these special malformations affect surgical positioning, thereby complicating both traditional and laparoscopic surgeries. Consequently, postoperative care becomes more challenging for these patients. Surgical procedures, intraoperative management, and perioperative treatment for individuals with kyphotic deformities differ significantly from those employed for standard patients. To ensure optimal patient rehabilitation, a comprehensive preoperative evaluation, functional exercises, and meticulous surgical techniques all play crucial roles.

3.7.4 Preoperative Evaluation and Functional Exercise

Kyphotic patients often experience thoracic deformation resulting from long-term spinal compression, which can be accompanied by restricted ventilation disorders. Postoperatively, these individuals are prone to pain, weakened expectoration, secondary pneumonia, and even respiratory failure [75, 76]. Hence, a collaborative assessment of surgical risks and lung function training should be conducted by the preoperative team and anesthesiologist. Lung function training may involve techniques such as deep breathing exercises and balloon blowing. Additionally, comprehensive health education and strict smoking cessation measures are recommended. Preoperative atomization inhalation and effective phlegm management should be implemented to encourage sputum discharge and reduce the incidence [77] of postoperative hypoxemia.

In cases of severe kyphosis, intraperitoneal anatomical variations can occur, leading to distortions of vital organs and blood vessels during malformation development. It has been reported that complex surgical procedures should be preceded by vascular reconstruction to identify major vessel variations and prevent vascular injuries [75, 78, 79].

3.7.5 Intraoperative Position and Operation

Severe kyphosis can pose challenges in positioning and securing patients for surgery, as well as in intubating the tracheal tube during anesthesia. Anesthesia management must not only consider potential cervical vertebra involvement that may restrict movement, but also be attentive to the possibility of joint fractures and dislocations. Given that these patients cannot lie flat like individuals without kyphosis, there are inherent risks of skin pressure injuries and joint fractures on prominent areas of the body following anesthesia. Therefore, it is recommended to provide patients with a soft neck cushion or pillow to maintain a proper angle during endotracheal intubation. Additionally, the use of visual laryngoscopy can help identify any uneven body contours and provide appropriate protection.

Furthermore, the abdominal organs may shift upward and backward due to kyphotic deformity, necessitating careful consideration when formulating the surgical plan. Additionally, it is important to note that most kyphotic patients tend to be of shorter stature, resulting in a reduced distance between the xiphoid process and symphysis pubis. Hence, the placement of surgical incisions should be adjusted accordingly to avoid instrument collisions.

3.7.6 Perioperative Management

Kyphotic deformity not only results in abnormalities in the chest and impaired lung function but also tends to be associated with nutritional issues and corresponding complications, demanding increased attention. Prior to surgery, the patient presented with multiple complications. Upon admission, blood glucose levels were regulated, and blood pressure was closely monitored. Given the patient's long history of smoking and the presence of severe restrictive ventilation dysfunction according to the lung function examination, preoperative health education was provided. This included smoking cessation measures, thrice-daily atomization therapy, encouragement of sputum expulsion following atomization, and lung function exercises such as balloon blowing. Considering the nutritional risk, interventions were implemented, and enteral nutrition preparations were adjusted accordingly. Clear and thorough communication regarding the patient's condition, alternative treatment options, and surgical risks was conducted.

Kyphosis is the most prevalent form of spinal deformity, commonly caused by spinal trauma, spondylitis, or spinal tuberculosis. It is characterized by the protrusion of the spine, leading to changes in the body's upright posture and resulting in a hunchback appearance. Patients with kyphosis often experience short stature and severe chest deformities, which can lead to varying degrees of pulmonary function impairment [80]. Additionally, the lateral scoliosis and chest changes associated with kyphosis can compress the abdominal space, thereby increasing the complexity of certain open surgeries. While laparoscopic cholecystectomy and laparoscopic appendectomy have been reported in numerous cases involving patients with severe kyphosis in China, reports of more complicated procedures are scarce.

After careful preoperative evaluation, the treatment team decided to perform a complete laparoscopic total gastrectomy for this particular case. It was recognized that although the patient's abdominal space was reduced, resembling that of a child, the advantages of laparoscopic surgery, which excels in narrow space operations, could be fully utilized. Notably, total endoscopy was employed for digestive tract reconstruction to avoid excessive downward movement of the thoracic cavity and the need for open surgery to address the deep positioning of the esophagojejunal anastomosis and the challenges associated with exposure. The use of small incisions helped minimize postoperative pain and proved beneficial for long-term smokers in overcoming psychological barriers associated with postoperative sputum discharge and pain, thereby expediting the recovery process.

3.7.7 Expert Comments

The distinctive anatomical variations associated with malformations often present challenges in traditional open surgery. However, the advantages of laparoscopic surgery, particularly its suitability for deep locations and operations in confined spaces, provide unique benefits over open surgery. The advancement of complete laparoscopy technology further minimizes tissue damage, making it particularly suitable for patients with multiple complications. As our understanding of laparoscopic technology continues to deepen, it is expected that endoscopic surgery will have a broader range of applications, expanding its prospects in the field.

Case provider: Tongbo Wang, Chunguang Guo.

Commentary: Chunguang Guo.

3.8 Case 15: Extended Multiorgan Resection for Advanced Gastric Carcinoma

3.8.1 Brief History

The patient, a 49-year-old male, presented with a chief complaint of abdominal distension following meals persisting for a period exceeding 2 months. Initially, the patient experienced episodic postprandial fullness without concurrent symptoms of nausea, acid regurgitation, or postprandial abdominal pain. Notably, there were no instances of melena or hematemesis. Seeking medical attention, the patient visited a local hospital where gastroscopy revealed the presence of a "gastric malignant tumor." Biopsy results confirmed the presence of "adenocarcinoma." Over the past month, the patient has experienced notable satiety and difficulty consuming solid foods, primarily relying on a liquid diet. Physical examination of the abdomen yielded unremarkable findings. The patient's tumor markers, including CEA, AFP, CA72–4, CA19–9, and CA24–2, all fell within the normal range. Subsequent gastroscopy identified invasive gastric cancer characterized by a leather-bottle stomach appearance, with lesions involving the cardia and a segment of the gastric antrum at the level of the gastric body (Fig. 3.20). Enhanced CT imaging revealed two significant findings: (1) diffuse irregular thickening of the gastric wall, consistent with gastric cancer, and (2) the presence of multiple lymph nodes surrounding the stomach, suggestive of possible metastasis (Fig. 3.21).

Diagnosis: Gastric cancer (cT4N + M0, stage III).

3.8.2 Treatment

No contraindications were identified following the comprehensive evaluations conducted at the hospital. Gastroscopy revealed the presence of linitis plastica, accompanied by symptoms indicative of obstruction. Based on these findings, surgical intervention was deemed necessary. Prior to the surgery, the patient was instructed to refrain from oral intake of food and water. Instead, total parenteral nutrition was administered, and the patient underwent gastric tube placement and gastric lavage using hypertonic saline.

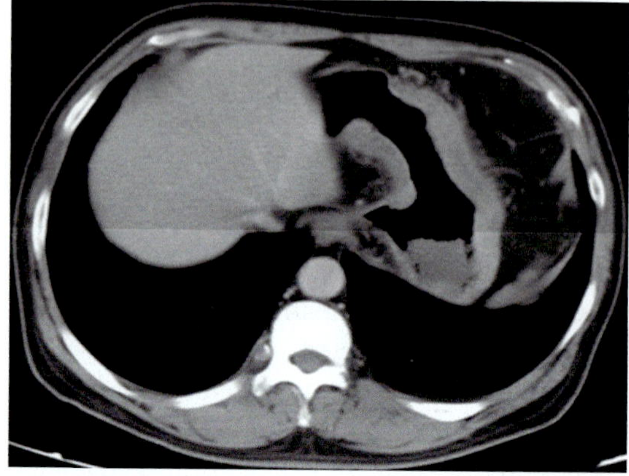

Fig. 3.21 CT imaging demonstrated diffuse and irregular thickening of the gastric wall within the gastric body, with the thickest segment measuring approximately 1.9 cm. The gastric wall exhibited stiffness, resulting in localized narrowing of the gastric cavity. Furthermore, the serosal surface displayed a blurred appearance, and the surrounding fat space exhibited multiple streaks and patchy shadows

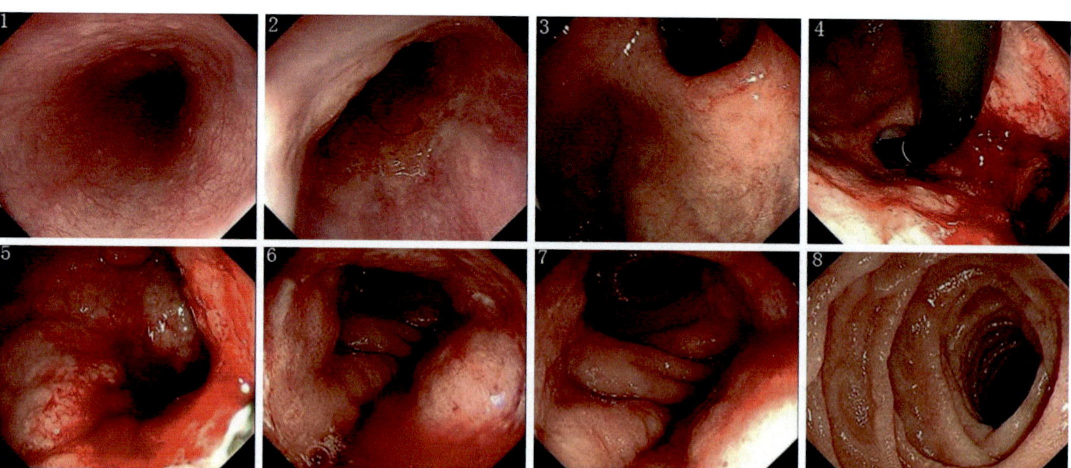

Fig. 3.20 Gastroscopy revealed the esophagogastric junction located approximately 42 cm from the incisors. Within the cardia region, both the anterior and posterior walls exhibited an ulcerated mass along the lesser curvature of the gastric body. Notably, the tumor affected the surrounding gastric body and a segment of the gastric antrum, resulting in swelling and elevation of these regions. The gastric wall displayed rigidity, impaired peristalsis, and the overall gastric cavity exhibited deformation and narrowing

A routine laparoscopic exploration was initially performed, during which intraoperative assessment revealed that the tumor was localized in the cardia and gastric body. Notably, it had penetrated the serosal layer and invaded the pancreas. However, no definite evidence of metastasis was observed in the liver or peritoneum (Fig. 3.22). Due to the extent of pancreatic involvement, the surgical approach was converted to an open procedure. The patient's postoperative recovery proceeded without complications.

A rapid recovery protocol was implemented to facilitate the patient's postoperative rehabilitation. On the fourth day post-surgery, the nasogastric tube was removed, and the patient commenced oral intake of drinking water while gradually mobilizing out of bed. Subsequently, on the ninth day, the abdominal drainage tube was safely removed, and the patient was discharged on the tenth day following the operation. Appropriate medical treatment was continued as part of the patient's post-discharge care.

Pathology: (Gross specimen) The total gastrectomy specimen exhibited the following measurements: the length of the lesser curve was 12 cm, the size of the greater curve was 19 cm, the length of the esophagus was 1 cm with a width of 2.5 cm, and the duodenum measured 1 cm in length and 4 cm in width. Notably, at the cardia region of the greater curve, a diffuse infiltrative mass measuring 8.5 × 8 × 1.5 cm was observed. The suspected pancreatic area measured 4 × 1 cm, and the surrounding gastric mucosa appeared gray-red and exhibited firm consistency. Additionally, pancreatic tissue and spleen were present within the specimen.

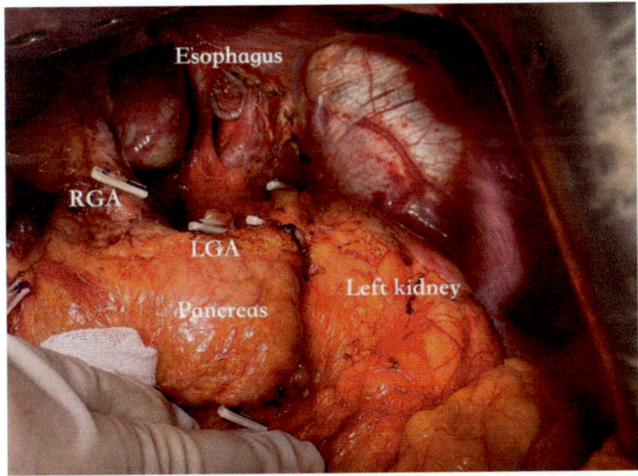

Fig. 3.22 The abdominal image depicts the postoperative outcome following total gastrectomy, distal pancreatec tomy, and splenectomy

(Microscopic diagnosis) Microscopic examination revealed diffusely infiltrating gastric poorly differentiated adenocarcinoma of the diffuse type. The tumor exhibited invasion of the serosa, presence of vascular tumor emboli, and invasion of nerves. However, the tumor did not involve the esophagus, pylorus, or duodenum. No evidence of cancer was detected in the greater omentum or at the upper and lower margins of the resected specimen.

(Pancreatic body and tail + spleen) Infiltration of poorly differentiated adenocarcinoma was observed in the peripancreatic adipose tissue and localized pancreatic parenchyma. However, no carcinoma was identified in the spleen. Moreover, no cancer was detected at the margin of the resected pancreatic tissue. Notably, metastatic carcinoma was found in 20 out of 34 examined lymph nodes. The metastasis involved the extracapsular adipose tissue of the lymph nodes, with multiple cancer nodules observed. The final pathological staging based on the pTNM classification is pT4bN3b, corresponding to stage IIIc.

3.8.3 Case Analysis

Combined organ resection for gastric cancer refers to an extensive surgical procedure aimed at achieving R0 resection by removing the primary gastric tumor that has invaded neighboring organs (T4b). Commonly involved organs in combined organ resection include the liver (partial hepatectomy), transverse mesocolon or part of the transverse colon, body and tail of the pancreas along with splenectomy or simple splenectomy, pancreaticoduodenectomy, among others. It is important to note that combined organ resection is not recommended in cases where the tumor has distant metastasis or when achieving R0 resection is not feasible.

Previously, combined organ resection was associated with significant trauma, high complication rates, and limited improvements in prognosis [81]. However, in recent years, advancements in surgical techniques and perioperative management have significantly improved the safety of combined organ resection, with reports even describing laparoscopic approaches [82, 83]. The anatomical relationships within the upper abdomen provide a theoretical basis for achieving R0 resection when gastric cancer is limited to the aforementioned local areas. The stomach, originating from the foregut, is surrounded by the transverse colon and mesentery below, with the pancreas and spleen located on the dorsal side and the liver on the ventral side. Carboni et al. [84] conducted a retrospective analysis of the long-term efficacy of combined viscera resection in treating T4 gastric cancer. Their findings demonstrated a 5-year overall survival rate of 21.8%, with the R0 resection group exhibiting superior outcomes compared to the R+ group (30.6% vs. 0, $P < 0.001$). Multivariate analysis identified R0 resection as the most significant prognostic protective factor ($P < 0.002$). Similar conclusions were reached by Maehara et al. [85] in Japan, who retrospectively analyzed 150 cases of multiple organ resection for gastric cancer and observed that R0 resection improved long-term patient survival. The fourth edition of the Japanese guidelines for treating gastric cancer also recommends extended resection combined with involved organs for cases where gastric cancer invades the body and tail of the pancreas [86].

Combined organ resection in gastric cancer plays a crucial role in achieving maximal tumor removal, alleviating symptoms such as bleeding and obstruction, improving the patient's quality of life, and facilitating subsequent adjuvant treatments. During the surgical procedure, meticulous attention should be paid to the anatomical planes, utilizing sharp tissue dissection to minimize intraoperative bleeding, prevent damage to surrounding tissues, and avoid tumor rupture. The principle of "no touch" and a stepwise approach should be followed, prioritizing ease of access and avoiding blind resection of the gastrointestinal tract before ensuring definitive R0 resection, thus preventing potential complications. Regarding lymph node dissection, extending the extent of dissection to the third station can be considered based on the second station of lymph node involvement, particularly in cases of combined organ resection. However, it is important to exercise caution and avoid unnecessary extension of lymph node dissection. The decision should be based on individual patient characteristics and surgical indications.

In summary, for T4b gastric cancer, adherence to strict surgical indications is crucial. Individualized treatment plans should be formulated based on the patient's specific condition, incorporating a multidisciplinary approach involving chemotherapy, radiotherapy, and surgery to optimize outcomes.

3.8.4 Expert Comments

Locally advanced gastric cancer with invasion of surrounding organs is generally associated with a poor prognosis. Preoperative neoadjuvant chemotherapy is often recommended as a treatment strategy to reduce tumor size and facilitate R0 resection. However, in cases where patients present with severe conditions such as obstruction, perforation, or bleeding, surgical resection becomes necessary to alleviate immediate life-threatening risks and create opportunities for further treatment interventions. The primary goal of surgical intervention is to achieve R0 resection, which refers to complete removal of the tumor with negative margins. It is important to note that patients who do not achieve R0 resection have a significantly worse prognosis.

Case provider: Hu Ren, Chunguang Guo.

Commentary: Xiaofeng Bai.

3.9 Case 16: Laparoscopic and Endoscopic Treatment for the Double Primary Gastric Carcinomas

3.9.1 Brief History

An octogenarian male presented with a 1-year history of mid-upper abdominal colic without an apparent underlying cause. The colic symptoms were aggravated after meals but were not radiating or severe in intensity and resolved spontaneously. Three months ago, the patient sought medical attention at a local hospital, where a gastroscopy was performed. The gastroscopic findings revealed an ulcer located in the lower part of the stomach, along with invasion of the gastric angle. The pathology report from the gastroscopy indicated high-grade intraepithelial neoplasia of the glandular epithelium in the lower portion of the gastric body.

The patient has a pre-existing medical history of chronic hepatitis B infection, which has not been systematically treated, as well as a diagnosis of Parkinson's disease for over a year. Furthermore, the patient underwent an appendectomy 20 years ago and bilateral inguinal hernia repair 5 years ago(Fig. 3.23).

3.9.2 Ultrasound Endoscopy

Localized mucosal roughness and erosion from the lower esophagus to the junction line about 35 cm from the incisor. The gastro-esophageal junction line is approximately 38 cm from the incisors. A superficial flat lesion (type 0-IIb, 40–48 cm from the incisor) was seen from the cardia of the residual gastric to the lesser curvature/posterior wall of the gastric body, with localized mucosal roughness and irregular surface microstructures visible on NBI+ magnification. The remaining residual gastric mucosa was congested and edematous.

Enhanced Abdominal CT:

1. No clear thickening and swelling shadow in the gastric wall, the combination with microscopic examination is recommended.
2. Enlarged lymph nodes in mediastinal area 7, which tend to be metastatic. Multiple small lymph nodes around the lower esophageal parietal and cardia, the nature of which is to be determined, are suggested to be followed up.

PET-CT:

1. Slightly thickened wall at the gastric angle near the pylorus with mildly increased metabolism; increased metabolism at the esophagogastric junction; it is recommended to combine the endoscopic findings. Multiple small nod-

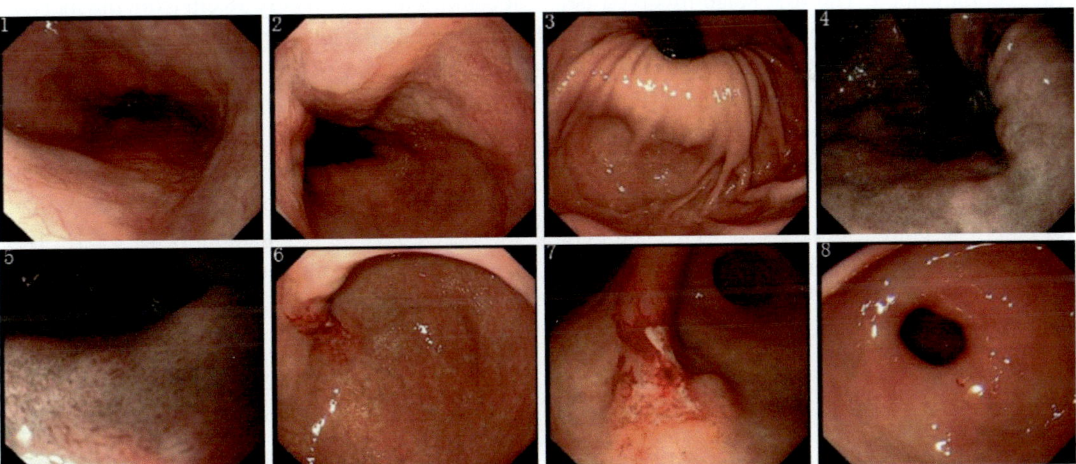

Fig. 3.23 Gastroscopy. A superficial flat lesion (type 0-IIb) was visible in the cardia, with localized mucosal roughness, and NBI+ magnification showed irregular surface microstructures visible in the lesion. An ulcerated swelling was seen in the anterior wall of the gastric angle, with a deep ulcerated base covered with sewage and an irregularly elevated ulcer dike, which was brittle and easily bleeding when touched. The mucosa of the remaining gastric sinus was congested and slightly rough. Diagnosis: gastric angle carcinoma, superficial flat lesion of the cardia (the nature needs to be pathologically clarified, type 0-IIb), considered as early gastric cancer or precancerous lesion, endoscopic treatment is recommended

ules next to the lower esophagus and next to the cardia, no metabolic increase seen; nature to be determined; please follow up closely. Small retroperitoneal lymph nodes with mildly increased metabolism.

2. Multiple microscopic nodules are seen in bilateral lungs, but no metabolic elevation, the nodules are currently small, the nature is to be determined, and follow-up is recommended. Multiple streak-like shadows in bilateral lungs with no significant metabolic elevation.

Diagnosis: Double primary gastric cancer (cT2N1M0), viral hepatitis B, Parkinson's disease.

3.9.3 Treatment

Following a comprehensive evaluation and case-based multidisciplinary discussion, a review of the PET-CT scan was conducted. Based on the discussion, it was determined that the patient's lymph node SUV of 8.4 ruled out metastatic lesions, suggesting the possibility of granuloma. Considering the patient's advanced age and other medical conditions, a staged treatment approach was recommended. The first stage involved performing radical resection of the distal gastric cancer, followed by endoscopic resection of the cardia lesion in the second stage. After thorough communication with the patient's family, laparoscopy-assisted radical distal gastrectomy (D2, Billroth II + Braun anastomosis) was performed. The patient progressed well postoperatively, resuming a liquid diet on the 6th day and a semi-liquid diet on the 9th day. Ultimately, the patient was discharged on the 13th day after surgery.

3.9.4 Postoperative Pathologic Report

The distal gastrectomy specimen was 11.5 cm long on the lesser curvature side of the stomach, 20 cm long on the greater curvature side, 1.5 cm long on the duodenum, 3 cm wide at the cut margin, and 6 cm from the end of the duodenum. An ulcerated mass, 1.5 cm × 1.5 cm × 0.3 cm in size, was seen in the gastric angle, with a gray, solid, hard cut surface that appeared to invade the submucosa, and the rest of the gastric mucosa was smooth with no obvious abnormalities, and no clear nodules in the perigastric fat.

(Microscopic diagnosis) Ulcerative-type medium-low differentiated adenocarcinoma of distal subtotal gastric, Lauren's staging: mixed type, choroidal tumor plugs were seen, and no clear nerve invasion was observed. The tumor invaded the submucosa but did not involve the pylorus, duodenum, or greater omentum. The peri-cancerous gastric mucosa showed chronic atrophic inflammation with intestinal epithelial metaplasia. No carcinoma was seen in the upper and lower cut margins. Metastatic carcinoma in lymph nodes (1/32) did not involve extra-peritoneal tissue of lymph nodes.

Two months after the initial surgery, the patient underwent ESD treatment. Preoperative gastroscopy revealed localized mucosal roughness and erosion from the lower esophagus to the junction line, approximately 35 cm from the incisors. The gastro-esophageal junction line was located at approximately 38 cm from the incisors. A superficial flat lesion of type 0-IIb was observed from the cardia of the residual stomach to the lesser curvature/posterior wall of the gastric body, measuring 40–48 cm from the incisor. The lesion exhibited localized mucosal roughness and irregular surface microstructures, as visualized through NBI+ magnification (Fig. 3.24). ESD was performed following appropriate preoperative preparation (Fig. 3.25). The postoperative recovery was smooth, and the patient was discharged on the 7th day after the procedure.

3.9.5 Pathologic Report of Post ESD Treatment

From the cardia to the lesser curvature/posterior wall of the gastric body, the glandular epithelium of the gastric mucosa showed mainly low-grade

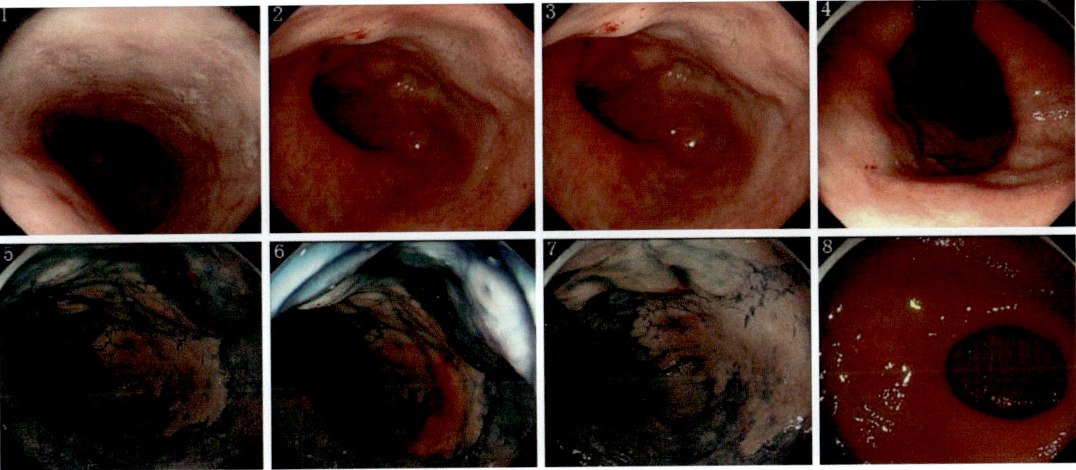

Fig. 3.24 Gastroscopy 2 months after distal gastrectomy

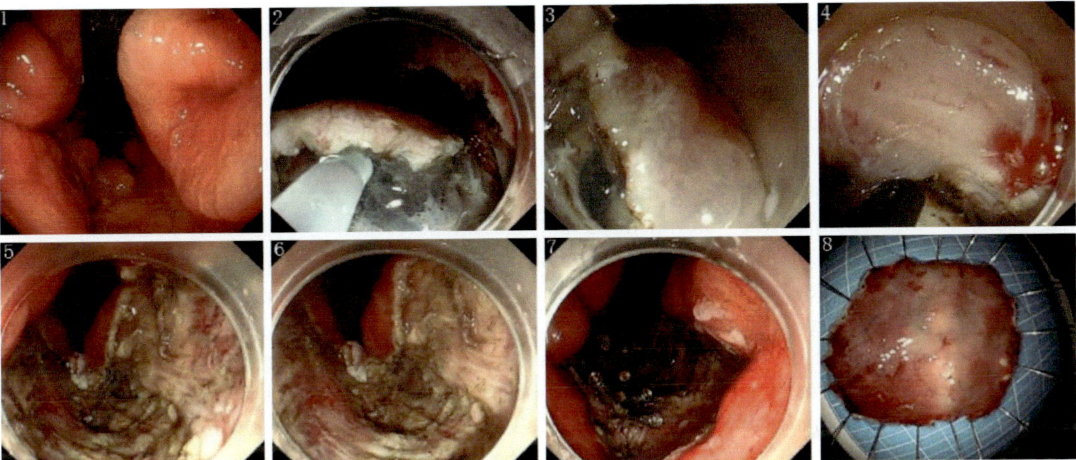

Fig. 3.25 ESD operation procedure

intraepithelial neoplasia and locally high-grade intraepithelial neoplasia, with a lesion area of 4.7 cm × 3.0 cm. The surrounding gastric mucosa showed mild chronic atrophic inflammation with mild intestinal epithelial metaplasia. Ultra-short segmental Barrett's esophagus could be seen. No tumor was seen at the lateral cut margin. The basal cut margin was localized to the lamina propria of the mucosa. Small foci of low-grade intraepithelial neoplasia were seen at the cautery margin. Immunohistochemical results: P53 (−), Ki-67 (40%).

Gastroscopy was repeated 1 year after surgery (Fig. 3.26): The local mucosa from the cardia of the remnant gastric to the lesser curvature/posterior wall of the gastric body showed scar-like changes, congested and rough, and no obvious swelling or ulcer was seen at the scar. There was no obvious narrowing of the canal lumen at the scar, so the endoscope passed smoothly. The gastrointestinal anastomosis was seen at about 51 cm from the incisor, the mucosa at the anastomosis was congested, no swelling or ulcer was seen, and there was no narrowing of the anastomosis. The interintestinal anastomosis was seen at about 70 cm from the incisor, no swelling or ulcer was seen, and there was no narrowing of the anastomosis.

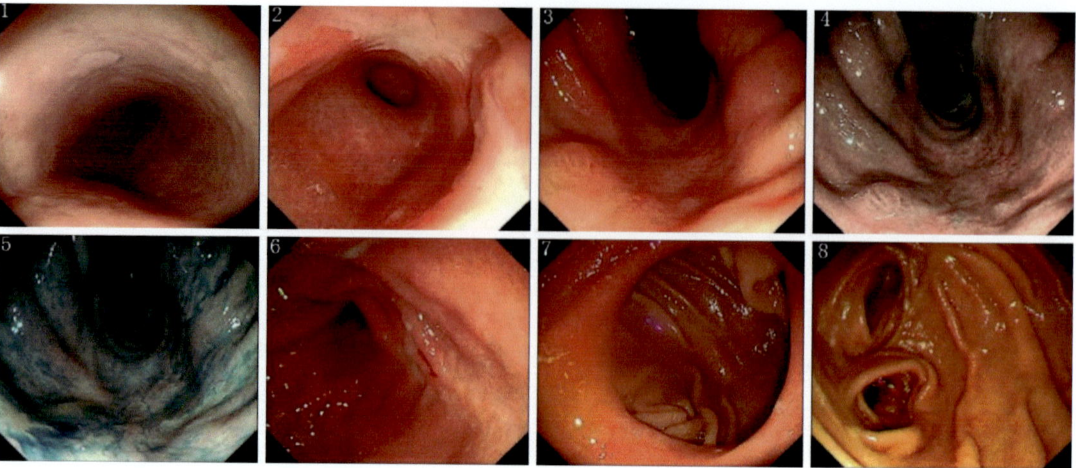

Fig. 3.26 A year after gastric cancer surgery, no abnormalities on repeat gastroscopy

3.9.6 Case Analysis

Multiple primary gastric cancer (MPGC), alternatively known as repetitive gastric cancer, denotes the presence of multiple distinct malignant lesions, each consisting of two or more gastric cancer foci within the stomach. The classification of MPGC depends on the time interval between the development of primary lesions. When two or more cancer lesions are detected simultaneously or within a span of 6 months, it is referred to as synchronous multiple primary gastric carcinoma (SMGC). On the other hand, if the interval exceeds 6 months, it is termed metachronous multiple primary gastric carcinoma (MMGC). The diagnosis of MPGC adheres to Moertel's criteria, which encompass the following aspects [25]: Firstly, there should be a presence of two or more tumors within the gastric cavity, and each tumor must exhibit malignant characteristics. Secondly, each tumor must possess a distinct pathological pattern, indicating its independence without extension or metastasis from another tumor. Lastly, the presence of normal tissues and migratory bands between the cancer foci is essential for the diagnosis of MPGC.

3.9.6.1 Clinical Features of MPGC

MPGC is less common, with an incidence of about 1.7% of the total incidence of gastric cancer. The incidence rate of SMGC is lower than that of MMGC, accounting for about 13% of MPGC. In recent years, the incidence of gastric cancer has been decreasing worldwide, on the other hand, the incidence of MPGC has been increasing year by year with the development of treatment technology, the aging of the population and the prolongation of the overall survival of gastric cancer. Epidemiological studies show that MPGC is generally seen at an older age, with a higher proportion of males than females, but the rate of missed diagnosis is high, up to 50% [87]. The largest tumor diameter is usually small, and the secondary lesions are often located near the main lesion. The pathological type is predominantly medium- and high-differentiated adenocarcinoma, which is mostly detected at an early stage [88]. The results of Matsuda et al. [89] showed that even early multiple primary gastric cancers can invade the duodenum.

The etiology of multiple primary gastric cancers is unclear, and relevant studies have shown that it may be related to genetic susceptibility, medical factors, immune deficiencies, and environmental and lifestyle factors [90–92]. It has also been suggested that gastric cancer is of polycentric origin. That is, gastric cancer appears multicentric in its early stages, as the cancer tissues grow, the cancer foci keep moving closer together and fusing. It is difficult to distinguish between single and multiple foci when the tumor progresses. It is difficult to distinguish whether the cancer foci are single or multiple fusion when the tumor progresses [93].

3.9.6.2 Diagnosis of Multiple Primary Gastric Cancer

In clinical diagnosis, attention should be paid to differentiate MPGC from recurrent metastatic gastric cancer. The treatment of metastatic gastric cancer is usually aimed at improving symptoms and relieving patients' pain, mostly with palliative treatment and poor prognosis. Palliative gastrectomy is not recommended unless it is used for symptomatic relief [94]. Studies have shown that there is no significant difference between MPGC and single gastric cancer in terms of various clinicopathological features including histological classification, pathological staging, degree of invasion of surrounding organs, and pTNM stage, indicating that their biological characteristics are similar to those of single gastric cancer [95]. Therefore, the treatment of MPGC should follow the principles of primary gastric cancer management, emphasizing a comprehensive treatment based on surgery. Early diagnosis is an important factor to improve the prognosis of MPGC. Detailed preoperative gastroscopy is an effective means to diagnose multifocal gastric cancers and reduce the misdiagnosis rate. In addition, other imaging examinations, such as enhanced CT and upper gastrointestinal imaging, can also help to detect multiple cancer foci, and the combined examination can effectively improve the detection rate of multiple cancer foci [96].

3.9.6.3 Choice of Surgical Approach for MPGC

The extent of surgical resection and the number of lymph node dissection for MPGC depend on the number, location, size, and histopathological staging of the cancer foci. Previously, total gastrectomy was thought to avoid residual lesions in MPGC and reduce the risk of gastric cancer recurrence. However, Otsuji et al. [97] found that prophylactic total gastrectomy did not improve the prognosis of patients with MPGC, and it resulted in greater surgical trauma and longer postoperative recovery time, so prophylactic total gastrectomy was not recommended. Hu et al. [98] found that multiple gastric cancer foci mostly occurred in the pyloric gland and the intermediate zone, and highly differentiated adenocarcinoma was predominant, and highly heterogeneous hyperplasia was often present along with it. Therefore, it is recommended to include the pyloric gland area and the intermediate zone containing the pyloric gland to avoid residual cancer and heterochronous multiple cancers.

Compared with single primary gastric cancer, MPGCs are located in different parts of the stomach, which makes surgical resection extensive and complicated. At present, among various common surgical methods, open surgery, laparoscopic surgery, and endoscopic surgery are combined or sequenced in different ways to treat MPGC. Endoscopic surgery is mainly applicable to early gastric cancer without lymph node metastasis, with tumor confined to the mucosal layer and less than 2 cm in diameter. Since the risk of lymph node metastasis in early MPGC is not significantly different from that in single primary gastric cancer, Kim et al. [99] suggested that endoscopic treatment could be considered for multiple cancer foci with tumors confined to the mucosal layer and without lymph node metastasis. Compared with open surgery, laparoscopic surgery has advantages such as less trauma and faster postoperative recovery. In particular, multiple anatomical sites can be completed without significantly increasing the number of skin incisions. When making treatment decisions, the advantages of various tools should be fully utilized to reduce trauma, preserve organ function, and improve the quality of life of patients. In this case, the patient was of advanced age and had two combined lesions. Although total gastrectomy is more in line with oncologic principles, excessive trauma may lead to a long-term reduction in the patient's quality of life. Therefore, according to the multidisciplinary review opinion, staged surgery was chosen to ensure the radical effect of the tumor and also to maximize the quality of life of the patient.

3.9.7 Expert Comments

The biological characteristics of MPGC exhibit no significant differences compared to solitary gastric cancers. However, MPGC poses challenges in terms of its numerous primary lesions and small maximum diameter of cancer foci, leading to high rates of underdiagnosis and misdiagnosis. Therefore, enhancing early detection of MPGC and promoting the concept of multidisciplinary comprehensive treatment are crucial for improving prognosis and enhancing patients' quality of life.

Case provider: Chunguang Guo, Penghui Niu.

Commentary: Dongbing Zhao.

3.10 Case 17:Prognostic Significance of Microscopic Positive Margins for Gastric Cancer Patients

3.10.1 Brief History

The patient, a 35-year-old male, was admitted to the hospital presenting with abdominal discomfort persisting for 2 weeks. The patient denied experiencing any specific triggers such as abdominal distension, acid reflux, heartburn, nausea, vomiting, abdominal pain, or diarrhea prior to the onset of symptoms. Gastroscopy revealed an ulcer in the gastric antrum pylorus, characterized by border swelling and a white moss-like covering on the base (see Fig. 3.27). Pathological analysis confirmed the presence of poorly differentiated adenocarcinoma, classified as mixed type according to the Lauren classification. Enhanced CT scan displayed irregular thickening of the gastric antrum and pylorus wall, evident enhancement of the mucosal surface, and slight blurring of the serous membrane surface. Multiple small lymph nodes surrounding the antrum were observed, with the largest lymph node exhibiting a short diameter of approximately 0.6 cm (see Fig. 3.28).

Diagnosis: Gastric cancer (cT2N0M0)

3.10.2 Treatment

Following appropriate preoperative preparation, a laparoscopic distal subtotal gastrectomy was performed, incorporating Billroth-II reconstruction with Braun anastomosis. Intraoperative exploration revealed a tumor located at the gastric antrum, measuring approximately 3 * 4 cm, with invasion into the pyloric ring. After excision, the specimens were sent for rapid frozen pathological examination, focusing on the incisal margin of the duodenum. The results indicated

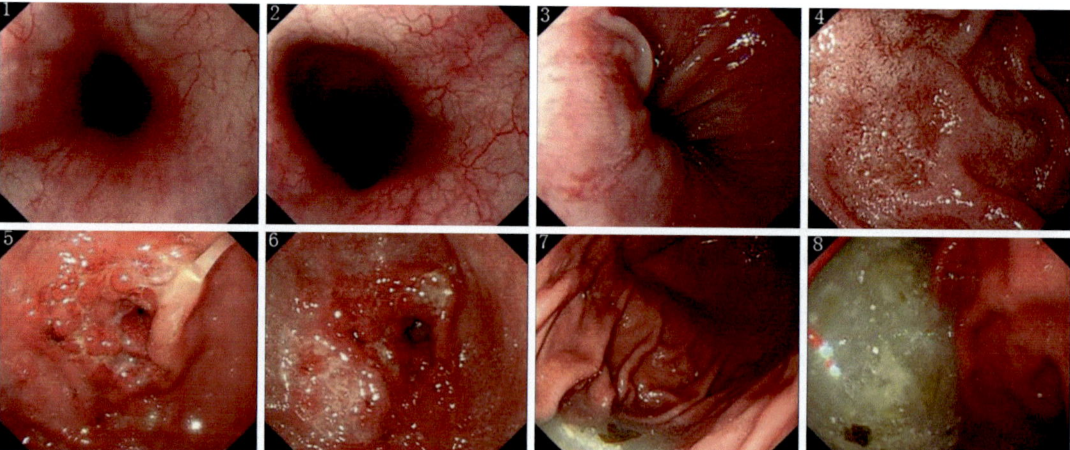

Fig. 3.27 Illustrates the findings from the gastroscopy, revealing a gastric antrum pylorus ulcer with border swelling. The base of the ulcer appears to be covered with a white moss-like substance

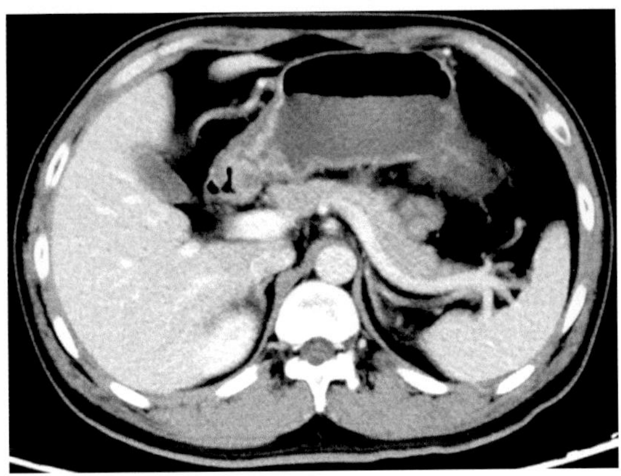

Fig. 3.28 Depicts the results of the enhanced CT scan, demonstrating a thickened wall of the gastric antrum, consistent with gastric cancer. Additionally, multiple small lymph nodes are observed in the vicinity of the antrum

the presence of anomalous cells at the incisal margin, and the possibility of signet-ring cell carcinoma could not be ruled out. Consequently, resection of the duodenal stump was performed once again, and heterotypic cells were identified at the pathological margin. Signet-ring cell carcinoma was still a possibility. Communication with the patient's family occurred during the operation to explain the situation and discuss the option of expanding the resection. Following consultation, the family declined to extend the resection and instead opted for postoperative radiotherapy targeted at the duodenal stump. The patient experienced a smooth recovery and was discharged on the 8th day after the surgery.

3.10.3 Pathology

The histopathological analysis revealed a superficial ulcerated gastric tumor characterized as poorly differentiated adenocarcinoma. According to Lauren's classification, it was classified as the diffuse type, with some components exhibiting features of signet-ring cell carcinoma. The tumor was observed to invade the submucosal layer without involvement of the muscularis propria. Anomalous cells were detected at the lower incisal margin, and the possibility of signet-ring cell carcinoma could not be ruled out. Furthermore, metastatic cancer was identified in 15 out of 39 examined lymph nodes. The pTNM staging for this case is determined as pT1bN3a.

3.10.4 Case Analysis

Gastric cancer, a prevalent malignancy of the digestive tract, necessitates a multidisciplinary comprehensive treatment approach that encompasses surgery, chemotherapy, radiotherapy, targeted therapy, and immunotherapy. Radical surgery aims to achieve negative surgical margins, as studies have established that positive surgical margins are significant contributors to poor prognoses in gastric cancer [100]. Positive margins can be further categorized into positive margins detected under microscopic examination (R1) and positive margins identified without magnification (R2) [100]. While advances in intraoperative freezing technology have led to a decrease in the incidence of postoperative positive margins, approximately 1.8–5.1% of gastric cancer patients still exhibit positive margins [101].

Previous investigations have indicated that positive margins can occur at proximal margins (42.8%), distal margins (45.7%), and bilateral margins (2.9%) [101]. A systematic review involving 19,355 patients revealed that positive margins were associated with larger tumor sizes, lymph node metastasis, advanced tumor stages, Borrmann type, and total gastrectomy [100].

Patients with positive margins tend to have a poor prognosis, with 5-year overall survival rates ranging from 13.3% to 51.9% [101–107]. There exists a significant variation in survival outcomes among patients with positive margins, possibly attributed to heterogeneity across studies. The impact of positive margins on prognosis slightly differs based on the specific type of gastric cancer. In the N0-N1 or T1-T2 subgroups, patients with positive margins generally exhibit worse prognoses compared to those with negative margins. However, in patients with N2-N3 or T3-T4 disease, positive incisal margins do not hold prognostic significance [108]. In certain special populations, such as those with positive cytology and highly unstable microsatellites (MSI-H), positive margins may not have prognostic significance [103, 109]. Furthermore, patients with positive margins experience significantly higher rates of postoperative recurrence and metastasis compared to those with negative margins, particularly in cases involving pT1-2, pN0-1, and stage I to II disease [110]. The postoperative recurrence and metastasis rates among patients with positive resection margins range from 63.6% to 76%, with distant metastasis being the predominant pattern of recurrence [101, 102, 108, 110].

Opinions regarding the follow-up treatment for patients with positive margins in gastric cancer are not unanimous among medical experts. The National Comprehensive Cancer Network (NCCN) guidelines recommend postoperative adjuvant chemoradiotherapy for patients with positive surgical margins although high-level evidence-based medical evidence to support this recommendation is lacking [111]. A study based on the National Cancer Database (NCDB) demonstrated that postoperative adjuvant chemoradiotherapy can significantly improve the prognosis of patients with positive margins compared to chemotherapy alone [112]. However, domestic retrospective studies conducted in certain countries did not find a beneficial effect of postoperative treatment, whether it was chemoradiotherapy or chemotherapy alone [102].

The question of whether patients with positive margins in gastric cancer should undergo a second operation remains a subject of debate. Some experts argue that surgery can be considered if a second operation can successfully remove the residual tumor. On the other hand, opponents of reoperation argue that for locally advanced gastric cancer patients in advanced tumor stages, the tumor stage itself is the most important factor influencing prognosis, and the impact of a positive incisal margin on survival is minimal. Therefore, they do not recommend reoperation in such cases.

It is important to note that treatment decisions for patients with positive margins in gastric cancer should be made on an individual basis, considering factors such as the patient's overall health, tumor characteristics, stage of disease, and the expertise of the medical team. Consultation with a multidisciplinary team of specialists, including surgeons, oncologists, and radiation oncologists, is crucial in determining the most appropriate course of treatment for each patient.

3.10.5 Expert Comments

Achieving a negative surgical margin is a critical aspect of maintaining surgical quality control in the management of resectable gastric cancer. This has significant practical implications for both long-term prognosis and current clinical practice. Considering the variations in prognosis associated with positive margins among different subtypes of gastric cancer, clinicians should adopt a nuanced approach and carefully evaluate the potential benefits of expanded surgical interventions for patients, particularly those with advanced tumor stages.

The decision to perform expanded surgery should be made on a case-by-case basis, taking into account various factors such as the specific subtype of gastric cancer, the stage of the tumor, and the overall condition of the patient. It is essential for clinicians to carefully weigh the potential benefits and risks associated with expanded surgery in order to optimize patient outcomes. This approach acknowledges the importance of tailoring treatment strategies to the individual needs and characteristics of each patient, ultimately striving to achieve the best possible clinical outcomes.

Case provider: Xiaojie Zhang, Chunguang Guo.

Commentary: Chunguang Guo.

3.11 Case 18: Foci Gastric Cancer Detected by Endoscopy

3.11.1 Brief History

The subject under examination is a 51-year-old female presenting with gastric cancer detected during a physical examination conducted over a month ago. The patient previously underwent gastroscopy at a local medical facility, revealing superficial lesions located at the junction of the gastric body and antrum. Subsequent pathological analysis confirmed the presence of adenocarcinoma. Seeking further treatment, the patient was subsequently referred to our institution. Notable findings from the abdominal physical examination were absent. Comprehensive tumor marker analysis, including CEA, AFP, CA724, CA199, and CA242, exhibited values within the normal range. Gastroscopy unveiled a superficial and flat gastric cancer situated along the larger curved aspect of the gastric body-antrum junction (refer to Fig. 3.29). Histopathological evaluation confirmed the diagnosis of locally poorly differentiated gastric adenocarcinoma with some signet-ring cell carcinoma components. Abdominal enhanced computed tomography (CT) revealed irregular thickening of the antrum region's gastric wall accompanied by an unpolished serosal surface (see Fig. 3.30a). Additionally, small lymph nodes were observed in the left gastric region and around the antrum, with the larger node measuring approximately 0.6 cm in short diameter, necessitating close monitoring. Moreover, a left renal mass exhibiting signs suggestive of malignancy was detected (refer to Fig. 3.30b). After multidisciplinary team (MDT) discussion, a sequential approach involving initial excision of the left renal mass followed by gastrectomy was recommended. Consequently, the patient was admitted to the urological department for left nephrectomy, and subsequent pathological analysis indicated the presence of an eosinophilic tumor. The patient's hospital admission pertains to the management of gastric cancer.

Diagnosis: Gastric cancer (cT1N0M0) after excision of eosinophilic tumor in left kidney.

3.11.2 Treatment

Following admission, the patient underwent comprehensive examinations, which revealed no contraindications. During the perioperative period, a rapid rehabilitation surgical approach was employed. Preoperative measures such as water fasting, skin preparation, and intestinal preparation were not performed on the day prior to the operation. Additionally, no gastric tube was inserted preoperatively. The patient underwent laparoscopic-assisted radical gastrectomy utilizing the Billroth II + Braun anastomosis technique. The surgical procedure was successful, and the patient was subsequently transferred to the ward.

Postoperatively, on the first day, the patient was encouraged to actively expectorate sputum

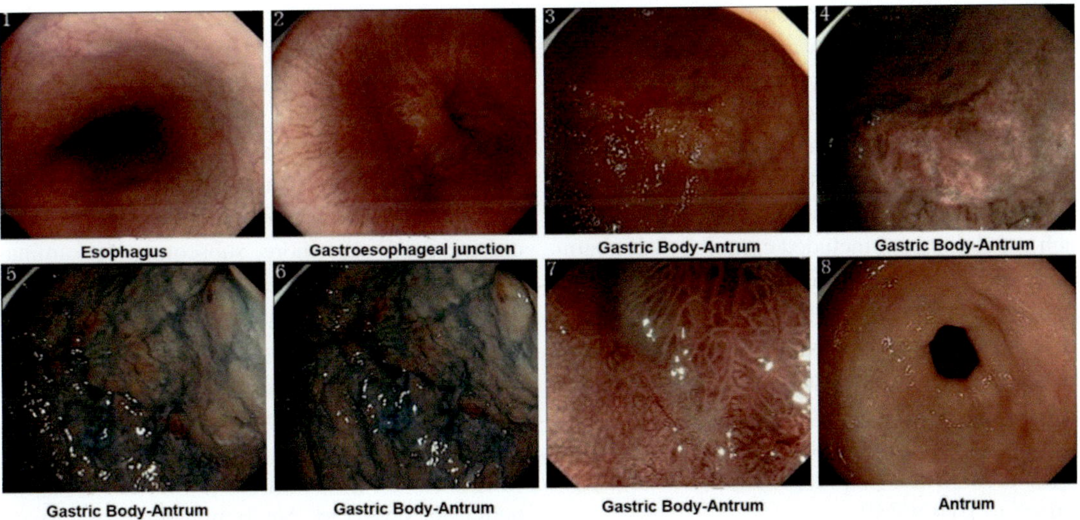

Fig. 3.29 Illustrates a gastroscopic examination revealing the presence of a superficial, flat gastric cancer situated along the greater curvature of the gastric body-antrum junction

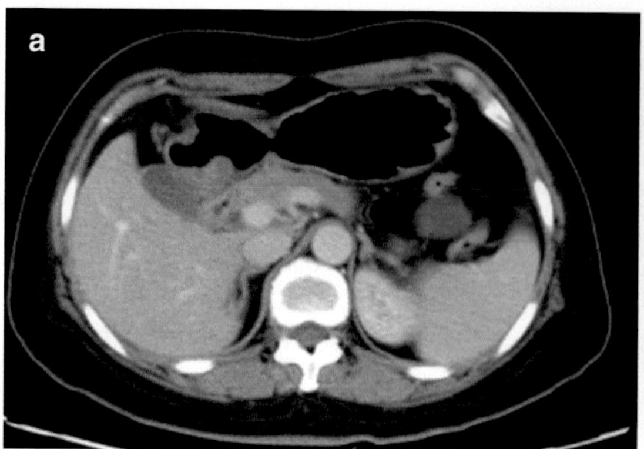

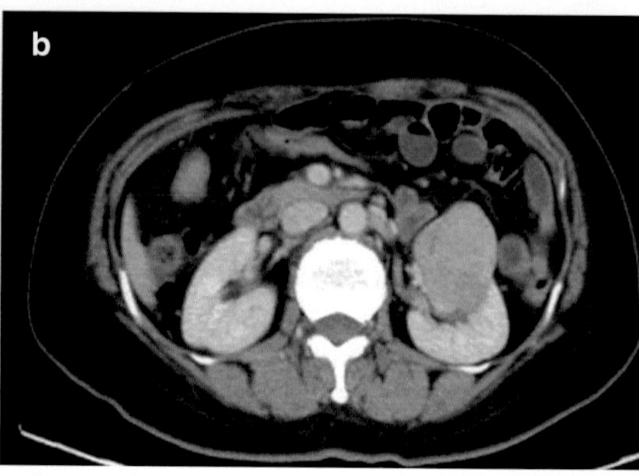

Fig. 3.30 Displays the initial abdominal computed tomography (CT) findings as follows: (**a**) Demonstrates irregular thickening of the gastric wall in the antrum region along with a less smooth serous surface, and (**b**) indicates a left kidney mass exhibiting features suggestive of malignancy

and engage in bed mobility. On the second day, the gastric tube was removed, and the patient was encouraged to begin oral fluid intake and initiate ambulation. On the third day, a clear liquid diet was initiated. By the fifth day, the patient advanced to passing flatus and consuming a semi-liquid diet. The abdominal drainage tube was removed on the seventh-day post-surgery. Ultimately, the patient was discharged from the hospital on the ninth day.

Pathological examination of the resected specimen revealed the following findings: The major curve measured 14 cm in length, while the minor curve measured 10 cm. The pyloric structure exhibited clarity, and the duodenum attached to its lower part measured 0.6 cm. Notably, at a distance of 5 cm from the pyloric region, there was a raised-type mass measuring 2 × 1 × 0.3 cm in size. The cut surface of the mass appeared gray, white, and firm, seemingly involving the muscular layer.

An endoscopic assessment of the distal stomach and duodenum included comprehensive sampling, revealing focal high-grade intraepithelial neoplasia (moderate to severe dysplasia) along with local atrophic gastritis and intestinal metaplasia. Lymph node examination did not detect any metastatic tumors among the sampled 32 lymph nodes (0/32). Based on the TNM staging system, the final pathological stage was determined as pTisN0M0.

3.11.3 Case Analysis

The concept of "one-spot cancer" was initially proposed by the Gastric Cancer Laboratory at China Medical University in 1984. It falls within the category of micro-gastric cancer, characterized by the presence of gastric mucosa biopsy and pathological diagnosis of cancer. However, in such cases, the surgically resected specimen does not exhibit any macroscopic tumor lesions (occasionally accompanied by benign ulcers or erosion), and extensive serial sections fail to identify cancerous tissue. Instead, the lesions primarily manifest as superficial ulcers and erosion.

In the present case, the diagnosis of gastric adenocarcinoma was confirmed through gastroscopy biopsy conducted at a foreign hospital, followed by pathological consultation at our institution. The biopsy area displayed poor differentiation, with a component of sigma-ring cell carcinoma. Furthermore, subsequent reexamination by our hospital under gastroscopy clearly identified lesions along the greater curvature of the gastric body-antrum junction. Consequently, a decision was made to proceed with laparoscopic radical gastrectomy for distal gastric cancer.

Postoperatively, no cancerous tissue was identified, with only focal high-grade intraepithelial neoplasia observed. No lymph node metastasis was detected. Therefore, the clinical presentation and pathological findings in this case are consistent with gastric carcinoma.

In recent years, the widespread implementation of endoscopic screening has led to an increasing detection rate of monocellular carcinoma, with reports indicating that monocellular carcinoma of the stomach comprises 4.2% of all detected early gastric cancers [113]. According to domestic literature, the gastric antrum is the most frequently affected site, followed by the minor curvature of the stomach, the anterior and posterior walls of the stomach body, the cardia, the angle of the stomach, and the fundus of the stomach. The majority of one-spot cancer foci have an average size of approximately 0.5 × 0.6 cm, although there are cases with larger foci exceeding 1 cm. Endoscopic examination reveals various manifestations of one-spot cancer, including superficial ulcers, erosions, and minor bleeding. Among them, erosions are the most commonly observed, followed by uplifted lesions, superficial ulcers, rough mucosa, and congested and edematous mucosa. Adenocarcinoma is the most prevalent histological type [114, 115].

Gastroscopic mucosal biopsy plays a pivotal role in the detection and diagnosis of early gastric cancer. Studies have reported that the accuracy of endoscopic biopsy for gastric mucosal lesions is 86.5%, while multipoint biopsy achieves an accuracy of 94.9%. When combined, the accuracy can reach as high as 98.8% [116]. However, due to their small size and atypical endoscopic appearance, one-spot cancer and early gastric cancer can often resemble gastritis-like carcinoma, small gastric cancer, small or flat erosions, or polypoid tumors. This poses a challenge in accurately determining the benign or malignant nature of one-spot cancer and increases the risk of misdiagnosis. Furthermore, one-spot cancer is frequently associated with atypical gastrointestinal symptoms such as upper abdominal discomfort, heartburn, and acid reflux. Conventional drug therapy aimed at acid suppression and gastric mucosal protection may lead to the reduction or even pseudo-healing of malignant ulcers, potentially delaying the diagnosis and treatment. Therefore, in cases where suspected lesions yield negative results on endoscopic biopsy, it is crucial to consider multiple excisions and deep tissue sampling, or to perform repeat sampling or biopsies within a short time frame. Caution should be exercised when deciding to administer proton pump inhibitors directly.

Pathological staging plays a pivotal role in assessing prognosis and guiding postoperative treatment strategies for patients with gastric cancer. Therefore, achieving precise and rigorous diagnosis requires a comprehensive approach that includes serial section pathological examinations of specimens obtained through gastroscopy, biopsy sampling, pathological assessment of biopsies, and surgical excision. Particularly, when obtaining mucosal specimens corresponding to the lesions observed during gastroscopy from surgical specimens, it has been recommended in the literature that no fewer than 30 sections should be taken to ensure diagnostic accuracy [117].

Currently, there is a lack of standardized guidelines for the treatment of one-spot cancer. Given that the diagnosis of one-spot cancer is made after the initial diagnosis, non-surgical approaches such as multiple biopsy forceps removal or microwave treatment can lead to lesion shrinkage or even apparent disappearance within a certain period. However, such approaches carry a higher risk of recurrence. Consequently, radical surgical excision remains the preferred treatment option. In recent years, with the increasing adoption of Endoscopic Submucosal Dissection (ESD) for early gastric cancer, the proportion of endoscopic treatment in our country has reached 24.3% [118]. Nevertheless, strict criteria should be applied when selecting patients for endoscopic treatment of primary cancer. However, for poorly differentiated cancers, such as poorly differentiated or signet ring cell carcinoma, and other specific pathological subtypes, as well as patients with suspiciously enlarged abdominal lymph nodes identified through preoperative CT evaluation, radical subtotal gastrectomy should be actively pursued to ensure the effectiveness of radical excision. In the present case, preoperative pathology indicated a poorly differentiated tumor with some signet ring cell components, and CT revealed the presence of small lymph nodes in the left gastric region and around the antrum, which did not meet the criteria for endoscopic resection. Therefore, radical gastrectomy (D2) was performed for distal gastric cancer.

3.11.4 Expert Comments

With the widespread implementation of gastroscopy screening, the detection rate of early gastric cancer has been gradually increasing. Among the various types of early gastric cancer, gastric "one-spot" cancer represents a unique entity where the focus is confined solely to the biopsy site. This distinct characteristic makes it susceptible to missed diagnoses and misdiagnoses. Therefore, in clinical practice, it is crucial for endoscopists to actively monitor all suspected lesions that yield negative biopsy results. Merely using medications to alleviate symptoms and delay treatment while suppressing acid and protecting the gastric mucosa should be avoided. Similarly, the diagnosis of "one-spot cancer" following surgical intervention should be made with great caution. A comprehensive pathological sampling approach and meticulous search for lesions are necessary to arrive at an accurate diagnosis.

Case provider: Tongbo Wang, Chunguang Guo.

Commentary: Chunguang Guo.

3.12 Case 19: Gastric Carcinomas in Young Patients

3.12.1 Brief History

The patient, a 23-year-old female, was admitted to the hospital due to persistent upper abdominal pain lasting for more than a month, which had worsened over the past 20 days. Prior to admission, the patient experienced intermittent upper abdominal pain for approximately 1 month. The pain was accompanied by symptoms such as nausea and acid reflux, but without vomiting. The patient initially sought treatment at a local hospital, where her symptoms improved following traditional Chinese medicine treatment. However, her condition deteriorated 20 days before admission. She began experiencing nocturnal awakening due to pain, along with acid reflux and episodes of vomiting, characterized by the presence of gastric juice in the vomitus. Gastroscopy performed at the local hospital revealed a deep gastric ulcer, and subsequent pathological examination confirmed a diagnosis of poorly differentiated adenocarcinoma. The patient's tumor markers, specifically CA199 and CEA, were within the normal range. Gastroscopy conducted at our hospital demonstrated the presence of gastric cancer primarily located at the junction of the gastric body and antrum (see Fig. 3.31). An enhanced CT scan revealed a prominent enhancement in the posterior wall of the gastric angle area near the pylorus, indicative of gastric cancer. The lesion measured approximately 3.2 cm × 3.0 cm and exhibited a rough serosal surface. Additionally, multiple cords and nodules were visible at the site of the lesion (see Fig. 3.32a). Multiple scattered small lymph nodes were observed in the mesentery and retroperitoneum, with the largest lymph node measuring 0.5 cm in short diameter (see Fig. 3.32b). The final diagnosis is gastric cancer, specifically stage IIb (cT4aN0M0).

3.12.2 Treatment

Upon admission, a comprehensive examination was conducted, revealing no contraindications to surgery. The patient underwent fast-track surgery, which included fasting, skin preparation, and bowel preparation abstention on the day prior to the operation. No gastric tube was inserted preoperatively. Elective laparoscopic-assisted radical distal gastrectomy was performed.

Pathological analysis of the resected specimen demonstrated an ulcerative and poorly differentiated gastric adenocarcinoma, characterized as diffuse type according to the Lauren classification, with a component of signet ring cells. Tumor infiltration was observed in the muscular layer,

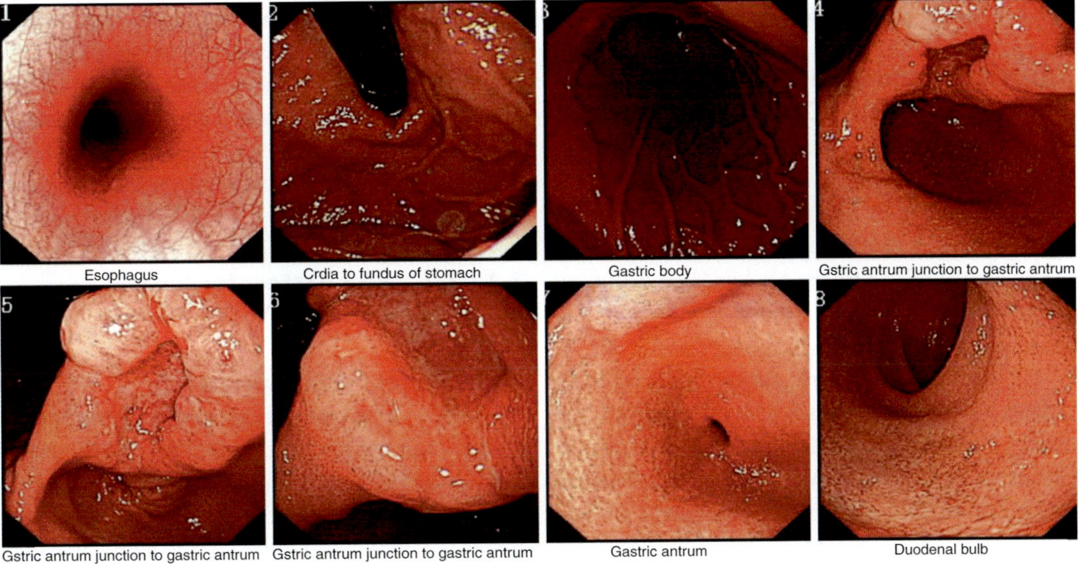

Fig. 3.31 Gastroscopic examination reveals the primary lesion predominantly situated at the junction between the gastric body and antrum

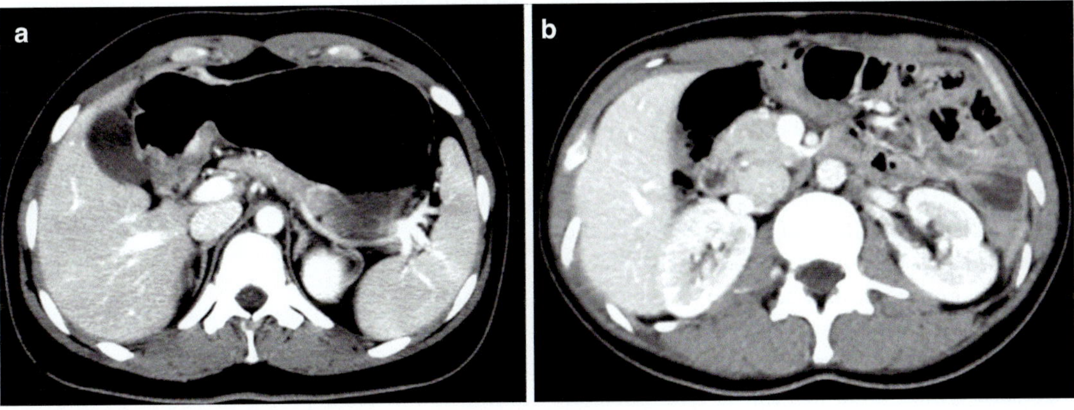

Fig. 3.32 (**a**) The posterior wall of the stomach near the pylorus exhibits a visible ulcerative mass. (**b**) Multiple small lymph nodes, measuring approximately 0.5 cm in short axis diameter, are scattered throughout the mesentery and retroperitoneum

with focal involvement of the serosa, while the pylorus, duodenum, and greater omentum remained unaffected. Margins were clear, and metastasis was detected in two out of thirty examined lymph nodes. The TNM staging indicated pT4aN1M0, corresponding to stage IIIA.

One-month post-surgery, adjuvant therapy was initiated with oxaliplatin and S1. However, due to gastrointestinal adverse reactions, the regimen was switched to oxaliplatin and 5-fluorouracil after three cycles. Subsequently, two cycles of 5-fluorouracil and cisplatin were administered following a platelet count reduction. The treatment plan was further adjusted to include oxaliplatin, 5-fluorouracil, and cisplatin for four cycles. Over the course of 3 years of follow-up after surgery, no recurrence of the tumor was detected.

3.12.3 Case Analysis

3.12.3.1 Trends and Characteristics of Gastric Cancer in Young People

Gastric cancer typically occurs in individuals between the ages of 55 and 70, with over 90% of cases diagnosed after the age of 40 [119]. However, the incidence of gastric cancer has been declining overall, while the incidence among young people has remained stable or slightly increased [120].

The definition of gastric cancer in young individuals varies among studies, with different age cutoffs used. Some studies define young gastric cancer as cases diagnosed in individuals under the age of 40, while others use age limits such as below 45 years old or even younger than 35 years old. Generally, the majority of studies consider individuals under 40 years old as having young-onset gastric cancer [121–123].

In young-onset gastric cancer, the male-to-female ratio is approximately 1:1, which is different from the higher ratio observed in older patients [124]. This gender distribution may be influenced by specific dietary and lifestyle habits of young women, as well as the potential correlation between female sex hormones and the occurrence of gastric cancer.

A meta-analysis [124] of retrospective studies revealed that young-onset gastric cancer tends to exhibit more aggressive behavior compared to older cases. It is associated with a higher proportion of advanced Bormann type IV tumors, increased lymph node metastasis rate, poor differentiation of cancer cells, and a higher proportion of signet ring cell carcinoma.

Furthermore, studies have found that young people with gastric cancer are more likely to be diagnosed at advanced stages, including stage IV [123–125]. This suggests that the diagnosis of young-onset gastric cancer is often delayed. Various factors contribute to this delay, including the hidden nature of clinical manifestations, which young individuals may not take seriously. Early-stage gastric cancer presents with nonspecific symptoms such as acid reflux, belching, upper abdominal pain, vomiting, and abdominal distension, which can easily be attributed to other conditions like gastric ulcers, chronic gastritis, or gastric spasms, leading to delayed diagnosis.

Overall, understanding the trends and characteristics of gastric cancer in young people is crucial for timely diagnosis and management of this condition in this particular age group. Increased awareness and vigilance are important in order to detect gastric cancer at earlier stages and improve patient outcomes.

3.12.3.2 Risk Factors for Gastric Cancer in Young People

Helicobacter pylori (Hp) Infection

There is a close correlation between young-onset gastric cancer and Hp infection [126]. After paired analysis, the incidence of Hp infection was found to be higher in gastric cancer patients under 30 years old than in the control group [127]. This correlation is particularly evident in poorly differentiated mucosal cancers [128].

Genetic Factors

Approximately 10% of gastric cancer cases exhibit familial aggregation, and the risk of gastric cancer is increased in first-degree relatives [129]. This familial aggregation is more common in young gastric cancer patients, suggesting a stronger genetic influence in this population [130–132].

Estrogen Effects

While the relationship between gastric cancer and estrogen receptor (ER) in the general population is not clear [133], in young people with gastric cancer, females are more commonly affected. This indicates that sex hormones, particularly estrogen, may play a role in the development of gastric cancer in young individuals. Studies have shown high expression of ERβ in young gastric cancer patients [134, 135]. Factors such as frequent use of oral contraceptives without progestin, older age at first childbirth, lack of lactation history, and infertility have also been associated with an increased risk of gastric cancer in young people, further supporting the potential role of estrogen in gastric cancer development [130].

These risk factors contribute to the understanding of the etiology of gastric cancer in young individuals and provide insights into the mechanisms underlying its development. However, it is important to note that the precise interactions and contributions of these factors in young-onset gastric cancer are still the subject of ongoing research.

3.12.3.3 Prognosis of Gastric Cancer in Young Adults

Gastric cancer in young adults is characterized by aggressive growth and often presents at an advanced stage, leading to a high rate of incurability and impacting prognosis [136]. Despite these factors, several studies suggest that the overall prognosis of gastric cancer in young adults is better compared to elderly patients although there may be variations depending on the study's publication year and geographic location [119, 137, 138].

However, it is important to note that in patients with stage III and IV gastric cancer, young adults tend to have a worse prognosis compared to older patients, even when diagnosed at the same stage [119, 137–139]. This difference in prognosis may be attributed to several factors. Young adults generally have higher metabolic rates and more rapid growth of tumor cells, which could contribute to more aggressive disease progression. Additionally, younger patients may have different physiological responses to treatments or may experience treatment-related side effects differently, which can affect their overall prognosis.

It is crucial to consider these factors when assessing the prognosis and planning treatment strategies for young adults with gastric cancer. Close monitoring, personalized treatment approaches, and comprehensive care are important in order to improve outcomes for this specific patient population. Further research is needed to better understand the underlying mechanisms and optimize management strategies for gastric cancer in young adults.

3.12.3.4 Treatment of Gastric Cancer in Young People

Surgical resection stands as the favored therapeutic modality for gastric cancer, representing the solitary curative approach presently available. The management strategy for gastric cancer in young adults generally mirrors that of their middle-aged and older counterparts, encompassing a comprehensive treatment plan comprising surgery as the primary therapeutic intervention. Additional adjunctive measures such as chemotherapy and radiation therapy are employed as deemed necessary. In select cases, targeted therapies and immunomodulatory agents may also be considered. Notably, landmark trials investigating gastric cancer treatment have included a relatively limited representation of patients under the age of 40. Therefore, extrapolating differential treatment responses from these findings remains challenging. Consequently, further research is warranted to corroborate these observations in subsequent investigations.

3.12.4 Expert Comments

Although the incidence of gastric cancer is declining overall, there is a concerning trend of increasing rates among young individuals. Gastric cancer has traditionally been viewed as a disease primarily affecting the elderly, with established associations to chronic factors such as lifestyle choices, dietary habits, and *H. pylori* infection. However, the rising occurrence of gastric cancer in the young population, constituting approximately 10% of cases, suggests a potential involvement of genetic factors, as evidenced by distinctive clinical and pathological features not commonly observed in older adults. This emerging understanding has spurred intensified research efforts aimed at unraveling the underlying etiology of early-onset gastric cancer, as novel tumor-driving factors have been identified through advancements in basic research.

Conversely, it is well-established that young individuals diagnosed with gastric cancer face a poor prognosis, posing a significant treatment challenge. Epidemiological analyses have suggested that the nonspecific symptoms of gastric cancer and a lack of cancer prevention awareness among young individuals may contribute to delayed diagnosis and unfavorable outcomes. This underscores the crucial importance of fostering cancer awareness among young people and implementing proactive screening measures for symptomatic patients in this age group. By enhancing awareness and promoting timely diagnosis and treatment, the current treatment landscape for gastric cancer in young individuals can be improved.

Case provider: Hong Zhou, Yingtai Chen.

Commentary: Dongbing Zhao.

3.13 Case 20: Neuroendocrine Carcinoma of the Stomach

3.13.1 Brief History

The male patient, aged 57, presented with a chief complaint of enduring upper abdominal pain and discomfort persisting for a duration exceeding 2 months. Approximately 2 months ago, the patient experienced intermittent upper abdominal discomfort without an identifiable cause, which was accompanied by episodes of nausea, acid regurgitation, and postprandial abdominal pain. Seeking medical attention, he visited a local hospital where he received irregular medication for a diagnosed gastric ulcer. Subsequently, the symptoms progressed and did not respond favorably to drug therapy, prompting the patient to seek further treatment at our hospital. During the abdominal examination, no positive signs were detected. The tumor markers, including CEA, AFP, CA72-4, CA19-9, and CA24-2, fell within the normal range. Gastroscopy revealed the presence of cardia cancer involving the junction, situated approximately 41–43 cm from the incisor (Fig. 3.33). Pathological examination confirmed the presence of adenocarcinoma. Computed tomography (CT) scans indicated the following: (1) Uneven thickening observed at the cardia and lesser curvature of the gastric body, suggestive of gastric cancer; (2) attention should be given to the possibility of metastasis to the cardiac lymph nodes (Fig. 3.34).

Diagnosis: gastric cancer (cT3N1M0, stage II B).

3.13.2 Treatment

Following the completion of pertinent examinations, a laparoscopic-assisted proximal subtotal gastrectomy was performed. The perioperative period involved the implementation of a fast-track surgery approach. Notably, no preoperative interventions such as water fasting, skin preparation, or bowel preparation were undertaken. Prior to the surgery, the placement of a gastric tube was not necessary. On the third day postoperatively, the patient underwent extubation and subsequent

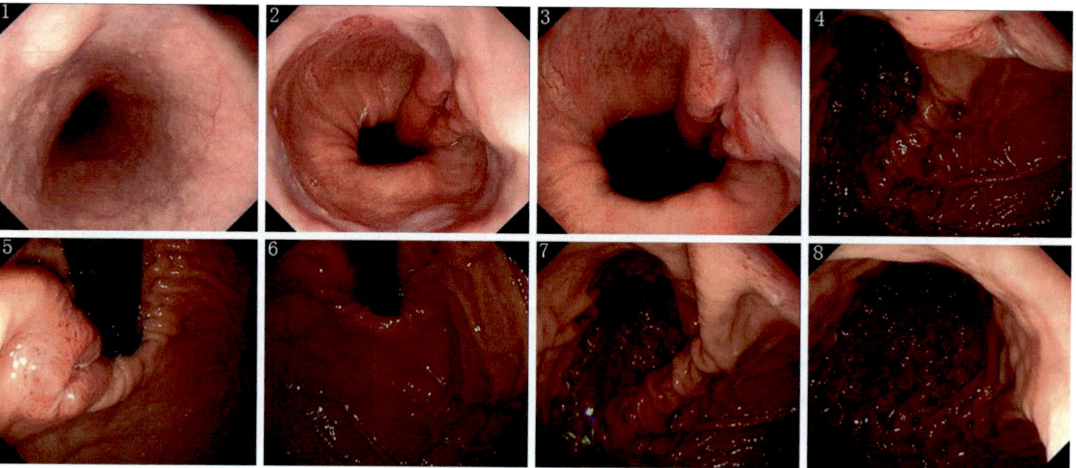

Fig. 3.33 Gastroscopic examination revealed the junction of the esophagus located 41 cm from the incisors. A profound, ulcerated mass spanning from 41 to 44 cm at the cardia was observed. The ulcerated area exhibited a coating of debris and white fibrinous exudates, while the ulcer edges displayed irregular contours

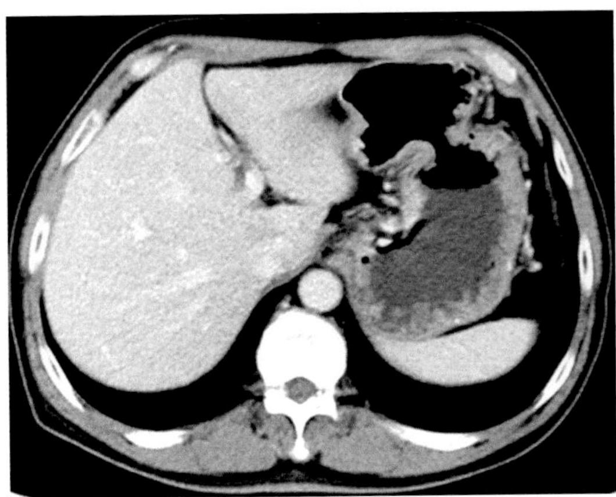

Fig. 3.34 Computed tomography (CT) findings demonstrated significant gastric cavity shrinkage, accompanied by uneven thickening of the cardia and the lesser curvature of the gastric body, with a maximum thickness measuring approximately 1.1 cm. Enhanced imaging revealed enhanced enhancement in the affected areas. Confluent lymph nodes were observed in the vicinity of the cardia, with the larger node exhibiting a short diameter of approximately 0.8 cm.

removal of the stomach tube. Encouraging early mobilization, water intake was initiated for the patient. Clear fluids were administered on the fourth day, followed by a transition to a liquid diet on the sixth day. The abdominal drainage tube was removed on the eighth day, and the patient was discharged from the hospital on the ninth day.

Pathological examination revealed the following findings on the gross specimen of the proximal gastrectomy specimen: the greater curvature of the stomach measured 18 cm, the lesser curvature measured 17 cm, and a free esophagus segment measuring 3.5 × 0.5 cm was also observed. At a distance of 2 cm from the upper resection margin, an elevated tumor was identified at the esophagus-gastric junction, measuring 3 × 1 × 0.6 cm. The tumor exhibited a gray-white, firm consistency with an indistinct cut surface, infiltrating the deep muscular layer.

Microscopic analysis provided the following diagnosis: a protuberant high-grade neuroendocrine carcinoma of the stomach, displaying a mixed morphology of small and large cell neuroendocrine carcinoma. The tumor invaded the middle muscular layer and involved the lower part of the esophagus, demonstrating vascular tumor emboli and nerve invasion. No cancerous involvement was detected at the upper and lower resection margins of the greater omentum. Lymph node metastasis was observed in 5 out of 21 examined lymph nodes, with partial involvement of the lymph node capsule. The final pathological staging was determined as pT2N2M0, corresponding to stage IIB.

Immunohistochemical analysis yielded the following results: AE1/AE3 (2+), Syno (3+), CD56 (3+), ChrA (2+), Ki-67 (60-70%+), P53 (80%+, displaying a missense mutant expression pattern), C-MET (focally weakly positive).

3.13.3 Case Analysis

Neuroendocrine Neoplasms (NENs) are relatively uncommon tumors arising from peptidergic neurons and neuroendocrine cells, with the ability to secrete bioactive amines and peptide hormones. They can manifest in various organs and regions of the human body. Among the diverse range of NENs, gastroenteropancreatic neuroendocrine tumors (GEP-NENs) are the most prevalent, comprising approximately 65–75% of all cases. Specifically, gastric neuroendocrine tumors (G-NENs) account for approximately 5.85% [140]. GEP-NENs can be categorized based on their morphological characteristics and proliferative activity into well-differentiated neuroendocrine tumors (NETs) of grades G1, G2, and G3, poorly differentiated neuroendocrine carcinomas (NECs) of grade G3, and a distinct mixed adenoneuroendocrine carcinoma (MiNEN) subtype. It is noteworthy that well-differentiated NET G3 and poorly differentiated NEC G3 exhibit mitotic figures and a Ki-67 index exceeding 20%, yet they possess significant prognostic differences. Consequently, the 2019 World Health Organization (WHO) classification classifies G3 GEP-NENs as either well-differentiated NET G3 or poorly differentiated NEC G3 [141] (Table 3.1) [142].

Based on the clinical characteristics and etiology of gastric neuroendocrine tumors (G-NENs) in China, they can be classified into four distinct

Table 3.1 2019 WHO classification of gastroenteropancreatic neuroendocrine

Type	Grading	Mitotic number (/2 mm^2)	Ki-67 index (%)
Well-differentiated NET	G1	<2	<3
Well-differentiated NET	G2	2~20	3~20
Well-differentiated NET	G3	>20	>20
Poorly-differentiated NEC	G3	>20	>20
• small cell type			
• large cell type			
MiNEN	uncertain	uncertain	uncertain

Table 3.2 Clinical features of G-NENs

Clinical features	Type 1	Type 2	Type 3	Type 4
Proportion of G-NENS	70~80	5~6	14~25	Rare
Tumor characteristics	1–2 cm, multiple, polypoid	1–2 cm, multiple, polypoid	>2 cm, solitary, with polyps and ulcers	Giant ulcer or spherical polyp
Related diseases	Chronic atrophic gastritis	Gastrinoma ZES/ MEN-1	None	None
Differentiation	High	High	High	High
Pathological grade	Mostly G1	G1, G2	G1, G2, G3	NECs, MiNEN
Serum gastrin level	Raised	Raised	Normal	Most normal
pH value in the stomach	Significantly increased	Obvious reduction	Normal	Most normal
Transfer ratio (%)	2~5	10~30	50~100	80~100
Cancer-related deaths (%)	0	<10	25~30	>50

types. Type 1 is the most prevalent and is primarily attributed to achlorhydria resulting from atrophic fundus inflammation. These tumors are predominantly well differentiated and generally have a favorable prognosis. Type 2 is predominantly associated with hypergastrinemia, commonly seen in individuals with Zollinger-Ellison syndrome and often accompanied by multiple endocrine neoplasia syndrome type 1. Most type 2 tumors exhibit good differentiation although a small proportion may present with metastases at the time of diagnosis. Type 3 G-NENs are primarily sporadic and not accompanied by elevated gastrin levels. Type 4, the rarest subtype, is characterized by the highest malignancy. Most type 4 tumors are poorly differentiated neuroendocrine carcinomas (NECs) or mixed adenoneuroendocrine carcinomas (MiNEN), and they carry the poorest prognosis (Table 3.2) [143].

The diagnosis of gastric neuroendocrine tumors (G-NENs) can present in various forms during endoscopic examination. Endoscopically, G-NENs may appear as raised lesions with smooth surfaces. The upper mucosa typically appears normal and firm, resembling polyps. The coloration of these lesions is often yellow or off-white, and there may be accompanying erosions or depressions. However, relying solely on endoscopic features for diagnosis carries a high risk of misdiagnosis. Therefore, obtaining pathological tissue samples through biopsy or puncture is essential. Immunohistochemistry and cell proliferation activity detection should be performed, and tumor classification and grading should be determined based on histological morphology, tumor differentiation degree, and cell proliferation activity [144]. Appropriate comprehensive treatment should be administered based on the pathological results to prevent the inadvertent resection of NENs as polyps, which could lead to recurrence and metastasis of residual tumor.

Gastrointestinal neuroendocrine carcinoma (G-NEC) is a rare tumor, accounting for less than 1% of gastric cancers. G-NEC exhibits deep invasion and a high likelihood of metastasis, with neuroendocrine cell growth patterns predominantly extending downward within the mucosa. Early-stage G-NEC often presents with surface erosion or non-erosion [145]. Due to the lack of effective early diagnostic methods, many G-NEC cases already have distant metastases, such as liver metastases, at the time of diagnosis. Studies have reported a low diagnostic rate of G-NEC in gastroscopic biopsy samples (11-27%) [146, 147], which often leads to delayed treatment. Given that most NEC tumors contain components of adenocarcinoma, they are frequently misdiagnosed as adenocarcinoma in biopsy diagnoses. In this case, the initial gastroscopic biopsy of the patient was also considered as adenocarcinoma, and it was only after surgery that the final diagnosis of high-grade neuroendocrine carcinoma was established based on histomorphology and immunohistochemical results.

Endoscopic ultrasonography (EUS) plays a crucial role in detecting gastric invasive tumors and can provide valuable assistance in the early diagnosis of gastric neuroendocrine carcinomas (G-NECs). EUS has high diagnostic accuracy and offers enhanced visualization of the gastric mucosa, submucosa, muscle layers, and muscular propria, allowing for a more precise assessment of lesion characteristics and facilitating the selection of optimal biopsy sites for accurate sampling. EUS-guided biopsies have proven effective in obtaining sufficient tissue samples, and the utilization of EUS-guided needles/biopsy techniques for deep submucosal tissue biopsies represents a safe and reliable diagnostic method for identifying gastric invasive tumors that yield negative results in conventional biopsies [145].

Pathological findings serve as the gold standard for diagnosing G-NECs. The primary distinction between neuroendocrine carcinoma (NEC) and neuroendocrine tumor (NET) lies in their histopathological morphology. Assessing the degree of histological differentiation is a critical step in NEN diagnosis. Typical poorly differentiated NEC encompasses small cell NEC and large cell NEC, sharing similar morphological features with corresponding lung tumors. In the present case, the patient exhibited a predominantly mixed morphology of small cell and large cell neuroendocrine carcinoma. Additionally, indicators of tumor proliferation activity, such as mitotic count and/or Ki-67 index, play a significant role in distinguishing NEC from NET. The mitotic count and/or Ki-67 index in NETs typically remain below 20%, while in NECs, it exceeds 20%. However, it is important to note that high-grade neuroendocrine tumors (NET G3) can display mitotic counts and/or Ki-67 indices exceeding 20%, necessitating differentiation from NEC. Most NET G3 cases exhibit distinct pathological morphology that distinguishes them from NEC. Immunohistochemistry aids in the differential diagnosis between NET G3 and NEC. Studies have reported that approximately 76% of patients with digestive system NECs exhibit mutant p53 expression, and around 1/5 to 3/5 of patients show loss of RB protein expression, while NET patients do not display abnormal TP53 and RB protein expression [148, 149]. Furthermore, factors such as ATRX, DAXX, SSTR2A, and CXCR4 contribute to the differential diagnosis of NET and NEC [150]. In this particular case of neuroendocrine carcinoma, the presence of Ki-67 (60–70%+), Syn (3+), ChA (2+), and P53 mutation aligns with the findings reported in the literature.

Tailored treatment strategies are implemented based on the type, size, pathological grade, and TNM stage of gastric neuroendocrine neoplasms (G-NENs). Generally, for type 1 neuroendocrine tumors (NETs) with G1, size < 2 cm, T1, and absence of regional lymphadenopathy and vascular invasion, endoscopic resection is recommended [151]. Type 2 G-NENs necessitate identification and surgical resection of the primary lesion causing hypergastrinemia. Type 3 and type 4 G-NENs primarily warrant radical surgery akin to gastric adenocarcinoma. Due to the high recurrence rate following radical surgery for neuroendocrine carcinoma (NEC) and high-grade NET G3, the ENETS guidelines propose the use of cisplatin or carboplatin in combination with etoposide as adjuvant or first-line therapy for advanced disease. Irinotecan or oxaliplatin-based regimens can be considered as second-line treatment [152]. In cases of NEC and NET G3 with advanced metastases, the ENETS guidelines do not recommend debulking surgery, metastasis resection, or radiofrequency ablation for liver metastases [152]. Currently, there is insufficient evidence supporting the use of somatostatin analogs or peptide receptor radionuclide therapy (PRRT) in the treatment of GEP NECs expressing somatostatin receptors.

3.13.4 Expert Comments

Gastric neuroendocrine carcinoma (G-NEC) is a rare malignancy of the stomach and belongs to the category of gastroenteropancreatic neuroendocrine tumors. It exhibits a high degree of malignancy and its incidence has been increasing in recent years. Early-stage diagnosis of gastric neuroendocrine carcinoma poses challenges, necessitating the use of gastroscopy for biopsy and pathological confirmation. Distinguishing between gastric adenocarcinoma and well-differentiated neuroendocrine tumors primarily relies on histomorphological and immunohistochemical findings. Comprehensive treatment approaches, predominantly surgical, are employed, following a similar surgical plan as that for gastric cancer. Adjuvant therapy is required for the majority of patients, and the overall prognosis is generally unfavorable.

Case provider: Hu Ren, Xiaofeng Bai.

Commentary: Xiaofeng Bai.

3.14 Case 21: Gastric Mixed Adenoneuroendocrine Carcinoma

3.14.1 Brief History

The patient, a 57-year-old male, was admitted to the hospital due to a persistent upper abdominal distension spanning a period of 6 months, with recent aggravation over the course of 1 month. Initial onset of upper abdominal distension occurred spontaneously 6 months ago, accompanied by belching and acid regurgitation, exacerbating following meals, and significantly diminishing appetite. Unfortunately, these symptoms were initially disregarded. However, their severity intensified within the past month, prompting the patient to seek medical attention. Gastroscopic examination conducted at an external healthcare facility revealed poorly differentiated adenocarcinoma at the antrum-body junction, measuring approximately 2.0 cm in diameter. Pathological analysis further demonstrated chronic atrophic gastritis with intestinal metaplasia. Notably, the patient experienced a weight loss of 5 kg since the onset of symptoms. Additionally, the patient's medical history includes a 12-year duration of diabetes mellitus, 5 years of hypertension, and 1 month of glaucoma. Physical and laboratory examinations did not reveal any abnormalities. Abdominal computed tomography (CT) imaging displayed slight thickening of the gastric wall near the gastric angle in the gastric antrum. The lesion's length measured approximately 1.5 cm, and the serous surface appeared smooth. Notably, no definitive evidence of enlarged lymph nodes was identified within the abdominal pelvic cavity or retroperitoneum (refer to Fig. 3.35).

Diagnosis: Gastric cancer (cT1N0M0), Diabetes, Hypertension, Glaucoma.

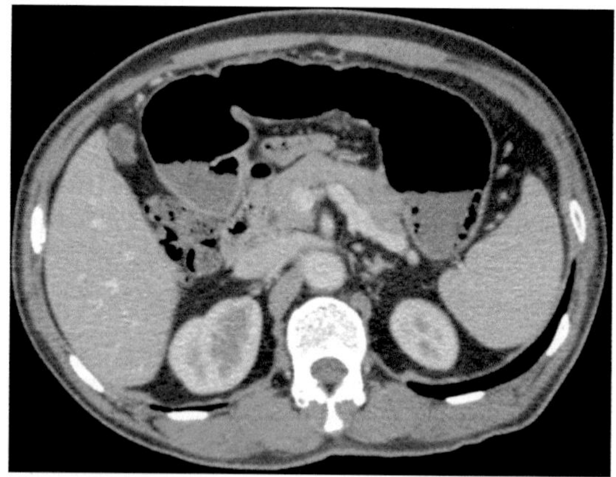

Fig. 3.35 Depicts an enhanced computed tomography (CT) scan showcasing the gastric wall near the gastric angle exhibiting a slight thickening. The length of the observed lesion measures approximately 1.5 cm, while the serous surface appears smooth

3.14.2 Treatment

Following adequate preoperative preparations, a laparoscopic distal subtotal gastrectomy with Billroth-I+Braun anastomosis was performed. Intraoperatively, the tumor was identified at the posterior gastric wall, precisely situated at the junction of the antrum-body, without evidence of serous membrane invasion. The tumor dimensions were approximately 2.0 * 1.8 cm, and no enlarged lymph nodes were detected in the vicinity of the stomach. The surgical procedure progressed smoothly. Subsequent to the surgery, the patient exhibited a seamless recovery, including the passage of flatus on the 4th postoperative day, removal of the gastric tube on the 5th day, removal of the drainage tube on the 8th day, and subsequent discharge on the 11th day.

3.14.3 Pathology

The pathological examination revealed a mixed adenoneuroendocrine carcinoma of the early gastric stage with a superficial concave type. Adenocarcinoma constituted 60% of the tumor and exhibited low differentiation, specifically classified as diffuse type according to Lauren classification. Neuroendocrine carcinoma accounted for 40% of the tumor, displaying a G3 grade with a Ki-67 index of 60%. The tumor infiltrated the submucosa without muscular involvement and exhibited nerve invasion. Notably, the pylorus remained unaffected by the tumor. Lymph node analysis did not reveal any evidence of metastatic cancer among the 39 examined nodes (0/39). Immunohistochemistry results indicated positive staining for AE1/AE3 (3+), CK18 (3+), CD56 (1+ for neuroendocrine carcinoma), CgA (2+ for neuroendocrine carcinoma), Syn (1+ for neuroendocrine carcinoma), EGFR (2+), HER2 (1+), MLH1 (+), MSH2 (+), MSH6 (+), PMS2 (+), and c-MET (1+). Additionally, the Ki-67 staining showed positivity with a 60% labeling index in the neuroendocrine carcinoma component (refer to Fig. 3.36a–c). The postoperative management included two cycles of adjuvant chemotherapy. Following regular postoperative reviews, no signs of tumor recurrence or metastasis were detected even after a 5-year follow-up period. The final pathological stage was determined as pT1bN0 according to the TNM staging system.

3.14.4 Case Analysis

Mixed adenoneuroendocrine tumor (MiNEN) is a rare pathological entity within the digestive system. According to the World Health Organization (WHO) classification, MiNEN primarily consists of two components, namely adenocarcinoma and neuroendocrine carcinoma, both of which account for more than 30% of the tumor composition [153]. Based on the specific tissue composition, MiNEN can be fur-

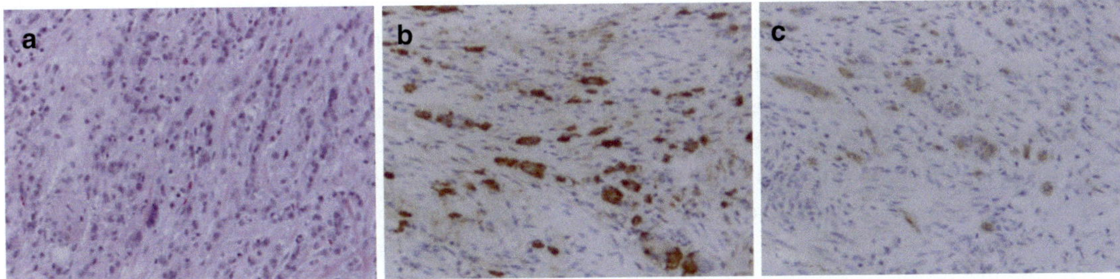

Fig. 3.36 Displays pathological images of mixed adenoneuroendocrine carcinoma. (**a**) The cancer cells exhibit a cord-like, poorly differentiated morphology with the absence of distinct glandular ducts. Locally, signet-ring cells are observed (HE staining, ×200). (**b**) Immunohistochemical staining reveals positive CgA expression in the cytoplasm of cancer cells. (**c**) Immunohistochemical staining demonstrates positive Syn expression in the cytoplasm of cancer cells

ther categorized into mixed adenoneuroendocrine carcinoma (where the two tissue types are intermixed), collision carcinoma (where the two tissue types are distinct and have clear boundaries), and amphicrine carcinoma (where both tissue characteristics are present within the same cell) [153].

MiNEN poses challenges in biopsy diagnosis as it can often be misdiagnosed as adenocarcinoma. Accurate diagnosis typically requires postoperative pathological examination and immunohistochemical staining. Immunohistochemical markers such as chromogranin A (CgA), synaptophysin (Syn), and CD56 are utilized to identify neuroendocrine carcinoma, with positive staining for at least two of these markers. Carcinoembryonic antigen (CEA) and cytokeratins (CKs) serve as diagnostic references for adenocarcinoma [154].

MiNEN primarily affects the gastrointestinal tract and certain specific anatomical sites, including the pancreas, gallbladder, bladder, and uterus. Colorectal involvement is particularly notable [155–157]. Analysis of the Surveillance, Epidemiology, and End Results (SEER) database revealed an increase in the incidence of gastrointestinal MiNEN from 0.23 cases per million in 2000 to 1.16 cases per million in 2016, corresponding to an annual percent change (APC) of 8.0% [158]. MiNEN can occur at any age although it is more common among middle-aged and elderly individuals between 50 and 70 years old [158].

MiNEN presents as a non-functional neuroendocrine tumor with insidious onset and late manifestation of clinical symptoms. These symptoms often include non-specific gastrointestinal symptoms or local tumor-related signs. Typically, MiNEN does not exhibit characteristic carcinoid syndrome manifestations such as facial flushing, bronchial asthma, or cardiac valvular disease [159].

The precise origin of MiNEN remains uncertain; however, it is hypothesized that both tissue components of MiNEN arise from pluripotent stem cells or result from the differentiation of adenocarcinoma cells into neuroendocrine cancer cells [160–162].

The incidence of mixed adenoneuroendocrine tumors (MiNEN) is relatively low, and limited research has been conducted on their clinicopathological features and prognosis. Existing literature predominantly focuses on colorectal MiNEN, while there is a lack of sufficient data on gastric MiNEN. Previous studies have reported widely varying prognosis for MiNEN, which may be attributed to the small number of cases available for analysis.

A study by Watanabe et al. [163] compared the survival outcomes of colorectal MiNEN with adenocarcinoma and found that patients with colorectal MiNEN had a poorer prognosis, primarily due to the neuroendocrine component. The 5-year disease-free survival rate for stage I patients was 100%, whereas stage II and III patients had lower rates (72.7% and 47.1%, respectively). Some studies have classified MiNEN into different risk groups, such as high risk, medium risk, and low risk, based on factors such as the Ki-67 index. Higher Ki-67 index in the high-risk group has been associated with increased tumor invasion and shorter survival time [164, 165].

Gastric MiNEN has shown characteristics of high invasiveness, easy metastasis, and low long-term survival rates, with 5-year overall survival rates ranging from 30 to 40% [166–170]. Studies have indicated that the depth of tumor invasion and tumor size are not the primary prognostic factors for MiNEN. Instead, lymph node invasion and distant metastasis have been found to be more significant [171]. Liver metastasis, abdominal metastasis, and lymph node metastasis are the main forms of recurrence in gastric MiNEN, accounting for over 60%, 30%, and 30% of recurrent cases, respectively [158, 172]. However, the underlying mechanisms of relapse and metastasis in MiNEN remain unclear.

Based on current reports, the primary treatments for gastrointestinal mixed adenoneuroendocrine tumors (MiNEN) consist of surgery and chemotherapy. Surgery remains the mainstay treatment modality with the potential for achieving curative outcomes. The 2015 National Comprehensive Cancer Network (NCCN) guidelines recommend surgical approaches such as gastrectomy and radical lymph node dissection for localized gastric neuroendocrine tumors. In cases where metastasis is present, a multimodal integrated therapy approach combining surgery, targeted therapy, chemotherapy, or biotherapy should be considered [173].

Within the domestic medical community, surgical intervention is considered the primary treatment for localized gastric MiNEN, following the same principles as those for adenocarcinoma. For advanced-stage MiNEN, a multidisciplinary treatment approach centered around surgery is recommended. This may involve the integration of adjuvant therapies such as chemotherapy and biological therapy to enhance overall survival rates [174].

3.14.5 Expert Comments

Mixed adenoneuroendocrine tumor (MiNEN) is a rare and poorly understood pathological type due to its low incidence. Currently, surgical intervention and chemotherapy remain the primary treatment modalities in clinical practice. However, the prognosis of MiNEN can be improved in the future through advancements in basic research, which can enhance our understanding of the disease and lead to the development of more effective therapeutic strategies. Continued research efforts are necessary to shed light on the underlying mechanisms, improve diagnostic accuracy, and identify novel targeted therapies for MiNEN.

Case provider: Xiaojie Zhang, Yingtai Chen.

Commentary: Chunguang Guo.

3.15 Case 22: Hepatoid Adenocarcinoma of the Stomach

3.15.1 Brief History

The subject under study is a 51-year-old male presenting with upper abdominal discomfort and concomitant heartburn persisting for over a period of 2 months, with an exacerbation noted in the past week. The patient experienced recurring episodes of upper abdominal discomfort, nausea, and acid regurgitation that commenced 2 months ago. These symptoms were intermittent in nature and not significantly associated with meal consumption. Gastroscopy revealed a notable gastric space occupation, as illustrated in Fig. 3.37. A PET-CT examination demonstrated thickening of the local mucosa along the greater curvature of the gastric body, with concurrent identification of metastatic lymph nodes surrounding the stomach. Notably, the patient had a prior medical history of multiple lung nodules. In 2014, he underwent surgical intervention for hemorrhoids. Additionally, he has an extensive smoking habit spanning two decades, amounting to a consumption of 10 cigarettes per day.

Diagnosis: Gastric cancer (cT4N+M0), Gastrointestinal bleeding, Anemia

3.15.2 Treatment

Following appropriate preoperative preparation, a total laparoscopic gastrectomy (D2, Roux-en-Y, π anastomosis, R0) was performed. Intraoperatively, it was observed that the tumor was situated along the greater curvature of the stomach body, measuring approximately 12 * 8 cm in size. Notably, it exhibited Borrmann III characteristics, penetrated the serous membrane, and exhibited the presence of multiple enlarged lymph nodes in its vicinity, as depicted in Fig. 3.38. On postoperative day 6, the gastric tube and the right abdominal drainage tube were both removed, while the left drainage tube was removed on postoperative day 7. The patient was subsequently discharged 9 days after the surgical procedure.

3.15.3 Pathology

The histopathological examination revealed the presence of gastric infiltrating ulcerative poorly differentiated adenocarcinoma (Lauren type: mixed type), accompanied by necrosis and increased infiltration of inflammatory cells. The

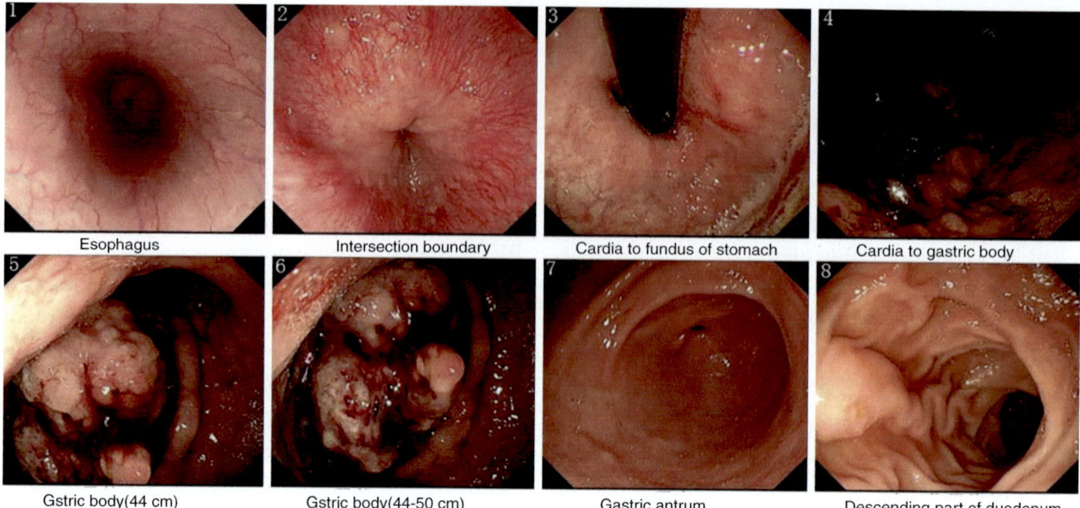

Fig. 3.37 Exhibits the gastroscopic findings, revealing the presence of an ulcerative mass situated on the greater curvature of the stomach body. The base of the ulcerative mass appears to be coated with debris and a white moss-like substance. The ulcerative ridge displays an irregularly elevated profile, which exhibits a friable nature, rendering it susceptible to bleeding. The gastric wall surrounding the lesion appears deformed and rigid, with the presence of dark red blood clots within the stomach. Notably, active bleeding is observed within the lesion

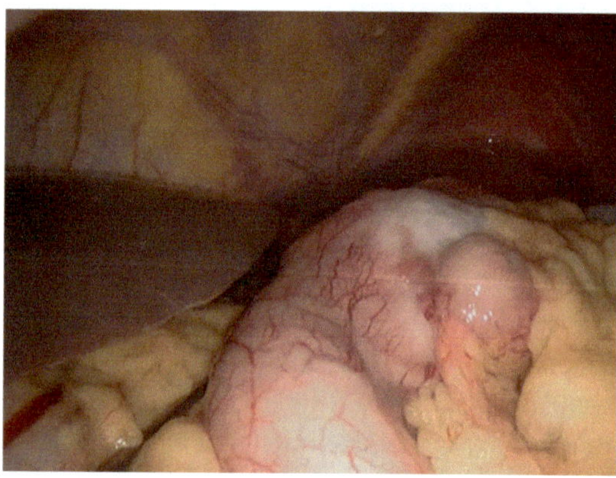

Fig. 3.38 Demonstrates the results of the abdominal exploration, revealing the absence of distant metastasis. The tumor was identified within the stomach body and fundus, with infiltration into the serous membrane. Its dimensions were approximately 6 × 8 cm, and the extent of mobility was found to be satisfactory

tumor predominantly exhibited a solid structure. Through immunohistochemical analysis, the tumor was determined to exhibit a primitive intestinal epithelial phenotype, with a tendency toward hepatoid adenocarcinoma. Penetration of the serous membrane by the tumor was observed, along with the presence of metastatic carcinoma in the lymph nodes (5 out of 70), with involvement of the capsular membrane in more extensive cases, as illustrated in Fig. 3.39a. The pTNM staging was determined as pT4aN2. Immunohistochemical results demonstrated the following: AFP (−), C-MET (1+), EGFR (1+), GPC3 (1+), HER2 (−), MLH1 (+), MSH2 (+), MSH6 (+), PMS2 (+), SALL4 (2+), AE1/AE3 (2+), CD56 (−), ChrA (in+), Ki-67 (+60%), P53 (+50%), Syno (1+), EBER (−), as depicted in Fig. 3.39b–d.

Postoperatively, the patient underwent adjuvant chemotherapy consisting of oxaliplatin and S1 for a duration of four cycles. Eight months after surgery, a CT examination revealed the presence of new soft tissue hyperplasia in the anterior spleen, with a maximum cross-section measuring 4.6 × 4.4 cm (Fig. 3.40a). Subsequently, at the 10th month after surgery, the patient experienced acute intestinal obstruction accompanied by gastrointestinal bleeding. CT imaging displayed a larger mass shadow anterior to the spleen, with a maximum cross-section of 8.0 × 5.7 cm. Enhanced scans revealed uneven enhancement, internal necrotic areas, multiple gas accumulations, and

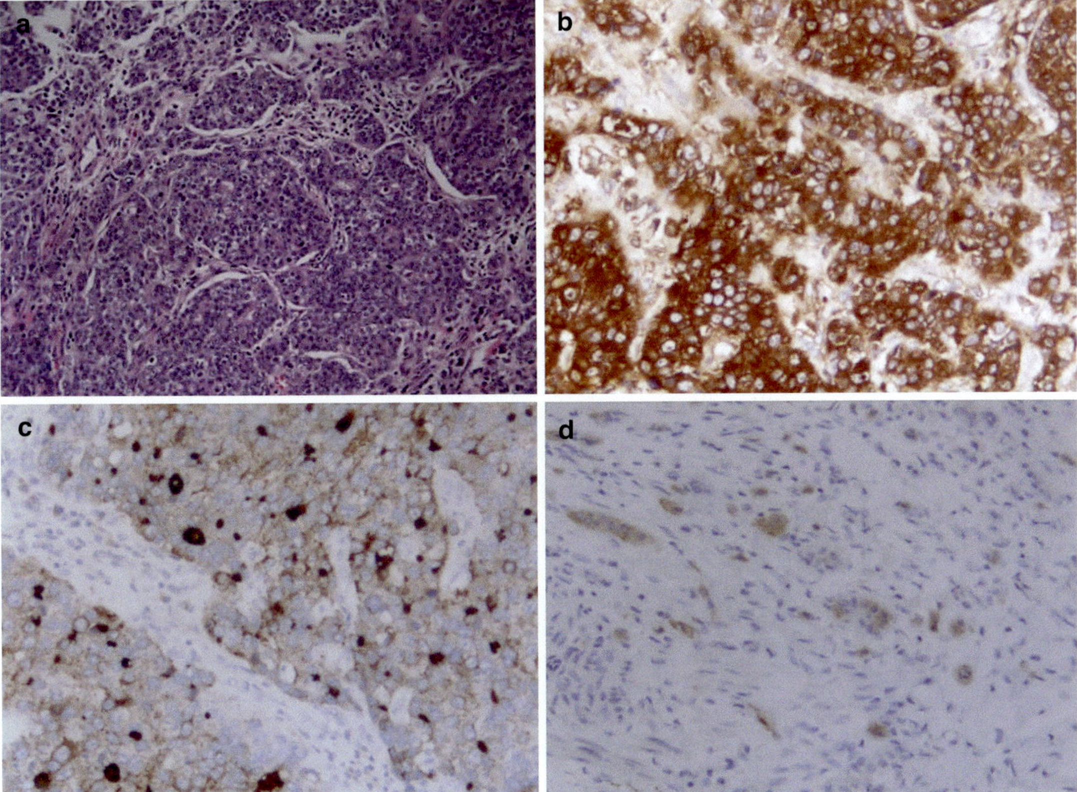

Fig. 3.39 Provides a pathological examination of hepatoid adenocarcinoma. (**a**) The cancer cells exhibited a poorly differentiated morphology, characterized by a solid or nest-like arrangement. They displayed abundant acidophilic cytoplasm, prominent nuclear atypia, and visible nucleoli, resembling the morphological features of hepatocellular carcinoma (HE, ×200). (**b**) Immunohistochemical staining demonstrated the presence of positive alpha-fetoprotein (AFP) in the cytoplasm of the cancer cells. (**c**) Immunohistochemical staining revealed positive glypican-3 (GPC) in the cytoplasm of the cancer cells. (**d**) Immunohistochemical staining demonstrated positive staining for SALL4 in the nuclei of the cancer cells

suspected local communication with the bowel, indicative of a metastatic tumor (Fig. 3.40b). Emergency abdominal exploration, abdominal tumor resection, and partial transverse colon resection were performed. Postoperative pathology confirmed abdominal metastasis. Two months following the second surgery, a CT examination identified a mass in the upper left abdominal cavity, measuring a maximum cross-section of 5.0 × 4.4 cm, consistent with a metastatic tumor. The patient then received two cycles of adjuvant chemotherapy utilizing albumin-paclitaxel and capecitabine. Four months after the second surgery, a follow-up CT scan revealed an enlargement of the upper left abdominal cavity mass, with a maximum cross-section of 9.9 × 7.4 cm. Due to the development of chemotherapy resistance, chemotherapy was discontinued. One month after discontinuation, the patient experienced acute intestinal obstruction. Further surgical exploration revealed that the intestinal obstruction was caused by metastatic tumor growth, which could not be resected. A jejune-jejunal short circuit procedure was performed, and subsequent treatment included albumin-paclitaxel, apatinib, and camrelizumab for a duration of two cycles. At the last follow-up, the patient had passed away, with an overall survival of 23 months.

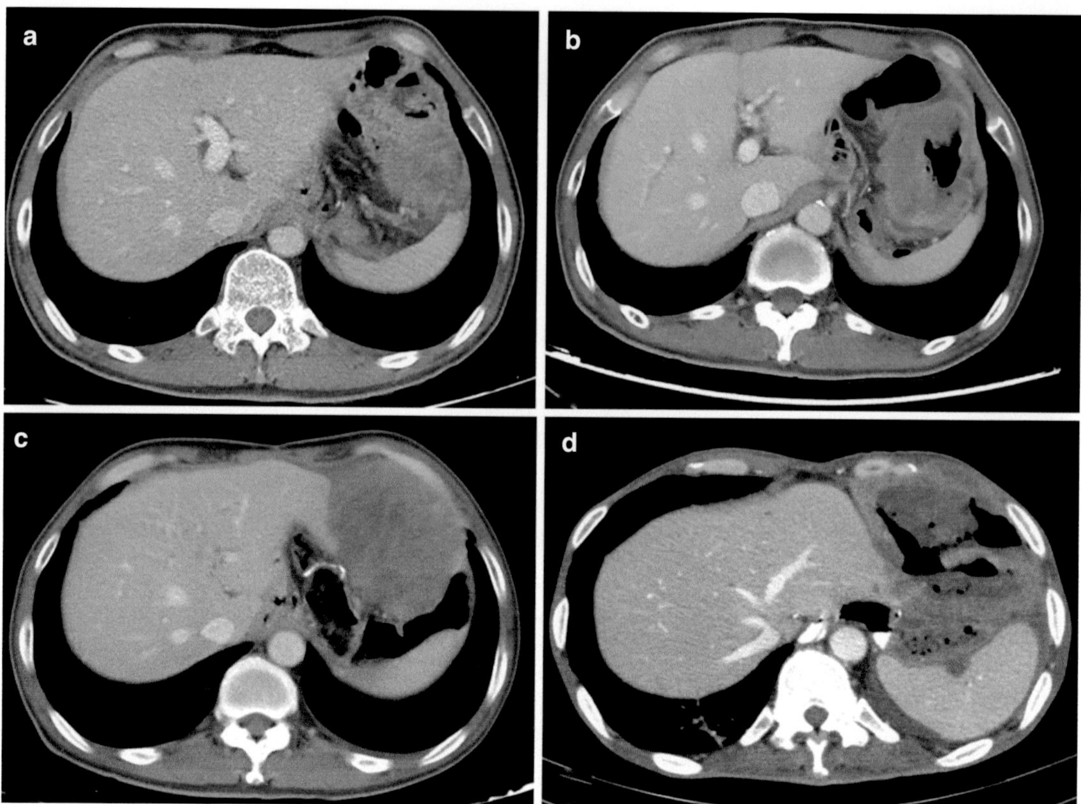

Fig. 3.40 Presents the following imaging findings: (**a**) Abdominal CT scan depicting the anterior spleen mass 8 months after surgery. (**b**) 10 months after surgery, the tumor exhibited enlargement and appeared to be connected to the bowel, indicating a metastatic tumor. (**c**) CT scan conducted 7 months after the second operation revealed the presence of a mass in the left upper abdomen and abdominal cavity. (**d**) CT findings obtained 4 months after the third operation displayed abdominal masses

3.15.4 Case Analysis

Hepatoid adenocarcinoma (HAC) is a rare tumor type characterized by a poor prognosis. Histologically, HACs exhibit similarities to hepatocellular carcinomas and often exhibit high expression of Alpha Fetal Protein (AFP). Confirming the diagnosis typically requires the use of multiple immunohistochemical markers [175, 176]. Since the initial report of gastric HAC in 1970, numerous cases of HAC have been documented [177]. Although gastric HAC is the most common type, cases have also been reported in other organs such as the lungs, pancreas, gallbladder, bladder, ovary, uterus, and more [178]. The incidence of gastric HAC accounts for only 0.3–1% of all gastric cancers.

The pathogenesis of gastric hepatoid adenocarcinoma (GHA) remains unclear. It is believed that both the stomach and liver originate from the foregut during development and share homology. In tumor cells, gastric adenocarcinomas can differentiate into liver-like cells, leading to the formation of GHA [179, 180]. Therefore, some researchers have suggested that GHA might originate from enteric gastric cancer [181]. At the molecular level, frequent gene copy number increases have been observed in the 20q11.21-13.12 region of GHA. It is speculated that potential driver genes located in this region might play a crucial role in the development and progression of GHA [182].

HAC is associated with poor prognosis, often characterized by lymph node and distant metastasis. The main contributing factor is the poor differentiation of the tumor. The 3-year survival rate for gastric HAC ranges from 17.2% to 22.6% [183, 184]. Data from the Surveillance, Epidemiology, and End Results (SEER) database indicate that the 1-year overall and tumor-specific survival rates for HAC are below 40%, while the 3-year rates are below 20%. Due to the low incidence of HAC, there is no consensus on prognostic factors. However, a meta-analysis of gastric HACs revealed that prognosis is associated with metastasis, but not with sex, tumor site, or differentiation [185]. Wang Yanfei et al. [186] identified elevated levels of tumor marker CA19-9, lymph node staging, radical surgery, and intensity of AFP staining as independent risk factors for poor prognosis. Another study by Wang et al. [182] found that preoperative serum AFP levels ≥500 ng/mL were significantly correlated with poor overall survival. Additionally, lymph node staging showed a significant correlation with survival, with patients classified as N0 or N1 demonstrating a better prognosis after R0 resection compared to those with lymph node stage N2 or above [187].

Surgery is the primary treatment for resectable HAC, and patients who undergo surgery generally have a significantly better prognosis compared to those who do not, with a 5-year overall survival rate of 34% [184]. Liver metastasis is the leading cause of death in HAC. Chemotherapy is recommended for patients with HAC who are not suitable for radical resection. Studies have indicated that neoadjuvant chemotherapy yields higher rates of disease-free and disease-specific survival compared to postoperative chemotherapy when the same chemotherapy regimen is administered [188]. Currently, there is no standardized chemotherapy regimen for HAC, and the tumor often exhibits poor response to conventional chemotherapy and is prone to developing drug resistance. However, notable results have been observed in epidermal growth factor receptor wild-type stage IV lung HAC, where a combination of sorafenib and platinum dual-drug chemotherapy achieved a partial response (PR), resulting in the longest survival reported in unresectable stage IV cases [189]. Similar outcomes have been reported in pancreatic HAC, with patients treated with sorafenib experiencing a progression-free survival of 8 months [190]. These findings suggest that anti-tumor angiogenesis targeting drugs may play a significant role in the treatment of HAC.

3.15.5 Expert Comments

HAC is a rare malignancy primarily affecting the stomach, characterized by a propensity for lymph node and liver metastasis, resulting in a poor prognosis and high mortality rate. Due to its rarity, clinical understanding of HAC remains limited, leading to frequent misdiagnosis and missed diagnoses. Early radical surgery remains the most effective treatment approach for HAC.

Case provider: Xiaojie Zhang, Chunguang Guo.

Commentary: Chunguang Guo.

3.16 Case 23: Epstein-Barr Virus-Associated Gastric Cancer

3.16.1 Brief History

The patient, a 51-year-old male, was admitted primarily due to "a persistent occurrence of melena spanning a period of three months and an episode of hematemesis approximately two weeks prior." The patient reported the onset of melena 3 months ago, which presented without associated abdominal pain, abdominal distension, or other related discomfort. The patient did not seek medical intervention for this matter. Approximately 2 weeks ago, the patient experienced three episodes of postprandial hematemesis characterized by bright red blood, accompanied by symptoms of dizziness and nausea. Subsequent esophagogastroduodenoscopy revealed the presence of a profound 3 × 3 cm ulcer located on the lesser curvature of the stomach. Histopathological examination of biopsied specimens confirmed the presence of adenocarcinoma. Symptomatic treatment measures, including hemostasis, were implemented, resulting in relief of the reported symptoms. The abdominal examination did not yield any positive clinical signs. Evaluation of tumor markers, namely CA199, CA724, AFP, cyfra211, NSE, SCC, and CEA, demonstrated levels within the normal range. Furthermore, abdominal contrast-enhanced computed tomography (CT) imaging unveiled an ulcerative lesion measuring approximately 3.5 × 2.3 cm, displaying significant enhancement at the site corresponding to the lesser curvature of the stomach (Fig. 3.41).

Diagnosis: gastric cancer (cT4aN0M0).

3.16.2 Treatment

Following admission, the patient underwent a series of pertinent examinations and subsequently underwent laparoscopic-assisted total gastrectomy with Roux-Y reconstruction. The postoperative course was uneventful, characterized by smooth recovery. Flatus was passed by the patient on the fifth day, and the gastric tube was removed on the sixth day. Ultimately, the patient was discharged on the ninth day.

Pathological analysis of the resected specimen revealed the following findings: The gross specimen consisted of a total gastrectomy specimen, with the lesser curvature measuring 14 cm and the greater curvature measuring 27 cm in length. The esophagus measured 0.5 cm in length and 1.5 cm in width, while the duodenum measured 0.6 cm in length and 3 cm in width. Microscopic examination demonstrated the presence of an infiltrating ulcerating tumor involving the serosa, located 3 cm away from the cut edge of the esophagus and measuring 3.5 × 3 × 1.3 cm. Histopathologically, the tumor was classified as a poorly differentiated adenocarcinoma of the gastric infiltrating ulcerative type, with the Lauren classification indicating an intestinal subtype. Based on the morphological features and results of in situ hybridization staining, the tumor was determined to be consistent with EBV-related gastric adenocarcinoma, accompanied by ulcer formation extending into the muscular layer. The tumor exhibited invasion into the serosa but did not involve the esophagogastric junction, pylorus, duodenum, or greater omentum. Nerve invasion was observed, while no definitive evidence of vascular tumor thrombus was identified. Clear resection margins were achieved both proximally and distally. The surrounding gastric mucosa exhibited chronic non-atrophic gastritis. Lymph node analysis revealed metastatic carcinoma in 1 out of 39 nodes examined. Immunohistochemical analysis demonstrated the following results: AFP (−), C-MET (1+), EGFR (2+), GPC3 (−), HER2 (1+), MLH1 (+), MSH2 (+), MSH6 (+), PMS2 (+), SALL4 (−). In situ hybridization results revealed EBER positivity (Fig. 3.42). Based on the TNM staging system, the final pathological stage was classified as pT4aN1M0, corresponding to stage IIIa.

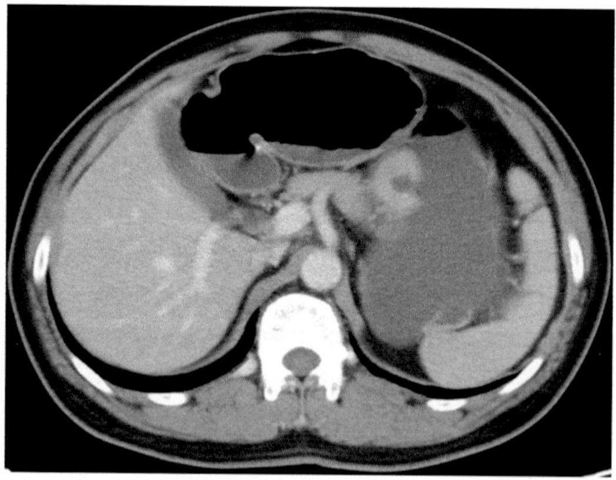

Fig. 3.41 Abdominal CT scan demonstrated the presence of a tumor situated along the lesser curvature of the stomach, exhibiting a notable ulcerative transformation measuring approximately 3.5 × 2.3 cm, characterized by substantial enhancement

Following the surgical intervention, the patient received three cycles of chemotherapy consisting of oxaliplatin in combination with S-1. Subsequently, 4 months postoperatively, a single cycle of chemotherapy comprising Sintilimab in combination with Albumin Paclitaxel was administered.

3.16.3 Case Analysis

EB virus, also known as human herpesvirus IV, is highly prevalent worldwide, infecting over 95% of the global population. Although the

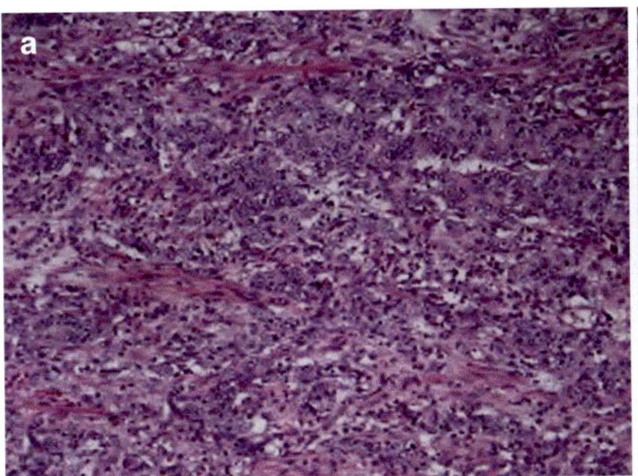

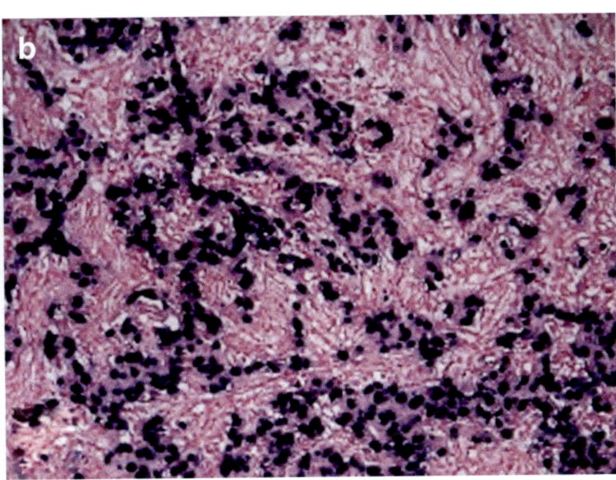

Fig. 3.42 (**a**) Cancer cells are observed in a poorly differentiated pattern, displaying syncytial-like features, abundant cytoplasm, and vesicular nuclei (HE staining, magnification ×200). (**b**) The results of in situ hybridization reveals positive nuclear staining for EBV-encoded RNA (EBER) in the cancer cells

majority of individuals remain asymptomatic, this virus can give rise to various diseases, including nasopharyngeal carcinoma, Burkitt's lymphoma, Hodgkin's lymphoma, and gastric cancer [191, 192]. In 1992, Akiba et al. first identified the presence of EB virus in gastric adenocarcinoma cells [193]. Direct infection of gastric mucosal cells by the EB virus through the digestive tract is challenging. Instead, it primarily infects B cells, subsequently entering gastric mucosal epithelial cells through interactions between B cells and gastric mucosal epithelial cells [194]. In 2014, the Cancer Genome Atlas (TCGA) proposed the molecular classification of gastric cancer, dividing it into four distinct types: Epstein-Barr virus-positive tumors, microsatellite unstable tumors, genomically stable tumors, and tumors with chromosomal instability [195].

EBV-associated gastric cancer (EBVaGC) accounts for approximately 2–18% of all gastric cancer cases [196], with the incidence varying across different countries and regions. In the Asian population, EBVaGC represents approximately 7.5% of all gastric cancer cases [197]. Notably, clinical studies conducted in China have indicated that the incidence of EBVaGC in Guangzhou, a high-incidence area for nasopharyngeal carcinoma, is not significantly higher compared to other regions. However, large-scale epidemiological data are still needed to confirm whether the regional distribution of EBVaGC parallels that of nasopharyngeal carcinoma [198, 199]. The incidence of EBVaGC is higher in men, with the fundus and body of the stomach being commonly affected sites [195]. Furthermore, patients with EBVaGC tend to be younger than those with other molecular subtypes of gastric cancer [200], and the average age of onset is around 60 years. Regarding Lauren's classification, EBVaGC is often classified as the intestinal type.

The latent form of EB virus in EBVaGC can be categorized as type I or type II. Type I is characterized by the expression of EB virus-encoded small RNAs (EBER), EBV nuclear antigen (EBNA), BamH I-A region rightward transcript (BART), and BART microRNA. Type II, based on type I, further expresses latent membrane protein 2A (LMP2A) [201].

EBVaGC exhibits distinctive molecular features, including a high prevalence of PIK3CA mutation and ARID1A mutation, DNA promoter CpG island methylation, overexpression of PD-L1/2, JAK2 amplification, low TP53 mutation frequency, HER2 amplification, and reduced expression of CDKN2A, among others [195]. The PIK3CA gene is involved in regulating the PI3K/AKT pathway. Abe et al. [202] have proposed that PIK3CA mutations may preexist before EB virus infection. Following EB virus infection, LMP2A further activates the PI3K/

AKT pathway, thereby promoting the progression of gastric cancer. The interplay between PIK3CA mutations, EB virus protein products, and the activation of the PI3K/AKT pathway may represent one of the mechanisms underlying EBVaGC. The AT-rich interactive domain 1A (ARID1A) gene encodes the nuclear protein BAF250a, a crucial component of the SWI/SNF chromatin remodeling complex (SWItch/Sucrose nonfermentable). ARID1A participates in tumor suppression by regulating chromatin structure and gene expression. In EBVaGC, the mutation rate of ARID1A is approximately 55%. It is worth noting that ARID1A mutations may also occur prior to EBV infection. Loss of ARID1A expression resulting from the mutation leads to alterations in chromatin structure, potentially facilitating EBV nuclear entry and subsequent gastric cancer development [203].

EB virus exerts its influence on gastric cells and immune microenvironment by secreting miRNA and virus-encoded proteins, thereby promoting the development of gastric cancer. The miRNA produced by EB virus can facilitate gastric cancer occurrence by targeting and degrading mRNA transcribed by tumor suppressor genes [204]. Additionally, miR-BART10-3p and miR-BART22 have been identified as contributors to the metastasis of EBVaGC through the activation of the classical Wnt signaling pathway [205]. Viral protein LMP2A can phosphorylate STAT3, leading to the activation of DNA methyltransferases 1 and 3b (DNMT1, DNMT3b) [206]. This, in turn, promotes promoter methylation, resulting in the downregulation of tumor suppressor gene expression [207]. Furthermore, EB virus has the ability to silence its own genes and conceal its antigens to evade host immune regulation [208]. In summary, potential mechanisms underlying EBVaGC encompass PIK3CA mutation-induced activation of the PI3K/AKT signaling pathway to facilitate tumor cell proliferation, ARID1A mutation-driven chromatin structural changes aiding EB virus nuclear entry, DNA hypermethylation-induced suppression of numerous tumor suppressor genes, and PD-L1 overexpression facilitating immune evasion by tumor cells [203].

Currently, the gold standard for diagnosing EBVaGC remains EBER in situ hybridization conducted on biopsy samples [209]. In recent years, quantitative analysis of EB virus load through DNA amplification in blood samples and tumor tissues has been proposed as a potential approach for early diagnosis of EBVaGC. This method holds promise for assessing virus latency, reactivation status, predicting chemotherapy efficacy, and estimating the likelihood of recurrence [210].

There is no specific treatment tailored for EBVaGC, and the treatment approach remains comprehensive, predominantly based on surgical intervention. EBVaGC is characterized by the molecular feature of PD-L1/2 overexpression. The overexpression of PD-L1 enables tumor cells to evade immune surveillance, making EBVaGC a potential candidate for immunotherapy. Several studies have demonstrated promising outcomes with immunotherapy for EBVaGC. However, most of these studies are limited to case reports and lack robust clinical evidence [211–213]. Besides, Schneider et al. [214] found that demethylation agents can enhance the therapeutic efficacy of chemotherapy in EBVaGC. Although the relatively low incidence of EBVaGC and the scarcity of clinical studies, its prognosis is generally considered to be more favorable [215, 216]. This improved prognosis may be attributed to the recruitment of lymphocytes in the immune microenvironment [217]. Such an immune-rich tumor microenvironment enhances the response to chemotherapy [218, 219].

3.16.4 Expert Comments

The treatment landscape of gastric cancer has transitioned into the era of molecular subtyping. EBVaGC represents a distinct molecular subtype with unique immune microenvironment and molecular characteristics. However, there is currently a dearth of specific treatment strategies for EBVaGC. Researchers are actively investigating the epidemiological aspects, vulnerable populations, and potential targeted therapies for this subtype. In the future, the development of precise and tailored treatments for gastric cancer, including EBVaGC, holds promise for significantly enhancing patient prognosis.

Case provider: Yuemin Sun, Zefeng Li.

Commentary: Yuemin Sun.

3.17 Case 24: Immunotherapy Therapy in MSI-H Gastric Cancer

3.17.1 Brief History

The admission of a 35-year-old female patient to the hospital was prompted by her persistent episodic epigastric pain spanning over a duration of more than 2 years. Initial manifestation of this discomfort occurred 2 years ago without any discernible cause, which led her to forgo medical intervention as she did not experience accompanying symptoms of nausea or vomiting. However, a recent diagnosis was made at a local hospital, revealing poorly differentiated adenocarcinoma situated in the upper posterior region of the stomach, as ascertained through gastroscopic examination and subsequent biopsy. An abdominal CT scan indicated an absence of evident gastric wall thickening, and no enlarged lymph nodes were detected within the abdominal cavity, retroperitoneum, or inguinal region (refer to Fig. 3.43). Further gastroscopic investigation exposed the presence of gastric cancer, primarily located in the upper and middle sections of the stomach, approximately 41–46 cm from the incisors (refer to Fig. 3.44). Preceding the patient's surgical intervention at our facility, genetic testing conducted at a different hospital revealed an MSI-H phenotype and a tumor mutational burden (TMB) of 42.03 mut/Mb. In response, she underwent a two-cycle course of immunotherapy, consisting of Toripalimab administered at a dosage of 240 mg on day 1 every 21 days, supplemented by Ipilimumab at a dosage of 50 mg on day 1 every 42 days. Following the completion of the immunotherapeutic regimen, the patient proceeded with surgical intervention at our hospital. Notably, her levels of CEA, AFP, CA72-4, CA19-9, and CA24-2 remained within the normal range. Subsequent gastroscopic evaluation unveiled scar-like alterations in the middle and posterior regions of the stomach, approximately 41–46 cm from the incisors, ostensibly attributable to the influence of immunotherapy (refer to Fig. 3.45). Final diagnosis: Gastric cancer (ycT2N1M0).

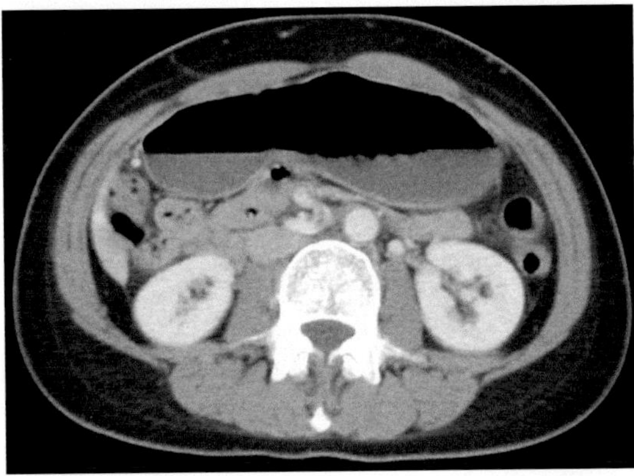

Fig. 3.43 Demonstrates the findings of an abdominal CT scan, revealing the gastric wall to be adequately filled, without any definitive evidence of thickening. Moreover, an absence of enlarged lymph nodes is observed within the abdomen, pelvis, or inguinal region

3.17.2 Treatment

Following the patient's selection for elective general anesthesia, a radical total gastrectomy procedure was performed, utilizing the D2 technique with Roux-en-Y reconstruction and overlap, resulting in complete tumor resection (R0).

The pathology report, titled "Post-immunotherapy (total gastrectomy)," provides insights into the histopathological examination. It reveals the presence of a small residual quantity of moderately to poorly differentiated adenocarcinoma (Lauren classification: mixed type) visible within the mucosa of the gastric body. The extent of the residual tumor is limited to the submucosal layer and exhibits significant cellular degeneration. Surrounding the residual tumor, there is a notable infiltration of inflammatory cells and the

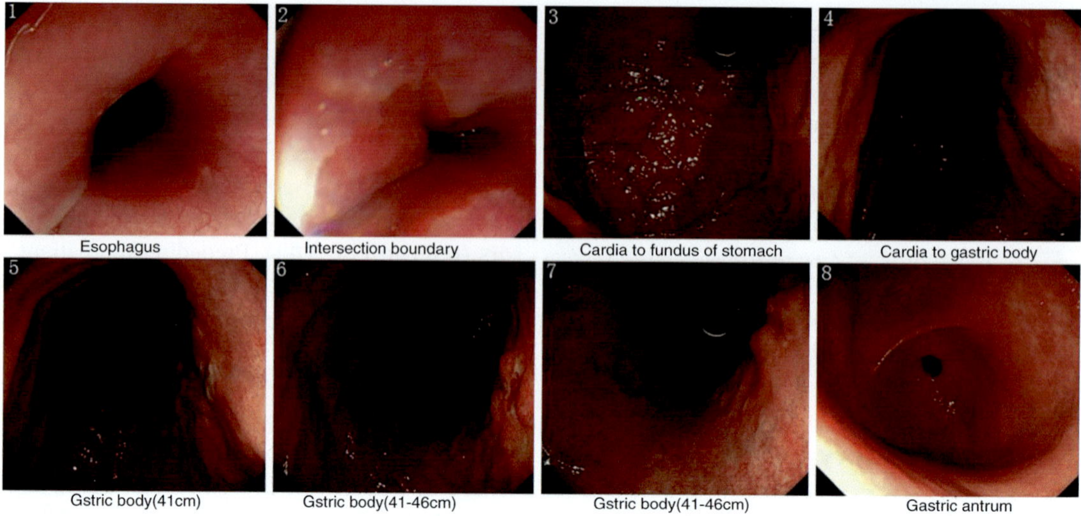

Fig. 3.44 Gastroscopic examination indicated the neoplasm located in the upper and middle sections of the stomach, approximately 41-46 cm from the incisors

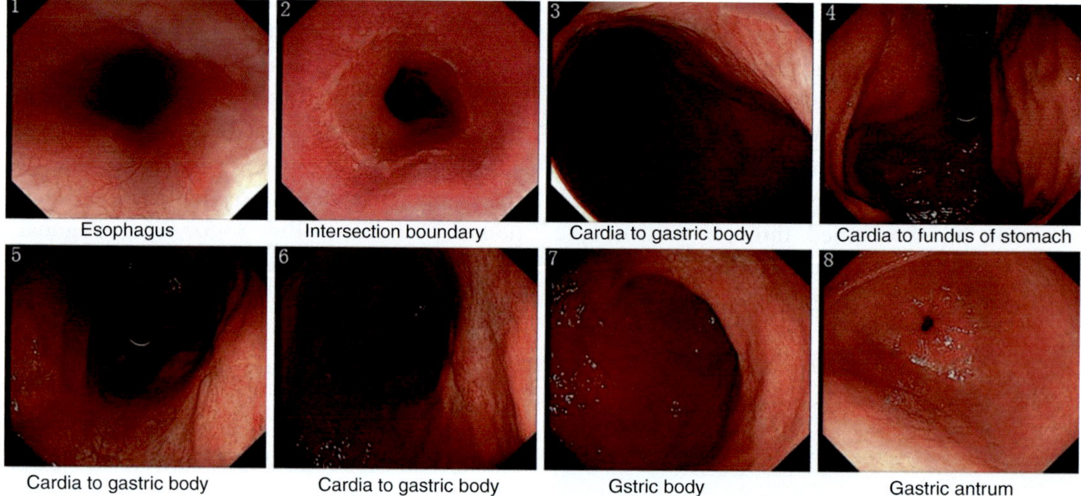

Fig. 3.45 Displays scar-like alterations detected in the posterior wall of the gastric body, adjacent to the lesser curvature. These changes, observed 1 month subsequent to immunotherapy administration, are indicative of post-immunotherapy effects

formation of lymphoid follicles, indicative of moderate post-treatment changes (Mandard TRG grade 3). Notably, no involvement of the gastroesophageal junction or pylorus duodenal area is observed. The surgical margins are free from malignant cells. Furthermore, thorough examination of 47 dissected lymph nodes reveals no evidence of metastatic carcinoma (0/47). According to ypTNM staging, the patient's condition is classified as ypT1aN0M0, corresponding to stage IA. Please refer to Fig. 3.46 for pathology images accompanying this report.

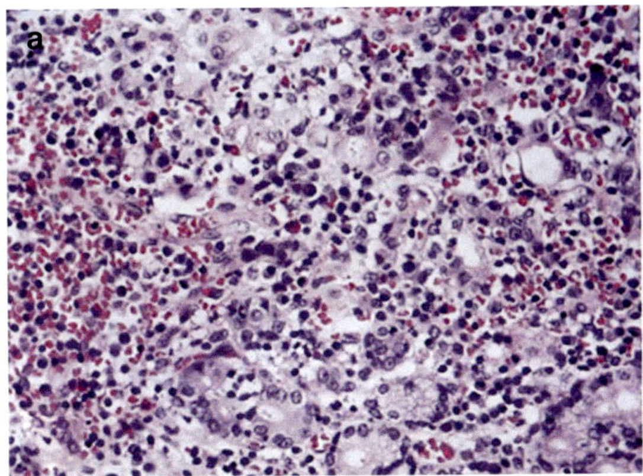
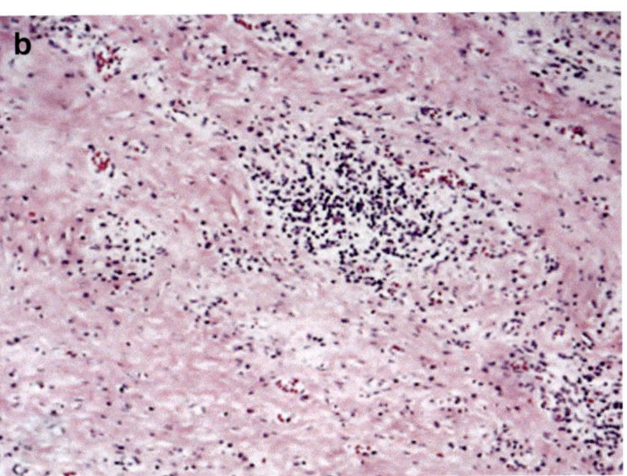

Fig. 3.46 (**a**) MSI-H Adenocarcinoma (HE ×200), a few cancer cells are mainly located in the lamina propria of the mucosa, and are scattered or strip shaped, surrounded by eosinophils, lymphocytes, and other inflammatory cells; (**b**) MSI-H adenocarcinoma (HE ×100) showing significant interstitial fibrosis in the submucosa, accompanied by more lymphocyte infiltration, consistent with the treatment response

3.17.3 Case Analysis

3.17.3.1 MSI-H Gastric Cancer: A Special Population in Gastric Cancer

Gastric cancer is a highly heterogeneous tumor, and current research focuses on individualized treatment based on accurate classification. One of the mechanisms of tumorigenesis is microsatellite instability (MSI), which refers to base pair insertion or loss in microsatellite fragments caused by deficiency in the DNA mismatch repair system (Mismatch repair deficiency or dMMR) [220].

In the analysis and classification of gastric cancer conducted by the Cancer Genome Atlas (TCGA), MSI-H (Microsatellite instability-high) gastric cancer accounts for approximately 22% of cases [221]. Patients with MSI-H gastric cancer exhibit distinct clinicopathological characteristics, including older age, female sex, distal gastric cancer, intestinal type according to the Lauren classification, fewer instances of lymph node metastasis, and earlier pathological stages (TNM stage II and III) [222].

Numerous studies have demonstrated that patients with MSI-H gastric cancer generally have a more favorable prognosis [223] A post-hoc analysis of the MAGIC trial in 2017 revealed the following [224]: Among gastric cancer patients who underwent surgical treatment alone, the overall survival of the MSI-H group was slightly better than that of the non-MSI-H group although the difference was not statistically significant. However, when MSI-H patients received perioperative chemotherapy, their survival outcomes were worse compared to the non-MSI-H group ($P = 0.03$). Similarly, post-hoc analyses of the CLASSIC trial in 2019 [225] and the ITACA-S trial in 2020 [226] both indicated a survival advantage for patients with MSI-H gastric cancer, regardless of whether they received radiotherapy or chemotherapy during the perioperative period. The favorable prognosis of MSI-H tumors may be attributed to their clinicopathological features. Several studies have revealed that more than 70% of MSI-H gastric cancers are of the intestinal type [227–230], which is associated with a good prognosis. Furthermore, compared to MSS (Microsatellite stability) gastric cancer, MSI-H tumors exhibit a higher mutation burden and greater infiltration of cytotoxic T lymphocytes [231]. Tumors with a high mutation burden have the potential to encode non-self-immunogenic neo-epitopes, thereby triggering recruitment of intratumoral lymphocytes and eliciting a robust immune response [231]. Excessive activation of intratumoral cytotoxic T lymphocytes may lead to tumor cell apoptosis, reducing postoperative residual micrometastasis and the risk of recurrence, thus explaining the favorable prognosis observed in MSI-H gastric cancer.

3.17.3.2 The Effect of Chemotherapy Is Controversial: MSI-H Gastric Cancer Is Not Sensitive to Chemotherapy

Limited studies have investigated the relationship between MSI-H gastric cancer and chemotherapy, and the findings have been inconsistent. An et al. conducted a retrospective study in 2012, involving 1722 patients with R0 resected gastric cancer in Korea [227]. The results demonstrated that non-MSI-H gastric cancer patients derived significant benefits from 5-fluorouracil (5-FU)-based adjuvant chemotherapy, whereas patients with MSI-H gastric cancer at stages II and III exhibited similar disease-free survival rates in both the postoperative chemotherapy group and the surgery-alone group. Subsequently, post-hoc analyses of the MAGIC trial in 2017 [224] and the CLASSIC trial in 2019 [232] yielded similar conclusions, indicating that MSI-H gastric cancer patients did not experience improved outcomes from perioperative or postoperative adjuvant chemotherapy. Notably, the post-hoc analysis of the MAGIC trial revealed that the prognosis of the surgery-alone group was superior to that of the perioperative chemotherapy group. It is worth mentioning that the perioperative chemotherapy regimen in the MAGIC trial involved the ECF regimen (Epirubicin, cisplatin, and fluorouracil), while the chemotherapy regimen in the CLASSIC trial consisted of capecitabine in combination with oxaliplatin; however, both trials incorporated 5-fluorouracil. Consequently, further exploration is warranted to determine the therapeutic sensitivity of MSI-H gastric cancer patients to 5-FU. Additionally, Miceli et al. presented the post-hoc analysis results from the ARTIST trial, which revealed no differences in overall survival (OS) and disease-free survival (DFS) between MSI-H and non-MSI-H populations among patients receiving chemotherapy or chemoradiotherapy after gastric cancer surgery [233]. These findings suggest that chemotherapy may attenuate the favorable prognosis associated with MSI-H gastric cancer, thereby eliminating the survival disparity between MSI-H and non-MSI-H gastric cancer patients.

3.17.3.3 The Era of Immunotherapy: New Prospects for the Treatment of MSI-H Gastric Cancer

Immunotherapy has shown remarkable advancements in the management of MSI-H solid tumors in recent years. In 2017, Le et al. conducted a study involving 86 patients with 12 different types of dMMR solid tumors who had previously failed chemotherapy. These patients were treated with pembrolizumab, and the results revealed an impressive objective response rate (ORR) of 53%, with a complete remission (CR) rate of 21% [234]. Based on these findings, the US Food and Drug Administration (FDA) granted approval for the use of pembrolizumab in children and adults with unresectable or metastatic solid tumors exhibiting microsatellite instability-high (MSI-H) or mismatch repair-deficient (dMMR) characteristics.

Since then, investigations into immunotherapy for MSI-H gastric cancer have continued, primarily focusing on advanced cases [235–240]. Regrettably, the current body of research in this area consists mainly of subgroup analyses with small sample sizes, and the treatment outcomes have not been as promising as those observed in colon cancer. Nonetheless, these studies have provided crucial insights and supportive evidence for exploring the potential of immunotherapy in MSI-H gastric cancer. However, the efficacy of immunotherapy in this context still needs to be confirmed through large-scale trials in the future.

3.17.4 Expert Comments

MSI-H gastric cancer represents a distinctive subgroup within the broader category of gastric cancer, characterized by specific clinical features, a favorable prognosis, a unique tumor microenvironment, and a distinct response to chemotherapy and immunotherapy. Given the molecular biological characteristics of MSI-H gastric cancer, immunotherapy offers a promising avenue for precision treatment and demonstrates unique advantages across all stages of gastric cancer management. Although the current research evidence remains limited, we recommend that patients with gastric cancer undergo molecular typing testing prior to treatment, and for those diagnosed with MSI-H gastric cancer, immunotherapy drugs should be incorporated into the optimal treatment plan. As large-scale clinical trials continue to unfold, we anticipate further advancements in the treatment landscape and improved outcomes for patients with MSI-H gastric cancer.

Case provider: Lulu Zhao, Yingtai Chen.

Expert comments: Dongbing Zhao.

References

1. Wu AW, Shan F, Xue WC, et al. Clinicopathological observation of gastric cancer with pathological complete response following neoadjuvant chemotherapy. Zhonghua Wei Chang Wai Ke Za Zhi. 2011;14(8):596–8. Chinese
2. Becker K, Mueller JD, Schulmacher C, et al. Histomorphology and grading of regression in gastric carcinoma treated with neoadjuvant chemotherapy. Cancer. 2003;98(7):1521–30.
3. Kitano S, Lso Y, Moriyama M, et al. Laparoscopy-assisted Billroth I gastrectomy. Surg Laparosc Endosc. 1994;4(2):146–8.
4. Yu J, Huang C, Sun Y, et al. Effect of laparoscopic vs open distal gastrectomy on 3-year disease-free survival in patients with locally advanced gastric cancer: the CLASS-01 randomized clinical trial. JAMA. 2019;321(20):1983–92.
5. Katai H, Mizusawa J, Katayama H, et al. Short-term surgical outcomes from a phase III study of laparoscopy-assisted versus open distal gastrectomy with nodal dissection for clinical stage IA/IB gastric cancer: Japan clinical oncology group study JCOG0912. Gastric Cancer. 2017;20(4):699–708.
6. Kim W, Kim HH, Han SU, et al. Decreased morbidity of laparoscopic distal gastrectomy compared with open distal gastrectomy for stage I gastric cancer: short-term outcomes from a multicenter randomized controlled trial (KLASS-01). Ann Surg. 2016;263(1):28–35.
7. Hu Y, Huang C, Sun Y, et al. Morbidity and mortality of laparoscopic versus open D2 distal gastrectomy for advanced gastric cancer: a randomized controlled trial. J Clin Oncol. 2016;34(12):1350–7.
8. Honda M, Hiki N, Kinoshita T, et al. Long-term outcomes of laparoscopic versus open surgery for clinical stage I gastric cancer: the LOC-1 study. Ann Surg. 2016;264(2):214–22.
9. Cho SY, Lee KS, Kim JH, et al. Effect of combined systematized behavioral modification education program with desmopressin in patients with nocturia: a prospective, multicenter, randomized, and parallel study. Int Neurourol J. 2014;18(4):213–20.
10. Kim HH, Hyung WJ, Cho GS, et al. Morbidity and mortality of laparoscopic gastrectomy versus open gastrectomy for gastric cancer: an interim report—a phase III multicenter, prospective, randomized trial (KLASS trial). Ann Surg. 2010;251(3):417–20.
11. Li Z, Shan F, Ying X, et al. Assessment of laparoscopic distal gastrectomy after neoadjuvant chemotherapy for locally advanced gastric cancer: a randomized clinical trial. JAMA Surg. 2019;154(12):1093–101.
12. Van Der Wielen N, Straatman J, Daams F, et al. Open versus minimally invasive total gastrectomy after neoadjuvant chemotherapy: results of a European randomized trial. Gastric Cancer. 2021;24(1):258–71.
13. Liao XL, Liang XW, Pang HY, et al. Safety and efficacy of laparoscopic versus open gastrectomy in patients with advanced gastric cancer following neoadjuvant chemotherapy: a meta-analysis. Front Oncol. 2021;11:704244.
14. Ajani JA, D'Amico TA, Almhanna K, et al. Gastric cancer, version 3.2016, NCCN clinical practice guidelines in oncology. J Natl Compr Cancer Netw. 2016;14(10):1286.
15. Ojima T, Nakamori M, Nakamura M, et al. Laparoscopic gastrojejunostomy for patients with unresectable gastric cancer with gastric outlet obstruction. J Gastrointest Surg. 2017;21(8):1220–5.
16. Jang S, Stevens T, Lopez R, et al. Superiority of gastrojejunostomy over endoscopic stenting for palliation of malignant gastric outlet obstruction. Clin Gastroenterol Hepatol. 2018;17(7):1295–1302.e1.
17. Kaminishi M, Yamaguchi H, Shimizu N, et al. Stomach partitioning gastrojejunostomy for unresectable gastric carcinoma. Arch Surg. 1997;132(2):184–7.
18. Tanaka T, Suda K, Satoh S, et al. Effectiveness of laparoscopic stomach-partitioning gastrojejunostomy for patients with gastric outlet obstruction caused by advanced gastric cancer. Surg Endosc. 2017;31(1):359–67.
19. O'regan PJ, Scarrow GD. Laparoscopic jejunostomy. Endoscopy. 1990;22(1):39–40.
20. Mohiuddin SS, Anderson CE. A novel application for single-incision laparoscopic surgery (SILS): SIL jejunostomy feeding tube placement. Surg Endosc. 2011;25(1):323–7.
21. Ramesh S, Dehn TC. Laparoscopic feeding jejunostomy. Br J Surg. 1996;83(8):1090.

22. Morris JB, Mullen JL, Yu JC, et al. Laparoscopic-guided jejunostomy. Surgery. 1992;112(1):96–9.
23. Ellis LM, Evans DB, Martin D, et al. Laparoscopic feeding jejunostomy tube in oncology patients. Surg Oncol. 1992;1(3):245–9.
24. Smyth EC, Nilsson M, Grabsch HI, et al. Gastric cancer. Lancet. 2020;396(10251):635–48.
25. Moertel CG, Bargen JA, Soule EH. Multiple gastric cancers; review of the literature and study of 42 cases. Gastroenterology. 1957;32(6):1095–103.
26. Oh SJ, Bae DS, Suh BJ. Synchronous triple primary cancers occurring in the stomach, kidney, and thyroid. Ann Surg Treat Res. 2015;88(6):345–8.
27. Demandante CG, Troyer DA, Miles TP. Multiple primary malignant neoplasms: case report and a comprehensive review of the literature. Am J Clin Oncol. 2003;26(1):79–83.
28. Jin F, Rao BQ, Ouyang XN, et al. The incidence of multiple carcinoma in 3292 cases of digestive system malignancy. Chin J Oncol. 2003;11:27–9.
29. Kong P, Wu R, Lan Y, et al. Association between mismatch-repair genetic variation and the risk of multiple primary cancers: a meta-analysis. J Cancer. 2017;8(16):3296–308.
30. Fan L, Yu Z, Ren J, et al. Distribution and prognosis of 61 cases with multiple primary carcinoma. J Fourth Mil Med Univ. 2002;01:95–6.
31. Park YK, Kim DY, Joo JK, et al. Clinicopathological features of gastric carcinoma patients with other primary carcinomas. Langenbeck Arch Surg. 2005;390(4):300–5.
32. Tokunaga M, Hiki N, Fukunaga T, et al. Laparoscopic surgery for synchronous gastric and colorectal cancer: a preliminary experience. Langenbeck Arch Surg. 2010;395(3):207–10.
33. Matsui H, Okamoto Y, Ishii A, et al. Laparoscopy-assisted combined resection for synchronous gastric and colorectal cancer: report of three cases. Surg Today. 2009;39(5):434–9.
34. Massironi S, Sciola V, Peracchi M, et al. Neuroendocrine tumors of the gastro-entero-pancreatic system. World J Gastroenterol. 2008;14(35):5377–84.
35. Guo LJ, Tang CW. Current status of clinical studies on gastrointestinal and pancreatic neuroendocrine tumors in China. Gastroenterology. 2012;17(05):276–8.
36. Liu Z, Li JQ, Tian DY, et al. Clinical analysis of 29 cases with neuroendocrine tumors of digestive system. Chin J Gastrointest Surg. 2013;16(11):1084–7.
37. Wang XY, Zeng Y, Liang H. Diagnosis, treatment and prognosis of gastroduodenal neuroendocrine tumor. Med J Chin Peoples Liberation Army. 2016;41(03):233–7.
38. Chen X. Application of endoscopic ultrasonography in diagnosis and treatment of gastrointestinal neuroendocrine tumors and analysis of clinical features. Zhejiang University; 2016.
39. Karagiannis S, Eshagzaiy K, Duecker C, et al. Endoscopic resection with the cap technique of a carcinoid tumor in the duodenal bulb. Endoscopy. 2009;41(Suppl 2):E288–9.
40. Han SL, Cheng J, Zhou HZ, et al. Surgically treated primary malignant tumor of small bowel: a clinical analysis. World J Gastroenterol. 2010;16(12):1527–32.
41. Li YQ, Sun DF, Xue XF. Clinical effect of laparoscopic resection and endoscopy in the treatment of gastrointestinal tumors. Clin Res Pract. 2018;3(33):11–2.
42. Guan LL, Li XH. Clinical analysis of minimally invasive treatment of gastrointestinal benign tumors by laparoscopy combined with endoscopy. Chi Hea Indu. 2014;11(03):166–7.
43. Toyonaga T, Nakamura K, Araki Y, et al. Laparoscopic treatment of duodenal carcinoid tumor. Wedge resection of the duodenal bulb under endoscopic control. Surg Endosc. 1998;12(8):1085–7.
44. Bowers SP, Smith CD. Laparoscopic resection of posterior duodenal bulb carcinoid tumor. Am Surg. 2003;69(9):792–5.
45. Balfour D. Factors influencing the life expectancy of patients operated on for gastric ulcer. Ann Surg. 1922;76(3):405–8.
46. Chen XP, Wang JP, Zhao JZ. Surgery. 9th ed. Beijing: People's Health Publishing House; 2018. p. 345.
47. Zhang SW, Sun KX, Zheng RS, et al. Cancer incidence and mortality in China, 2015. JNCC. 2020;1(1):2–11.
48. Tanigawa N, Nomura E, Lee S, et al. Current state of gastric stump carcinoma in Japan: based on the results of a nationwide survey. World J Surg. 2010;34(7):1540–7.
49. Kidokoro T, Hayashida Y, Urabe M. Long-term surgical results of carcinoma of the gastric remnant: a statistical analysis of 613 patients from 98 institutions. World J Surg. 1985;9(6):966–71.
50. Gao ZD, Jiang KW, Ye YJ, et al. Interpretation on Chinese surgeons' consensus opinion for the definition of gastric stump cancer (version 2018). Chin J Gastrointest Surg. 2018;21(5):486–90.
51. Hu X, Zhang C. Excerpt of Japanese classification of gastric carcinoma (the 15th edition). Chin J Pract Surg. 2018;38(05):520–8.
52. China Cooperation Group for the Diagnosis and Treatment of Gastric Remnant Cancer. Chinese surgeons' consensus opinion for the definition of gastric stump cancer (version 2018). Chin J Gastrointest Surg. 2018;21(5):483–5.
53. Li F, Zhang R, Liang H, et al. The pattern of lymph node metastasis and the suitability of 7th UICC N stage in predicting prognosis of remnant gastric cancer. J Cancer Res Clin Oncol. 2012;138(1):111–7.
54. Japanese Gastric Cancer Association. Japanese classification of gastric carcinoma-2nd English edition. Gastric Cancer. 1998;1(1):10–24.
55. Han S, Hua Y, Wang C, et al. Metastatic pattern of lymph node and surgery for gastric stump cancer. J Surg Oncol. 2003;82(4):241–6.

56. Liang H. Advertent problems about gastric stump cancer surgery. Chin J Gastrointest Surg. 2018;21(5):502–6.
57. Kitano S, Iso Y, Moriyama M, et al. Laparoscopy-assisted Billroth I gastrectomy. Surg Laparosc Endosc. 1994;4(2):146–8.
58. Yamada H, Kojima K, Yamashita T, et al. Laparoscopy-assisted resection of gastric remnant cancer. Surg Laparosc Endosc Percutan Tech. 2005;15(4):226–9.
59. Tsunoda S, Okabe H, Tanaka E, et al. Laparoscopic gastrectomy for remnant gastric cancer: a comprehensive review and case series. Gastric Cancer. 2016;19(1):287–92.
60. Booka E, Kaihara M, Mihara K, et al. Laparoscopic total gastrectomy for remnant gastric cancer: a single-institution experience. Asian J Endosc Surg. 2019;12(1):58–63.
61. Kitadani J, Ojima T, Nakamura M, et al. Safety and feasibility of laparoscopic gastrectomy for remnant gastric cancer compared with open gastrectomy: single-center experience. Medicine (Baltimore). 2021;100(4):e23932.
62. Zhang RC, Xu XW, Mou YP, et al. Laparoscopic gastrectomy for gastric stump cancer: analysis of 7 cases. Chin J Gastrointest Surg. 2016;19(5):553–6.
63. Shimada H, Fukagawa T, Haga Y, et al. Does remnant gastric cancer really differ from primary gastric cancer? A systematic review of the literature by the Task Force of Japanese Gastric Cancer Association. Gastric Cancer. 2015;19(2):339–49.
64. Omori T, Oyama T, Akamatsu H, et al. Transumbilical single-incision laparoscopic distal gastrectomy for early gastric cancer. Surg Endosc. 2011;25(7):2400–4.
65. Ertem M, Ozveri E, Gok H, et al. Single incision laparoscopic total gastrectomy and D2 lymph node dissection for gastric cancer using a four-access single port: the first experience. Case Rep Surg. 2013;2013:504549.
66. Ahn SH, Park DJ, Son SY, et al. Single-incision laparoscopic total gastrectomy with D1+beta lymph node dissection for proximal early gastric cancer. Gastric Cancer. 2014;17(2):392–6.
67. Lee CM, Park DW, Jung DH, et al. Single-port laparoscopic proximal gastrectomy with double tract reconstruction for early gastric cancer: report of a case. J Gastric Cancer. 2016;16(3):200–6.
68. Kunisaki C, Makino H, Yamaguchi N, et al. Surgical advantages of reduced-port laparoscopic gastrectomy in gastric cancer. Surg Endosc. 2016;30(12):5520–8.
69. Omori T, Fujiwara Y, Yamamoto K, et al. The safety and feasibility of single-port laparoscopic gastrectomy for advanced gastric cancer. J Gastrointest Surg. 2019;23(7):1329–39.
70. Inaki N, Tsuji T, Doden K, et al. Reduced port laparoscopic gastrectomy for gastric cancer. Transl Gastroenterol Hepatol. 2016;1:38.
71. Surgical Single Hole Group of Minimally Noninvasive Professional Committee of Chinese Medical Doctor Association. Expert consensus on single-port plus laparoscopic gastric cancer surgery (2020 edition). J Laparosc Surg. 2021;26(1):7–12.
72. Lee S, Kim JK, Kim YN, et al. Safety and feasibility of reduced-port robotic distal gastrectomy for gastric cancer: a phase I/II clinical trial. Surg Endosc. 2017;31(10):4002–9.
73. Seo WJ, Son T, Shin H, et al. Reduced-port totally robotic distal subtotal gastrectomy for gastric cancer: 100 consecutive cases in comparison with conventional robotic and laparoscopic distal subtotal gastrectomy. Sci Rep. 2020;10(1):16015.
74. Yan S, Xinfu M, Kang Z, et al. Technical difficulties of single-port and reduced-hole laparoscopic radical gastrectomy. Chin J Dig Surg. 2019;18(03):222–8.
75. Zhicheng Y, Wei X, Xingwang Z, et al. Three cases of laparoscopic abdominal surgery in patients with severe kyphotic deformity. Chin J Endosc Surg. 2020;13(6):377–80.
76. Zhengqian W, Yangwen L, Deqian K. Laparoscopic cholecystectomy for patients with benign gallbladder diseases and kyphosis. Minim Invasive Med. 2009;4(1):15–6.
77. Raw DA, Beattie JK, Hunter JM. Anaesthesia for spinal surgery in adults. Br J Anaesth. 2003;6:886–904.
78. Zakoji H, Miyamoto T, Kira S, et al. Complete laparoscopic nephroureterectomy for the upper urinary tract urothelial carcinoma in a female patient with severe senile kyphosis: an initial case report. J Endourol Case Rep. 2015;1(1):56–8.
79. Yao SY, Ikeda A, Tada Y. Reduced port laparoscopic surgery for colon cancer in a patient with tuberculous kyphosis and dwarfism: a rare case and literature review. Wideochir Inne Tech Maloinwazyjne. 2015;10(2):275–81.
80. Yifei Z, Yi S, Haile P. Research progress of kyphotic deformity. Med Rev. 2016;22(08):69–72.
81. Zhang M, Zhang H, Ma Y, et al. Prognosis and surgical treatment of gastric cancer invasive adjacent organs. ANZ J Surg. 2010;80(7–8):510–4.
82. Azagra JS, Goergen M, De Simone P, et al. Minimally invasive surgery for gastric cancer. Surg Endosc. 1999;13(4):351–7.
83. Uyama I, Sugioka A, Fujita J, et al. Laparoscopic total gastrectomy with distal pancreatosplenectomy and D2 lymphadenectomy for advanced gastric cancer. Gastric Cancer. 1999;2(4):230–4.
84. Carboni F, Lepiane P, Santoro R, et al. Extended multiorgan resection for T4 gastric carcinoma: 25-year experience. J Surg Oncol. 2005;90(2):95–100.
85. Maehara Y, Oiwa H, Tomisaki S, et al. Prognosis and surgical treatment of gastric cancer invasive the pancreas. Oncology. 2000;59(1):1–6.
86. Japanese Gastric Cancer Association. Japanese gastric cancer treatment guidelines 2014 (ver. 4). Gastric Cancer. 2017;20(1):1–19.
87. Guo L, Yang TF, Zhang M, et al. Diagnosis and treatment of 11 cases with multiple gastric carcinoma. Chin Med J. 2013;03:338–40.

88. Kosaka T, Miwa K, Yonemura Y, et al. A clinicopathologic study on multiple gastric cancers with special reference to distal gastrectomy. Cancer. 1990;65(11):2602–5.
89. Matsuda A, Kato S, Furuya M, et al. Multiple early gastric cancer with duodenal invasion. World J Gastroenterol. 2007;5:125.
90. Hamm A, Veeck J, Bektas N, et al. Frequent expression loss of Inter-alpha-trypsin inhibitor heavy chain (ITIH) genes in multiple human solid tumors: a systematic expression analysis. BMC Cancer. 2008;8:25.
91. Yuan L, Liu LX, Che GW. The advancement of predictive diagnosis and molecular mechanism in multiple primary lung cancer. Chin J Cancer. 2010;29(5):575–8.
92. Feng RM, Zong YN, Cao SM, et al. Current cancer situation in China: good or bad news from the 2018 Global Cancer Statistics? Cancer Commun (London, England). 2019;39(1):22.
93. Ji YB, Ji CF, Yue L. Human gastric cancer cell line SGC-7901 apoptosis induced by SFPS-B2 via a mitochondrial-mediated pathway. Bio-med Mater Eng. 2014;24(1):1141–7.
94. Zhou MT, He WH, Lv NH. Interpretation of practice guidelines for gastric cancer in Korea, 2018 edition. Chin J Dig. 2020;03:212–6.
95. Sun XW, Zhan YQ, Li W, et al. Analysis of 58 cases with multiple primary gastric cancer. Chin J Cli Onco. 2007;05:261–5.
96. Gweon TG, Park JM, Lim CH, et al. Trimodal imaging endoscopy reduces the risk of synchronous gastric neoplasia. Eur J Gastroenterol Hepatol. 2015;27(3):215–20.
97. Otsuji E, Kuriu Y, Ichikawa D, et al. Clinicopathologic characteristics and prognosis of synchronous multifocal gastric carcinomas. Am J Surg. 2005;189(1):116–9.
98. Hu X, Bi W, An WD, et al. Study on the scope of gastrectomy for multiple gastric cancers. Chin J Gastrointestinal Surg. 2002;01:17–9.
99. Kim HG, Ryu SY, Lee JH, et al. Clinicopathologic features and prognosis of synchronous multiple gastric carcinomas. Acta chirurgica Belgica. 2012;112(2):148–53.
100. Raziee HR, Cardoso R, Seevaratnam R, et al. Systematic review of the predictors of positive margins in gastric cancer surgery and the effect on survival. Gastric Cancer. 2012;15(Suppl 1):S116–24.
101. Woo JW, Ryu KW, Park JY, et al. Prognostic impact of microscopic tumor involved resection margin in advanced gastric cancer patients after gastric resection. World J Surg. 2014;38(2):439–46.
102. Ma LX, Espin-Garcia O, Lim CH, et al. Impact of adjuvant therapy in patients with a microscopically positive margin after resection for gastric and esophageal cancers. J Gastrointest Oncol. 2020;11(2):356–65.
103. Endo S, Fujiwara Y, Yamatsuji T, et al. Is it necessary to confirm negative margins in gastrectomy for peritoneal lavage cytology-positive gastric cancer? Anticancer Res. 2020;40(10):5807–13.
104. Liang Y, Ding X, Wang X, et al. Prognostic value of surgical margin status in gastric cancer patients. ANZ J Surg. 2015;85(9):678–84.
105. Nagata T, Ichikawa D, Komatsu S, et al. Prognostic impact of microscopic positive margin in gastric cancer patients. J Surg Oncol. 2011;104(6):592–7.
106. Cho BC, Jeung HC, Choi HJ, et al. Prognostic impact of resection margin involvement after extended (D2/D3) gastrectomy for advanced gastric cancer: a 15-year experience at a single institute. J Surg Oncol. 2007;95(6):461–8.
107. Shen JG, Cheong JH, Hyung WJ, et al. Influence of a microscopic positive proximal margin in the treatment of gastric adenocarcinoma of the cardia. World J Gastroenterol. 2006;12(24):3883–6.
108. Bickenbach KA, Gonen M, Strong V, et al. Association of positive transection margins with gastric cancer survival and local recurrence. Ann Surg Oncol. 2013;20(8):2663–8.
109. Polom K, Marrelli D, Smyth EC, et al. The role of microsatellite instability in positive margin gastric cancer patients. Surg Innov. 2018;25(2):99–104.
110. Sun Z, Li DM, Wang ZN, et al. Prognostic significance of microscopic positive margins for gastric cancer patients with potentially curative resection. Ann Surg Oncol. 2009;16(11):3028–37.
111. Ajani JA, D'Amico TA, Almhanna K, et al. Gastric cancer, version 3.2016, NCCN clinical practice guidelines in oncology. J Natl Compreh Cancer Netw JNCCN. 2016;14(10):1286–312.
112. Rhome RM, Moshier E, Sarpel U, et al. Predictors of positive margins after definitive resection for gastric adenocarcinoma and impact of adjuvant therapies. Int J Radiat Oncol Biol Phys. 2017;98(5):1106–15.
113. Peifan Z, Mengchang. Special types in early gastric cancer. Chin J Cancer. 1990;012(001):52–5.
114. Hongying C, Guowei L, Jianying L, et al. Three cases of one point gastric carcinoma and review of domestic literature. Chin J Endosc. 2005;011(007):772–4.
115. Wenzhen Y, Ruchao M, Xiaoyun Z, et al. Two cases of one spot gastric carcinoma and literature review. J Lanzhou Univ (Med Edition). 2015;41(005):68–70.
116. Llanos O, Guzman S, Duarte I. Accuracy of the first endoscopic procedure in the differential diagnosis of gastric lesions. Ann Surg. 1982;195(2):224–6.
117. Honghua Z, Xiaoling X, Chao S, et al. One case of gastric poorly differentiated adenocarcinoma with one spot cancer in the posterior wall of the stomach body. J Gastroenterol. 2015;5:317–8.
118. Rulin M, Ziyu L, Jiafu J. The diagnosis and treatment status and development trend of early gastric cancer in China were analyzed based on the data of gastrointestinal Cancer Surgical Association in China. Chin J Pract Surg. 2019;39(05):419–23.
119. De B, Rhome R, Jairam V, et al. Gastric adenocarcinoma in young adult patients: patterns of care and survival in the United States. Gastric Cancer. 2018;21(6):889–99.

120. Merchant SJ, Kim J, Choi AH, et al. A rising trend in the incidence of advanced gastric cancer in young Hispanic men. Gastric Cancer. 2017;20(2):226–34.
121. Keegan TH, Ries LA, Barr RD, et al. Comparison of cancer survival trends in the United States of adolescents and young adults with those in children and older adults. Cancer. 2016;122(7):1009–16.
122. Parsons HM, Harlan LC, Lynch CF, et al. Impact of cancer on work and education among adolescent and young adult cancer survivors. J Clin Oncol. 2012;30(19):2393–400.
123. Li J. Gastric cancer in young adults: a different clinical entity from carcinogenesis to prognosis. Gastroenterol Res Pract. 2020;2020:9512707.
124. Clinicopathological characteristics and survival outcomes of younger patients with gastric cancer: a systematic review and meta-analysis. Transl Cancer Res. 2020;9(10):6026–38.
125. Kulig J, Popiela T, Kolodziejczyk P, et al. Clinicopathological profile and long-term outcome in young adults with gastric cancer: multicenter evaluation of 214 patients. Langenbecks Arch Surg. 2008;393(1):37–43.
126. Pisanu A, Podda M, Cois A, et al. Gastric cancer in the young: is it a different clinical entity? A retrospective cohort study. Gastroenterol Res Pract. 2014;2014:125038.
127. Koshida Y, Koizumi W, Sasabe M, et al. Association of Helicobacter pylori-dependent gastritis with gastric carcinomas in young Japanese patients: histopathological comparison of diffuse and intestinal type cancer cases. Histopathology. 2000;37(2):124–30.
128. Hirahashi M, Yao T, Matsumoto T, et al. Intramucosal gastric adenocarcinoma of poorly differentiated type in the young is characterized by Helicobacter pylori infection and antral lymphoid hyperplasia. Mod Pathol. 2007;20(1):29–34.
129. Yaghoobi M, Rakhshani N, Sadr F, et al. Hereditary risk factors for the development of gastric cancer in younger patients. BMC Gastroenterol. 2004;4:28.
130. Chung HW, Noh SH, Lim JB. Analysis of demographic characteristics in 3242 young age gastric cancer patients in Korea. World J Gastroenterol. 2010;16(2):256–63.
131. Medina-Franco H, Heslin MJ, Cortes-Gonzalez R. Clinicopathological characteristics of gastric carcinoma in young and elderly patients: a comparative study. Ann Surg Oncol. 2000;7(7):515–9.
132. Zhou F, Shi J, Fang C, et al. Gastric carcinomas in young (younger than 40 years) Chinese patients: clinicopathology, family history, and postresection survival. Medicine (Baltimore). 2016;95(9):e2873.
133. Wesołowska M, Pawlik P, Jagodziński PP. The clinicopathologic significance of estrogen receptors in human gastric carcinoma. Biomed Pharmacother. 2016;83:314–22.
134. Zhou F, Xu Y, Shi J, et al. Expression profile of E-cadherin, estrogen receptors, and P53 in early-onset gastric cancers. Cancer Med. 2016;9(12):3403–11.
135. Matsuyama S, Ohkura Y, Eguchi H, et al. Estrogen receptor beta is expressed in human stomach adenocarcinoma. J Cancer Res Clin Oncol. 2002;128(6):319–24.
136. Tekesin K, Emin Gunes M, Tural D, et al. Clinicopathological characteristics, prognosis and survival outcome of gastric cancer in young patients: a large cohort retrospective study. JBUON. 2019;24(2):672–8.
137. Isobe T, Hashimoto K, Kizaki J, et al. Characteristics and prognosis of gastric cancer in young patients. Oncol Rep. 2013;30(1):43–9.
138. Cormedi MCV, Katayama MLH, Guindalini RSC, et al. Survival and prognosis of young adults with gastric cancer. Clinics (Sao Paulo, Brazil). 2018;73(suppl 1):e651s.
139. Tavares A, Gandra A, Viveiros F, et al. Analysis of clinicopathologic characteristics and prognosis of gastric cancer in young and older patients. Pathol Oncol Res POR. 2013;19(1):111–7.
140. Modlin IM, Lye KD, Kidd M. A 5-decade analysis of 13,715 carcinomas. Cancer. 2003;97(4):934–59.
141. Nagtegaal ID, Odze RD, Klimstra D, et al. The 2019 WHO classification of tumors of the digestive system. Histopathology. 2020;76(2):182–8.
142. Pavel M, Öberg K, Falconi M, et al. Gastroenteropancreatic neuroendocrine neoplasms: ESMO Clinical Practice Guidelines for diagnosis, treatment and follow-up. Ann Oncol. 2020;202(7):844–60.
143. Chinese expert consensus on gastroenteropancreatic neuroendocrine tumors (2016 edition). J Clin Oncol. 2016;21(Chinese Society of Clinical Oncology Neuroendocrine Tumor Expert Committee, 10):927–46.
144. Hua G, Xin W, Xiaowei W, et al. Endoscopic manifestations and treatment of gastrointestinal neuroendocrine tumors. Chin J Digest Endosc. 2015;9:608–12.
145. Kulke MH, Anthony LB, Bushnell DL, et al. NANETS treatment guidelines: well-differentiated neuroendocrine tumors of the stomach and pancreas. Pancreas. 2010;39(6):735–52.
146. Tanemura H, Ohshita H, Kanno A, et al. A patient with small-cell carcinoma of the stomach with long survival after percutaneous microwave coagulating therapy (PMCT) for liver metastasis. Int J Clin Oncol. 2002;7(2):128–32.
147. Okita NT, Kato K, Takahari D, et al. Neuroendocrine tumors of the stomach: chemotherapy with cisplatin plus irinotecan is effective for gastric poorly-differentiated neuroendocrine carcinoma. Gastric Cancer. 2011;14(2):161–5.
148. Tang LH, Untch BR, Reidy DL, et al. Well-differentiated neuroendocrine tumors with a morphologically apparent high-grade component: a pathway distinct from poorly differentiated neuroendocrine carcinomas. Clin Cancer Res. 2016;22(11):1101–7.
149. Tang LH, Basturk O, Sue JJ, et al. A practical approach to the classification of WHO Grade

3 (G3) Well-differentiated Neuroendocrine Tumor (WD-NET) and Poorly Differentiated Neuroendocrine Carcinoma (PD-NEC) of the pancreas. Am J Surg Pathol. 2016;40(9):1192–202.
150. Chinese consensus on pathological diagnosis of gastrointestinal neuroendocrine tumors (2020 edition). Chin J Pathol. 2021;50(1):14–20.
151. Delle Fave G, O'toole D, Sundin A, et al. ENETS consensus guidelines update for gastroduodenal neuroendocrine neoplasms. Neuroendocrinology. 2016;103(2):119–24.
152. Garcia-Carbonero R, Sorbye H, Baudin E, et al. ENETS consensus guidelines for high-grade gastroenteropancreatic neuroendocrine tumors and neuroendocrine carcinomas. Neuroendocrinology. 2016;103(2):186–94.
153. Rindi G, Petrone G, Inzani F. The 2010 WHO classification of digestive neuroendocrine neoplasms: a critical appraisal four years after its introduction. Endocrine Pathol. 2014;25(2):186–92.
154. Rindi G, Bordi C, La Rosa S, et al. Gastroenteropancreatic (neuro)endocrine neoplasms: the histology report. Digest Liver Dis. 2011;43(Suppl 4):S356–60.
155. Nishimura C, Naoe H, Hashigo S, et al. Pancreatic metastasis from mixed adenoneuroendocrine carcinoma of the uterine cervix: a case report. Case Reports Oncol. 2013;6(2):256–62.
156. Shintaku M, Kataoka K, Kawabata K. Mixed adenoneuroendocrine carcinoma of the gallbladder with squamous cell carcinomatous and osteosarcomatous differentiation: report of a case. Pathol Int. 2013;63(2):113–9.
157. Volante M, Birocco N, Gatti G, et al. Extrapulmonary neuroendocrine small and large cell carcinomas: a review of controversial diagnostic and therapeutic issues. Human Pathol. 2014;45(4):665–73.
158. Wang J, He A, Feng Q, et al. Gastrointestinal mixed adenoneuroendocrine carcinoma: a population level analysis of epidemiological trends. J Transl Med. 2020;18(1):128.
159. Dulskas A, Pilvelis A. Oncologic outcome of mixed adenoneuroendocrine carcinoma (MANEC): a single center case series. Eur J Surg Oncol. 2020;46(1):105–7.
160. Mixed adenoneuroendocrine carcinoma (MANEC) of the gallbladder: a possible stem cell tumor? J Pathol Int 2011;61(10):608–14.
161. Domori K, Nishikura K, Ajioka Y, et al. Mucin phenotype expression of gastric neuroendocrine neoplasms: analysis of histopathology and carcinogenesis. Gastric Cancer. 2014;17(2):263–72.
162. Furlan D, Cerutti R, Genasetti A, et al. Microallelotyping defines the monoclonal or the polyclonal origin of mixed and collision endocrine-exocrine tumors of the gut. Lab Investig J Tech Methods Pathol. 2003;83(7):963–71.
163. Watanabe J, Suwa Y, Ota M, et al. Clinicopathological and prognostic evaluations of mixed adenoneuroendocrine carcinoma of the colon and rectum: a case-matched study. Dis Colon Rectum. 2016;59(12):1160–7.
164. La Rosa S, Marando A, Sessa F, et al. Mixed adenoneuroendocrine carcinomas (MANECs) of the gastrointestinal tract: an update. Cancers. 2012;4(1):11–30.
165. Scholzen T, Gerdes J. The Ki-67 protein: from the known and the unknown. J Cell Physiol. 2000;182(3):311–22.
166. Furukawa K, Miyahara R, Funasaka K, et al. Gastrointestinal: gastric mixed adenoneuroendocrine carcinoma. J Gastroenterol Hepatol. 2016;31(7):1236.
167. Nie L, Li M, He X, et al. Gastric mixed adenoneuroendocrine carcinoma: correlation of histologic characteristics with prognosis. Ann Diagn Pathol. 2016;25:48–53.
168. Fang C, Wang W, Feng X, et al. Nomogram individually predicts the overall survival of patients with gastroenteropancreatic neuroendocrine neoplasms. Br J Cancer. 2017;117(10):1544–50.
169. Xie JW, Lu J, Wang JB, et al. Prognostic factors for survival after curative resection of gastric mixed adenoneuroendocrine carcinoma: a series of 80 patients. BMC Cancer. 2018;18(1):1021.
170. Gurzu S, Fetyko A, Bara T, et al. Gastrointestinal mixed adenoneuroendocrine carcinoma (MANEC): an immunohistochemistry study of 13 microsatellite stable cases. Pathol Res Pract. 2019;215(12):152697.
171. Brathwaite S, Rock J, Yearsley MM, et al. Mixed adeno-neuroendocrine carcinoma: an aggressive clinical entity. Ann Surg Oncol. 2016;23(7):2281–6.
172. Brathwaite S, Yearsley MM, Bekaii-Saab T, et al. Appendiceal mixed adeno-neuroendocrine carcinoma: a population-based study of the surveillance, epidemiology, and end results registry. Front Oncol. 2016;6:148.
173. Chen L, Chen J, Zhou Z. Interpretation of the latest guidelines in the treatment of gastrointestinal neuroendocrine neoplasms. Zhonghua Wei Chang Wai Ke Za Zhi. 2016;19(11):1201–4.
174. Expert Committee of Neuroendocrine Oncology, Chinese Society of Clinical Oncology. Chinese expert consensus on gastrointestinal and pancreatic neuroendocrine tumors (2016 edition). Chin Clin Oncol. 2016;21(10):927–46.
175. Zhao M, Sun L, Lai JZ, et al. Expression of RNA-binding protein LIN28 in classic gastric hepatoid carcinomas, gastric fetal type gastrointestinal adenocarcinomas, and hepatocellular carcinomas: an immunohistochemical study with comparison to SALL4, alpha-fetoprotein, glypican-3, and Hep Par1. Pathol Res Pract. 2018;214(10):1707–12.
176. Ushiku T, Shinozaki A, Shibahara J, et al. SALL4 represents fetal gut differentiation of gastric cancer, and is diagnostically useful in distinguishing hepatoid gastric carcinoma from hepatocellular carcinoma. Am J Surg Pathol. 2010;34(4):533–40.
177. Bourreille J, Metayer P, Sauger F, et al. Existence of alpha feto protein during gastric-origin sec-

ondary cancer of the liver. La Presse Medicale. 1970;78(28):1277–8.
178. Su JS, Chen YT, Wang RC, et al. Clinicopathological characteristics in the differential diagnosis of hepatoid adenocarcinoma: a literature review. World J Gastroenterol. 2013;19(3):321–7.
179. Zhou RU, Cai Y, Yang YI, et al. Hepatoid adenocarcinoma of the stomach: a case report and review of the literature. Oncol Lett. 2015;9(5):2126–8.
180. Ishikura H, Fukasawa Y, Ogasawara K, et al. An AFP-producing gastric carcinoma with features of hepatic differentiation. A case report. Cancer. 1985;56(4):840–8.
181. Kumashiro Y, Yao T, Aishima S, et al. Hepatoid adenocarcinoma of the stomach: histogenesis and progression in association with intestinal phenotype. Human Pathol. 2007;38(6):857–63.
182. Wang Y, Sun L, Li Z, et al. Hepatoid adenocarcinoma of the stomach: a unique subgroup with distinct clinicopathological and molecular features. Gastric Cancer. 2019;22(6):1183–92.
183. Yang J, Wang R, Zhang W, et al. Clinicopathological and prognostic characteristics of hepatoid adenocarcinoma of the stomach. Gastroenterol Res Pract. 2014;2014:140587.
184. Inoue M, Sano T, Kuchiba A, et al. Long-term results of gastrectomy for alpha-fetoprotein-producing gastric cancer. Br J Surg. 2010;97(7):1056–61.
185. Qu BG, Bi WM, Qu BT, et al. PRISMA-compliant article: clinical characteristics and factors influencing prognosis of patients with hepatoid adenocarcinoma of the stomach in China. Medicine. 2016;95(15):e3399.
186. Wang YF, Lai YM, Kou F, et al. Clinicopathological characteristics and prognosis of 30 patients with gastric hepatoid adenocarcinoma. Chin Clin Oncol. 2018;45(07):37–43.
187. Xie Y, Zhao Z, Li P, et al. Hepatoid adenocarcinoma of the stomach is a special and easily misdiagnosed or missed diagnosed subtype of gastric cancer with poor prognosis but curative for patients of pN0/1: the experience of a single center. Int J Clin Exp Med. 2015;8(5):6762–72.
188. Zeng XY, Yin YP, Xiao H, et al. Clinicopathological Characteristics and prognosis of hepatoid adenocarcinoma of the stomach: evaluation of a pooled case series. Curr Med Sci. 2018;38(6):1054–61.
189. Gavrancic T, Park YH. A novel approach using sorafenib in alpha fetoprotein-producing hepatoid adenocarcinoma of the lung. J Natl Comprehen Cancer Netw JNCCN. 2015;13(4):387–91; quiz 91.
190. Petrelli F, Ghilardi M, Colombo S, et al. A rare case of metastatic pancreatic hepatoid carcinoma treated with sorafenib. J Gastrointest Cancer. 2012;43(1):97–102.
191. Kliszczewska E, Jarzyński A, Boguszewska A, et al. Epstein-Barr virus—pathogenesis, latency and cancers. J Pre-Clin Clin Res. 2017;11(2):142–6.
192. Chew MM, Gan SY, Khoo AS, et al. Interleukins, laminin and Epstein–Barr virus latent membrane protein 1 (EBV LMP1) promote metastatic phenotype in nasopharyngeal carcinoma. BMC Cancer. 2010;10:574.
193. Shibata D, Weiss LM. Epstein-Barr virus-associated gastric adenocarcinoma. Am J Pathol. 1992;140(4):769–74.
194. Imai S, Nishikawa J, Takada K. Cell-to-cell contact as an efficient mode of Epstein-Barr virus infection of diverse human epithelial cells. J Virol. 1998;72(5):4371–8.
195. Cancer Genome Atlas Research N. Comprehensive molecular characterization of gastric adenocarcinoma. Nature. 2014;513(7517):202–9.
196. Akiba S, Koriyama C, Herrera-Goepfert R, et al. Epstein-Barr virus associated gastric carcinoma: epidemiological and clinicopathological features. Cancer Sci. 2008;99(2):195–201.
197. Camargo MC, Kim WH, Chiaravalli AM, et al. Improved survival of gastric cancer with tumour Epstein-Barr virus positivity: an international pooled analysis. Gut. 2014;63(2):236–43.
198. Han J, He D, Feng ZY, et al. Clinicopathologic features and protein expression study of Epstein-Barr virus-associated gastric carcinoma in Guangzhou. Chin J Pathol. 2010;39(12):798–803.
199. Li SY, Hu JH, Zhou TJ. Analysis of the correlation between Epstein-Barr virus infection and gastric cancer in Tangshan area. Chin J Gerontol. 2007;27(23):2323–5.
200. Yanagi A, Nishikawa J, Shimokuri K, et al. Clinicopathologic characteristics of Epstein-Barr virus-associated gastric cancer over the past decade in Japan. Microorganisms. 2019;7(9).
201. Sugiura M, Imai S, Tokunaga M, et al. Transcriptional analysis of Epstein-Barr virus gene expression in EBV-positive gastric carcinoma: unique viral latency in the tumour cells. Br J Cancer. 1996;74(4):625–31.
202. Abe H, Kaneda A, Fukayama M. Epstein-Barr virus-associated gastric carcinoma: use of host cell machineries and somatic gene mutations. Pathobiology. 2015;82(5):212–23.
203. Zhang MQ, Gao J. Molecular characterizations and possible treatment strategies for Epstein-Barr virus-associated gastric cancer. Chin J Clin Oncol. 2018;45(10):525–8.
204. Kang D, Skalsky RL, Cullen BR. EBV BART microRNAs target multiple pro-apoptotic cellular genes to promote epithelial cell survival. PLoS Pathog. 2015;11(6):e1004979.
205. Dong M, Gong L, Chen J, et al. EBV-miR-BART10-3p and EBV-miR-BART22 promote metastasis of EBV-associated gastric carcinoma by activating the canonical Wnt signaling pathway. Cell Oncol (Dordrecht). 2020;43(5):901–13.
206. Hino R, Uozaki H, Murakami N, et al. Activation of DNA methyltransferase 1 by EBV latent membrane protein 2A leads to promoter hypermethylation of PTEN gene in gastric carcinoma. Cancer Res. 2009;69(7):2766–74.

207. Shinozaki-Ushiku AYA, Kunita A, Fukayama M. Update on Epstein-Barr virus and gastric cancer (Review). Int J Oncol. 2015;46(4):1421–34.
208. Li W, He C, Wu J, et al. Epstein barr virus encodes miRNAs to assist host immune escape. J Cancer. 2020;11(8):2091–100.
209. Yoon SJ, Kim JY, Long NP, et al. Comprehensive multi-omics analysis reveals aberrant metabolism of Epstein-Barr-virus-associated gastric carcinoma. Cells. 2019;8(10).
210. Qiu M, He C, Lu S, et al. Prospective observation: clinical utility of plasma Epstein-Barr virus DNA load in EBV-associated gastric carcinoma patients. Int J Cancer. 2020;146(1):272–80.
211. Xie T, Liu Y, Zhang Z, et al. Positive status of Epstein-Barr virus as a biomarker for gastric cancer immunotherapy: a prospective observational study. J Immunother (Hagerstown, Md:1997). 2020;43(4):139–44.
212. Kim ST, Cristescu R, Bass AJ, et al. Comprehensive molecular characterization of clinical responses to PD-1 inhibition in metastatic gastric cancer. Nat Med. 2018;24(9):1449–58.
213. Panda A, Mehnert JM, Hirshfield KM, et al. Immune activation and benefit from avelumab in EBV-positive gastric cancer. J Natl Cancer Inst. 2018;110(3):316–20.
214. Schneider B, Shah M, Klute K, et al. Phase I Study of epigenetic priming with azacitidine prior to standard neoadjuvant chemotherapy for patients with resectable gastric and esophageal adenocarcinoma: evidence of tumor hypomethylation as an indicator of major histopathologic response. Clin Cancer Res. 2017;23(11):2673–80.
215. Cristescu R, Lee J, Nebozhyn M, et al. Molecular analysis of gastric cancer identifies subtypes associated with distinct clinical outcomes. Nat Med. 2015;21(5):449–56.
216. Sohn BH, Hwang JE, Jang HJ, et al. Clinical significance of four molecular subtypes of gastric cancer identified by the cancer genome atlas project. Clin Cancer Res. 2017;23:4441–9.
217. Jia X, Guo T, Li Z, et al. Clinicopathological and immunomicroenvironment characteristics of Epstein-Barr virus-associated gastric cancer in a Chinese population. Front Oncol. 2020;10:586752.
218. Kohlruss M, Grosser B, Krenauer M, et al. Prognostic implication of molecular subtypes and response to neoadjuvant chemotherapy in 760 gastric carcinomas: role of Epstein-Barr virus infection and high- and low-microsatellite instability. J Pathol Clin Res. 2019;5(4):227–39.
219. Corallo S, Fuca G, Morano F, et al. Clinical behavior and treatment response of Epstein-Barr virus-positive metastatic gastric cancer: implications for the development of future trials. Oncologist. 2020;25(9):780–6.
220. Accordino G, Lettieri S, Bortolotto C, et al. From interconnection between genes and microenvironment to novel immunotherapeutic approaches in upper gastro-intestinal cancers—a multidisciplinary perspective. Cancers. 2020;12(8).
221. Comprehensive molecular characterization of gastric adenocarcinoma. Nature. 2014;513(7517):202–9.
222. Pietrantonio F, Miceli R, Raimondi A, et al. Individual patient data meta-analysis of the value of microsatellite instability as a biomarker in gastric cancer. J Clin Oncol. 2019;37(35):3392–400.
223. Polom K, Marano L, Marrelli D, et al. Meta-analysis of microsatellite instability in relation to clinicopathological characteristics and overall survival in gastric cancer. Br J Surg. 2018;105(3):159–67.
224. Smyth EC, Wotherspoon A, Peckitt C, et al. Mismatch repair deficiency, microsatellite instability, and survival: an exploratory analysis of the medical research council adjuvant gastric infusional chemotherapy (MAGIC) trial. JAMA Oncol. 2017;3(9):1197–203.
225. Roh CK, Choi YY, Choi S, et al. Single patient classifier assay, microsatellite instability, and Epstein-Barr virus status predict clinical outcomes in stage II/III gastric cancer: results from CLASSIC trial. Yonsei Med J. 2019;60(2):132–9.
226. Di Bartolomeo M, Morano F, Raimondi A, et al. Prognostic and predictive value of microsatellite instability, inflammatory reaction and PD-L1 in gastric cancer patients treated with either adjuvant 5-FU/LV or sequential FOLFIRI followed by cisplatin and docetaxel: a translational analysis from the ITACA-S trial. Oncol. 2020;25(3):e460–8.
227. An JY, Kim H, Cheong JH, et al. Microsatellite instability in sporadic gastric cancer: its prognostic role and guidance for 5-FU based chemotherapy after R0 resection. Int J Cancer. 2012;131(2):505–11.
228. Fang WL, Chang SC, Lan YT, et al. Microsatellite instability is associated with a better prognosis for gastric cancer patients after curative surgery. World J Surg. 2012;36(9):2131–8.
229. Choi J, Nam SK, Park DJ, et al. Correlation between microsatellite instability-high phenotype and occult lymph node metastasis in gastric carcinoma. APMIS. 2015;123(3):215–22.
230. Marrelli D, Polom K, Pascale V, et al. Strong prognostic value of microsatellite instability in intestinal type non-cardia gastric cancer. Ann Surg Oncol. 2016;23(3):943–50.
231. Mandal R, Samstein RM, Lee KW, et al. Genetic diversity of tumors with mismatch repair deficiency influences anti-PD-1 immunotherapy response. Science (New York, NY). 2019;364(6439):485–91.
232. Choi YY, Kim H, Shin SJ, et al. Microsatellite instability and programmed cell death-ligand 1 expression in stage II/III gastric cancer: post hoc analysis of the CLASSIC randomized controlled study. Ann Surg. 2019;270(2):309–16.
233. Miceli R, An J, Di Bartolomeo M, et al. Prognostic impact of microsatellite instability in Asian gastric cancer patients enrolled in the ARTIST Trial. Oncology. 2019;97(1):38–43.

234. Le DT, Durham JN, Smith KN, et al. Mismatch repair deficiency predicts response of solid tumors to PD-1 blockade. Science (New York, NY). 2017;357(6349):409–13.
235. Pietrantonio F, Randon G, Di Bartolomeo M, et al. Predictive role of microsatellite instability for PD-1 blockade in patients with advanced gastric cancer: a meta-analysis of randomized clinical trials. ESMO Open. 2021;6(1):100036.
236. Janjigian YY, Bendell J, Calvo E, et al. CheckMate-032 study: efficacy and safety of nivolumab and nivolumab plus ipilimumab in patients with metastatic esophagogastric cancer. J Clin Oncol. 2018;36(28):2836–44.
237. Fuchs CS, Doi T, Jang RW, et al. Safety and efficacy of pembrolizumab monotherapy in patients with previously treated advanced gastric and gastroesophageal junction cancer: phase 2 clinical KEYNOTE-059 trial. JAMA Oncol. 2018;4(5):e180013.
238. Marabelle A, Le DT, Ascierto PA, et al. Efficacy of pembrolizumab in patients with noncolorectal high microsatellite instability/mismatch repair-deficient cancer: results from the phase II KEYNOTE-158 study. J Clin Oncol. 2020;38(1):1–10.
239. Shitara K, Özgüroğlu M, Bang YJ, et al. Pembrolizumab versus paclitaxel for previously treated, advanced gastric or gastro-oesophageal junction cancer (KEYNOTE-061): a randomised, open-label, controlled, phase 3 trial. Lancet (London, England). 2018;392(10142):123–33.
240. Shitara K, Van Cutsem E, Bang YJ, et al. Efficacy and safety of pembrolizumab or pembrolizumab plus chemotherapy vs chemotherapy alone for patients with first-line, advanced gastric cancer: the KEYNOTE-062 phase 3 randomized clinical trial. JAMA Oncol. 2020;6(10):1571–80.

4 The Management for the Complications Associated with Gastrectomy

Chongyuan Sun, Chunguang Guo, Xiaofeng Bai, Yuemin Sun, Dongbing Zhao, Yingtai Chen, and Hong Zhou

4.1 Case 25: The Postoperative Bleeding After Gastrectomy

4.1.1 Brief History

The patient is a 49-year-old male admitted due to intermittent upper abdominal pain for 15 months. The patient had recurrent upper abdominal pain 15 months ago, with poor response to medication. Gastroscopy showed an ulcerative mass located in the gastric body and partially extending to the gastric antrum (distance measured from the incisor teeth was 50–56 cm), mainly on the greater curvature and anterior wall. The ulcer base was deep and covered with debris, and the ulcer edge was irregular, fragile, and prone to bleeding (Fig. 4.1). Endoscopic ultrasound examination revealed a hypoechoic mass within the gastric wall, with uneven echoes and indistinct boundaries. The focal lesion primarily infiltrated the intrinsic muscle layer of the gastric wall, with partial involvement of the serosal layer. Scattered lymph nodes were visible in the left gastric region, with the largest measuring about 11.0 mm × 8.9 mm (Fig. 4.2). Pathological examination confirmed the presence of signet-ring cell carcinoma. Abdominal enhanced CT showed a thickening of the gastric wall in the gastric body, with the thickest segment measuring approximately 1.8 cm, rough serosal surface, and multiple lymph nodes of varying sizes between the left gastric region and the portal vein. The patient underwent three cycles of chemotherapy with the DOS regimen chemotherapy (comprising oxaliplatin + S-1+ docetaxel) prior to surgery. Additionally, the patient's medical history revealed a cholecystectomy performed 20 years ago, as well as a prolonged history of tobacco and alcohol consumption.

Diagnosis: gastric cancer (cT4N+M0).

4.1.2 Treatment

Following appropriate preoperative preparations, the patient underwent an open distal gastrectomy with D2 lymph node dissection (Billroth II + Braun anastomosis), and the surgery went smoothly. However, on the fourth day after surgery, the patient experienced melena and exhibited a hemoglobin level of 71 g/L, indicating the

C. Sun · C. Guo (✉) · X. Bai · Y. Sun
D. Zhao · Y. Chen
Department of Pancreatic and Gastric Surgical Oncology, National Cancer Center/National Clinical Research for Cancer/Cancer Hospital, Chinese Academy of Medical Sciences and Peking Union Medical College, Beijing, China

H. Zhou
Department of Breast Surgical Oncology, National Cancer Center/National Clinical Research Center for Cancer/Cancer Hospital and Shenzhen Hospital, Chinese Academy of Medical Science and peking Union Medical College, Shenzhen, China

J. Cai (ed.), *Interpretation of Gastric Cancer Cases*, Experts' Perspectives on Medical Advances,
https://doi.org/10.1007/978-981-99-5302-8_4

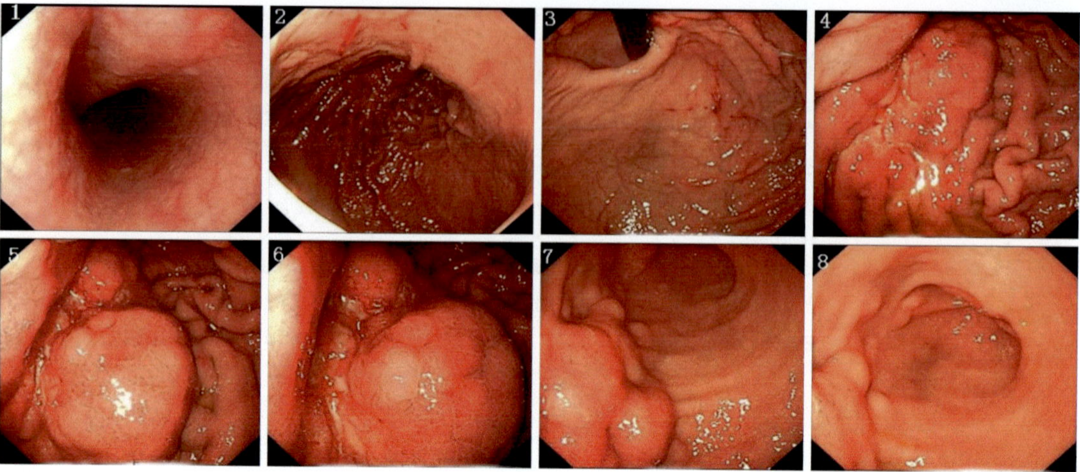

Fig. 4.1 Pre-treatment gastric endoscopy examination

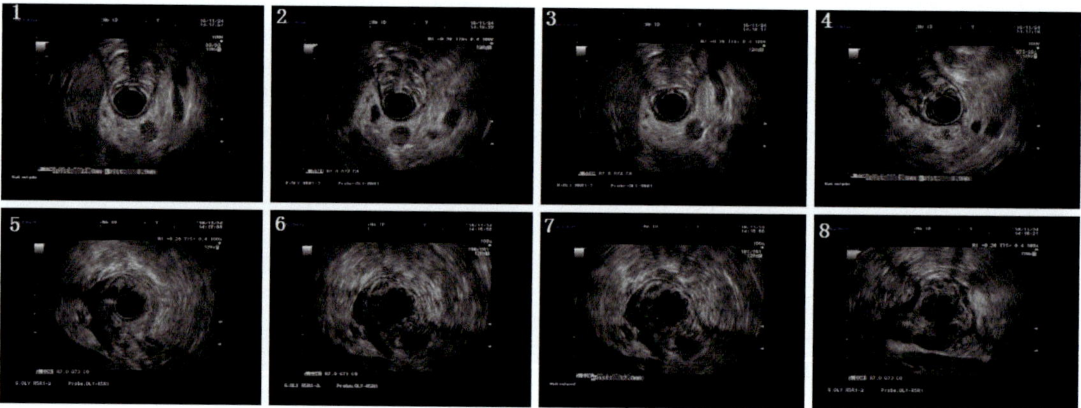

Fig. 4.2 Pre-treatment endoscopic ultrasound: The lesion is mainly located in the muscularis propria, with a partial invasion of the serosa. Scattered lymph nodes can be seen in the left region of the stomach, indicating metastasis

likelihood of postoperative intestinal blood accumulation. Symptomatic management was administered, consisting of blood transfusion and hemostatic medications. By the seventh postoperative day, the drainage volume decreased and the abdominal drainage tube was removed. On the eighth postoperative day, the patient encountered hematemesis with an estimated volume of 300 mL and a hemoglobin level of 64 g/L. Intravenous infusion of suspended red blood cells was initiated, and routine blood tests were repeated, showing a hemoglobin level of 77 g/L. Nevertheless, the hemoglobin levels continued to decline progressively, measuring 69 and 59 g/L at intervals of 4 and 8 h, respectively. Consequently, an urgent consultation was sought from the gastroenterology department and gastroscopy showed intermittent seepage at the intestinal anastomotic site located about 65 cm from the incisor teeth. Hemostasis was performed using electrocoagulation forceps (Fig. 4.3), and no active bleeding was observed following the intervention. The patient was safely transferred to the general ward and ultimately discharged on the 19th postoperative day.

4.1.3 Case Analysis

Postoperative bleeding following radical gastrectomy for gastric cancer is an infrequent complication, with reported incidences ranging from 0.3% to 6% [1, 2]. However, patients experiencing such bleeding episodes often present with

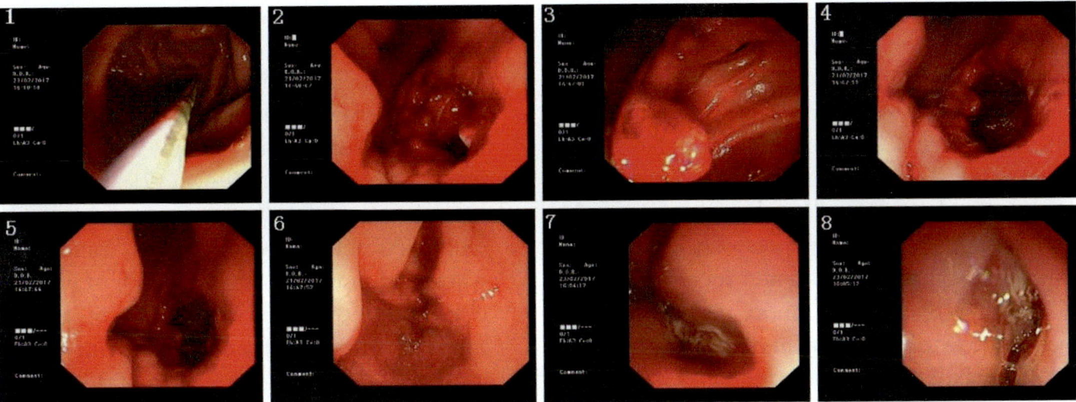

Fig. 4.3 Emergency gastroscopy shows active oozing at the intestinal anastomotic site, which was treated with electrocoagulation

severe conditions and rapid disease progression. Without prompt and appropriate intervention, severe consequences can ensue, leading to mortality rates as high as 10% to 20% [3]. Given the concealed nature of the bleeding source, identifying the underlying cause and implementing suitable treatment methods have vital clinical significance.

The presence of fresh blood in gastric decompression tubes or abdominal drainage tubes serves as a crucial indicator for early diagnosis of postoperative bleeding. As the peripheral circulatory blood volume decreases to a level where compensatory mechanisms become inadequate, patients may manifest initial signs of shock, including dizziness, palpitations, fatigue, cold and clammy skin, and an elevated heart rate. In severe cases, shock and even fatality may occur. During this process, hemoglobin and hematocrit levels progressively decrease, and the circulatory system gradually loses its compensatory ability.

Postoperative bleeding of gastric cancer can be divided into two types: early and delayed bleeding [4–6]. Early bleeding typically occurs within 24 h after surgery and is more frequently observed at the anastomotic site. It is often related to incomplete intraoperative hemostasis or improper surgical technique, such as improper use of anastomotic instruments, inadequate vascular ligation, or postoperative wound oozing. Delayed bleeding occurs between 24 h and 2 weeks post-surgery and encompasses various causes, including pseudoaneurysm rupture bleeding in major blood vessels (such as the hepatic artery, splenic artery, and abdominal aorta), duodenal stump fistula, and secondary bleeding from anastomotic fistulas [7]. During lymph node dissection around blood vessels, the high temperature generated by energy instruments can result in thermal injury to the blood vessel wall, leading to the formation of pseudoaneurysms. Temporary increases in blood pressure due to stress or physical activity may trigger the rupture of these pseudoaneurysms [8]. In addition, anastomotic fistula and abdominal infections after surgery can corrode the blood vessel ends and arterial walls, resulting in life-threatening intra-abdominal bleeding. It is important to note that early and delayed bleeding are not exclusively associated with gastrointestinal or intra-abdominal bleeding. A study reported that 71% of anastomotic bleeding is early bleeding, and 58% of abdominal arterial bleeding manifests as delayed bleeding [3].

Postoperative bleeding in gastric cancer cases can present with various symptoms, necessitating comprehensive assessment for accurate diagnosis. The following indicators should raise a high suspicion of bleeding [9]: (1) Observation of fresh blood in the gastric tube or abdominal drainage tube, with a drainage volume exceeding 100 mL/h; (2) symptoms of gastrointestinal bleeding, such as profuse vomiting or the presence of melena (black, tarry stool); (3) non-cardiogenic hemodynamic instability or signs of shock in patients; (4) significant decline in hemoglobin levels compared to preoperative measurements.

According to the consensus of domestic experts [10], the severity of postoperative bleeding following gastrectomy for gastric cancer is classified based on the intervention method. The grading system is as follows: Grade I: No special intervention (except for intravenous hemostatic drugs); Grade II: Blood transfusion or hemodynamic support with vasopressors; Grade IIIa: Interventional procedure under local anesthesia; Grade IIIb: Intervention under general anesthesia; Grade IVa: Development of at least one organ function failure due to bleeding; Grade IVb: Presence of multiple organ function failures; Grade V: Patient mortality.

Once the diagnosis of postoperative bleeding is established, prompt intervention and vigilant monitoring of hemodynamic parameters become imperative. The following measures should be considered:

1. General treatment: When bleeding signs are found in patients, monitor heart rate, blood pressure, bleeding volume, and urine output. Establish and maintain clear intravenous access for rapidly supplement. Ensure airway patency and minimize coughing induced by vomiting. Patients with gastrointestinal bleeding should refrain from oral intake to prevent exacerbation of bleeding or interference with subsequent treatment.
2. Drug treatment: Administration of hemostatic drugs orally or via gastric tube, such as thrombin and epinephrine. Intravenous administration of coagulation-promoting medications like vitamin K, tranexamic acid, and snake venom thrombin. H2 receptor blockers and proton pump inhibitors can effectively reduce gastric acid secretion, prevent mucosal damage, and promote hemostasis. Other drugs, such as somatostatin analogs and vasopressin, can effectively slow bleeding by reducing portal blood flow and constricting small blood vessels, and maintaining blood pressure.
3. Endoscopic treatment: Emergency endoscopic examination and direct endoscopic hemostasis provide a valuable approach to treating postoperative anastomotic bleeding. At the same time as identifying the bleeding site, effective intervention can be performed [11], including the following methods: (1) Metal clip hemostasis: Utilizing the mechanical force produced by the hemostatic clip to ligate the surrounding tissue and bleeding vessels to block blood flow [12]. (2) Electric coagulation hemostasis is a commonly employed technique. However, caution is warranted in controlling the depth of electrocoagulation to minimize the risk of anastomotic fistula formation, necessitating safety evaluation. (3) Local injection of adrenaline or sclerosant is a relatively common method of hemostasis with a definite effect. (4) Local spraying of hemostatic drugs, such as epinephrine and thrombin [13].
4. Angiography and interventional treatment: Angiography plays a vital role in both diagnosing and treating postoperative bleeding. By injecting contrast agent into the blood vessel, the condition of the vasculature can be visualized, aiding in the identification of the bleeding site. Administration of hemostatic agents (e.g., gelatin sponge) into the blood vessels proximal to the bleeding site can effectively achieve hemostasis. This approach is particularly suitable for elderly patients who are not suitable candidates for reoperation or those with significant abdominal adhesions. Even if vascular embolization fails, it can provide valuable information for subsequent surgical interventions. However, interventional vascular therapy is not appropriate for cases involving venous bleeding, diffuse bleeding, or intermittent bleeding.
5. Surgical treatment: Most patients with upper gastrointestinal bleeding can be improved with conservative treatment. However, if conventional therapy fails to yield improvement, vital signs remain unstable, or hemoglobin levels continue to decline, active bleeding should be suspected. In such cases, while implementing standard treatments such as blood transfusion, hemostasis, and fluid resuscitation, prompt open surgery should be considered to identify the underlying cause of bleeding.

4.1.4 Expert Comments

Postoperative bleeding is a severe complication following gastrectomy for gastric cancer, characterized by a relatively low incidence rate but with potential life-threatening consequences. Several factors, including preoperative hypoalbuminemia, prolonged surgical duration, intraoperative vascular calcification, extent of lymph node dissection, and postoperative intra-abdominal infection, significantly influence the occurrence of postoperative bleeding. High-risk patients with these factors should be given special attention. Compared with early bleeding, delayed bleeding is more dangerous, with common causes including digestive tract fistula and pseudoaneurysm. This underscores the importance of meticulous attention to the quality of digestive tract reconstruction and judicious use of energy devices during surgery. While modern imaging and interventional techniques offer effective management options for most cases of postoperative bleeding, it is crucial to highlight the need for timely re-exploration surgery in patients who do not respond to conservative treatment.

Case provider: Chongyuan Sun, Yingtai Chen.

Commentary: Chunguang Guo.

4.2 Case 26: Duodenal Stump Fistula After Gastrectomy for Gastric Cancer

4.2.1 Brief History

The patient is a 56-year-old male admitted due to the "discovery of gastric cancer during the physical examination for over 20 days." Approximately 20 days ago, the patient underwent a physical examination, during which a gastric antral mass was incidentally detected, leading to the suspicion of gastric antral carcinoma. Subsequent gastroscopy at our institution revealed an ulcerated mass predominantly situated on the lesser curvature and posterior wall of the gastric antrum, with deep ulceration covered by debris (Fig. 4.4). Pathological examination confirmed the presence of adenocarcinoma with high-grade intraepithelial neoplasia. Further assessment through abdominal enhanced CT scan disclosed irregular thickening of the gastric antral wall, reaching a maximum thickness of approximately 1.4 cm, accompanied by uneven enhancement and nodular high-density lesions in select areas, exhibiting a smooth outer surface (Fig. 4.5). Tumor markers, including CEA, AFP, CA724, CA199, and CA242, were within

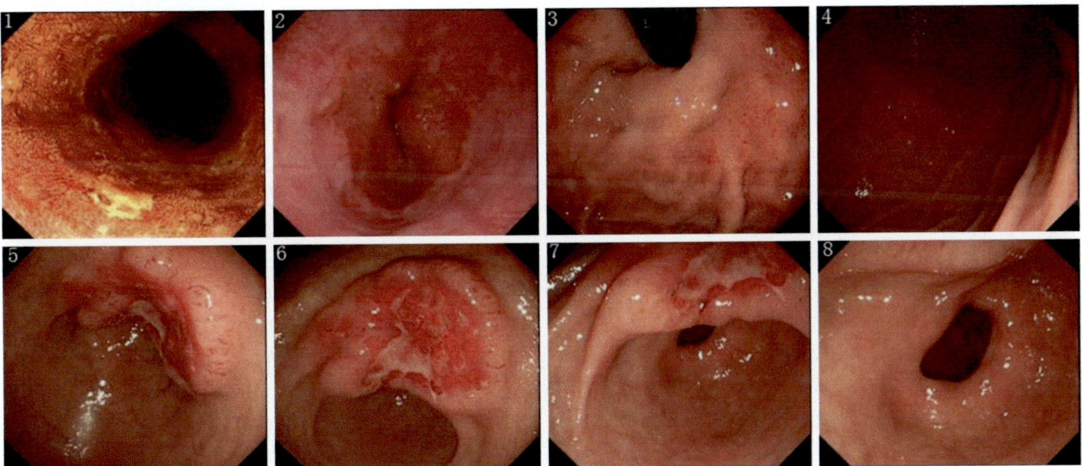

Fig. 4.4 Gastroscopy: The gastric antrum cancer is mainly located on the lesser curvature side and posterior wall

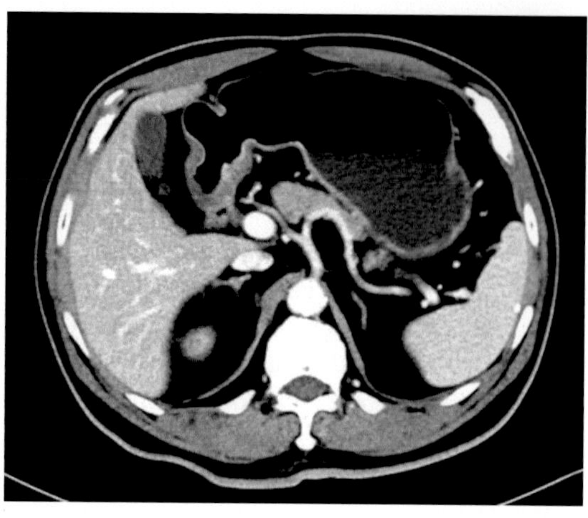

Fig. 4.5 Abdominal enhanced CT: Irregular thickening of the gastric wall in the gastric antrum

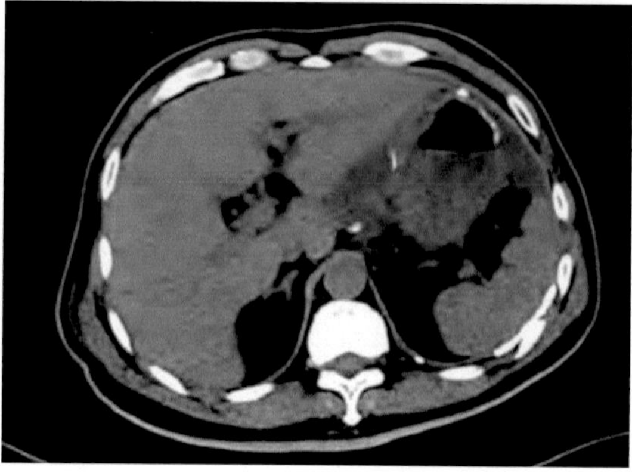

Fig. 4.6 Abdominal CT scan: thickening of the soft tissue at the anastomosis, accumulation of gas in the surrounding adipose interspace and porta hepatis, as well as increased fluid accumulation in the abdomen and pelvis

normal limits. The patient's medical history revealed a 1-year duration of well-controlled diabetes, managed through regular administration of acarbose, metformin, and subcutaneous injections of insulin aspart. Additionally, 4 months ago, the patient underwent coronary artery stent placement for coronary heart disease and had been consistently taking aspirin and clopidogrel until discontinuation over 2 weeks ago. The patient had a smoking history spanning two decades, with a consumption of 40 cigarettes per day, but ceased smoking 4 months ago. Furthermore, the patient had been consuming 200 mL of white liquor daily for the past 20 years but has remained abstinent for the last 4 months.

Diagnosis: gastric cancer (cT4N+M0), diabetes mellitus, and post-coronary stent implantation.

4.2.2 Treatment

After completing relevant examinations, the patient underwent laparoscopic distal gastrectomy with D2 lymph node dissection (Billroth II reconstruction plus Braun anastomosis). Intraoperative exploration revealed the presence of an ulcerative tumor measuring 3 cm × 3 cm in the gastric antrum without serosal invasion or enlarged lymph nodes surrounding the stomach. The patient recovered well and was discharged on the seventh day after surgery.

However, on the ninth day post-surgery, the patient complained of abdominal pain and exhibited a high fever, necessitating admission to the emergency department. Abdominal CT imaging showed thickening of the soft tissue at the anastomosis, accumulation of gas in the surrounding adipose interspace and porta hepatis, as well as increased fluid accumulation in the abdomen and pelvis (Fig. 4.6). Despite fluid resuscitation and administration of anti-infection treatment, the patient's symptoms failed to demonstrate significant improvement. Owing to unstable vital signs and evident indications of peritonitis, the patient was urgently readmitted to the hospital and underwent an exploratory operation. During the operation, a substantial volume of yellowish fluid was observed within the abdominal and pelvic cavities, as well as the mesentery. Additionally, a small quantity of bile-like fluid was observed leaking from the residual duodenum. No bleeding or fistulas were found at the anastomosis sites or the Braun anastomosis. The abdominal secretions were collected for bacterial culture, and the adhesions were meticulously released. The wound was thoroughly irrigated with copious amounts of iodine and warm saline to remove residual purulent secretions. Drainage tubes were placed adjacent to the anastomosis sites, duodenal stump, and pelvic cavity, while an enteric nutrition tube was inserted through the oral cavity. After the operation, the patient was transferred to the intensive care unit (ICU) for close monitoring and initiated on a regimen of meropenem in combination with vancomycin for anti-infection therapy. The patient was transferred to a general ward on the third day and was discharged 59 days later.

4.2.3 Case Analysis

Duodenal stump fistula (DSF) is one of the most severe complications of gastric cancer surgery and remains a major cause of perioperative death in gastric cancer patients. DSF is a high-output intestinal fistula and commonly arises within the postoperative period of 1–7 days, with reported incidence rates ranging from 1 to 6% and associated mortality rates spanning from 7 to 67% [14]. Notably, the leakage of duodenal contents, such as bile and pancreatic juice, can precipitate severe intra-abdominal infection, shock, and potentially life-threatening conditions. Therefore, the prevention, early detection, and appropriate management of DSF are pivotal for ensuring postoperative safety.

DSF after gastric cancer surgery is related to multiple factors, encompassing both preoperative health status and intraoperative procedures. Key aspects contributing to DSF development include the following: (1)Patient factors: Preoperative malnutrition, hypoalbuminemia, hypertension, diabetes, and other comorbidities have been identified as high-risk factors for DSF [15, 16]; (2) Tumor factors: DSF is more likely to occur in cases where the tumor is located in the gastric antrum and involves the duodenum. Furthermore, emergency surgeries performed to address conditions such as bleeding, perforation, or pyloric obstruction pose an increased risk of DSF due to the associated edema and fragility of the intestinal wall; (3) Surgical factors: excessive mobilization of the duodenum during surgery may compromise the blood supply to the stump, leading to intestinal ischemic necrosis; excessive tension during linear cutting and closure of the duodenum can result in suture detachment; Inappropriate suture height can contribute to suboptimal closure; additionally, forcefully closing or burying the residual duodenal stump can also predispose to DSF [17].

The early diagnosis of DSF is pivotal for determining the prognosis and instituting timely interventions. Suspicions of DSF should arise when the following conditions are observed [18]: (1) Sudden onset of severe upper abdominal pain occurring 2–5 days after surgery, accompanied by localized or diffuse peritonitis in the right upper abdomen, high fever, tachycardia, elevated white blood cell count and procalcitonin levels; (2) Aspiration of bile-like or turbid purulent drainage fluid from the abdominal drainage tube or the surgical incision site; (3) Identification of fluid accumulation in the right upper abdomen through abdominal ultrasound or CT scan; (4) Overflow of contrast agent from the duodenal stump observed during upper gastrointestinal contrast examination. Alternatively, the administration of orally ingested methylene blue or other dyes can result in the rapid drainage of the dye from the side drainage tube situated at the duodenal stump.

Once DSF is diagnosed, immediate and comprehensive treatment is essential. The treatment approach revolves around several principles, including ensuring unobstructed drainage of the duodenal stump, controlling infection, providing adequate nutritional support, correcting internal environment disturbances, and considering exploratory surgery if necessary [19]. The treatment includes the following key aspects:

1. General treatment: In cases of localized DSF, conservative treatment should be given first, which entail strictly prohibiting water intake and continuing gastrointestinal decompression. For instances where there is inadequate drainage of locally accumulated encapsulated fluid or abscess, ultrasound-guided puncture and drainage can be attempted.
2. Nutritional support treatment: DSF patients experience a heightened catabolic state following gastric cancer surgery, and prolonged fasting can rapidly lead to malnutrition and imbalances in the internal environment. Thus,

nutritional support plays a vital role in the treatment approach. Initially, total parenteral nutrition is preferred to meet the immediate nutritional needs. However, long-term use of parenteral nutrition may compromise the integrity of the intestinal mucosal barrier and increase the risk of microbial translocation [20]. Therefore, a timely transition to a combination of enteral and parenteral nutrition is recommended, with a gradual shift towards full enteral nutrition. This approach helps preserve the integrity of the intestinal barrier, prevent microbial translocation, and promote healing of the DSF.

3. Drug therapy: Empirical administration of antibiotics should be initiated, followed by drainage fluid culture to guide appropriate antibiotic selection based on sensitivity results, thus preventing bacterial dysbiosis. Prompt adjustment of medication should be based on infection control indicators such as body temperature, white blood cell count, and C-reactive protein (CRP) levels. Additionally, antifungal drugs may be added when necessary to address fungal infections [21]. Furthermore, the use of somatostatin and its analogs (e.g., octreotide), proton pump inhibitors, or H2 receptor blockers can effectively inhibit the secretion of pancreatic juice, bile, and gastric juice, thereby alleviating infection-related symptoms. (4) Surgical treatment: Patients with diffuse peritonitis, abdominal bleeding, or those who fail to achieve unobstructed drainage after catheterization may require surgical intervention [22]. It is important to note that direct repair of severely damaged duodenal stump fistulas, which have been corroded by digestive juices, yields poor efficacy. Therefore, the primary objective of surgical treatment is to evacuate abdominal effusion, perform thorough irrigation of the abdominal cavity using a large volume of warm saline or diluted iodine solution to reduce toxin absorption, and establish adequate drainage and enteral nutrition pathways, such as a nasoenteric tube or jejunal fistula.

4.2.4 Expert Comments

Duodenal stump fistula is a severe complication following gastric cancer surgery, often accompanied by abdominal infection, secondary bleeding, multiple organ failure, and shock, resulting in a high mortality rate. Familiarity with the risk factors associated with DSF is essential for preventing its occurrence and improving patient prognosis. Preoperative nutritional assessment, treatment of comorbidities, proper handling of the duodenal stump, and placement of abdominal drainage tubes are vital to preventing duodenal stump fistula. In the event that DSF does occur, the establishment of adequate drainage, administration of appropriate anti-infection treatment, provision of optimal nutritional support, and maintenance of internal environment balance can effectively improve the overall cure rate of DSF.

Case provider: Chongyuan Sun, Chunguang Guo.

Commentary: Chunguang Guo.

4.3 Case 27: Postoperative Gastroparesis Syndrome

4.3.1 Brief History

A patient, 46-year-old male, was admitted due to persistent upper abdominal distension and pain extending beyond a 6-month duration, which has exhibited a progressive exacerbation within the past month. Throughout the preceding 6 months, the patient experienced intermittent upper abdominal pain unaccompanied by nausea, regurgitation, or any discernible association with food intake. Approximately 1 month ago, the patient underwent gastroscopy at a local medical facility, which disclosed the presence of a gastric mass. Subsequent histopathological examination substantiated the existence of signet-ring cell carcinoma located in the gastric body. The patient exhibited elevated levels of tumor markers CA724 and cytokeratin 19 fragment, although within the normal range for CEA, AFP, and

CA242. Abdominal enhanced computed tomography (CT) exhibited thickening of the gastric wall along the greater curvature of the gastric body, measuring approximately 0.9 cm, with uneven enhancement and a smooth serosal surface. No enlarged lymph nodes were identified within the abdominal or retroperitoneal cavities (Fig. 4.7).

Diagnosis: gastric cancer (cT3N0M0).

4.3.2 Treatment

After admission, the patient underwent a laparoscopic-assisted distal gastrectomy with D2 lymph node dissection (Billroth II). A gastric tube and a nasojejunal nutrition tube were placed during the surgery, and the operation was successful. Following the surgery, the patient received symptomatic supportive treatments, including fluid supplementation, acid suppression, pain relief, and antiemetics.

On the third day after the operation, the patient complained of mild abdominal distension. From the sixth day onwards, the gastric tube drained approximately 1000 mL/day, and the patient experienced intolerable abdominal distension after enteral nutrition. This was attributed to anastomotic stenosis caused by postoperative edema, and enteral nutrition was administered through the nasojejunal nutrition tube. Upper gastrointestinal contrast imaging conducted on the 12th day after the surgery revealed the entry of contrast agent into the residual stomach; however, the residual stomach exhibited weak peristalsis, and no contrast agent was observed in the distal intestinal lumen (Fig. 4.8). On the eighteenth day after the surgery, the patient was advised to consume a small liquid diet while clamping the gastric tube. However, the patient still complained of abdominal distension and nausea after eating. These symptoms improved upon unclamping the gastric tube. On the 27th day after the surgery, the gastric tube drained about 750 mL of gastric juice daily, and there was no significant improvement in delayed gastric emptying. Given the patient's stable condition, the patient was discharged for rest.

The pathological examination indicated the presence of a limited ulcerative poorly differentiated adenocarcinoma in the stomach, classified according to the Lauren classification as diffuse type. The tumor infiltrated the deep muscle layer and exhibited visible nerve invasion. No definite vascular tumor embolus was observed, and there

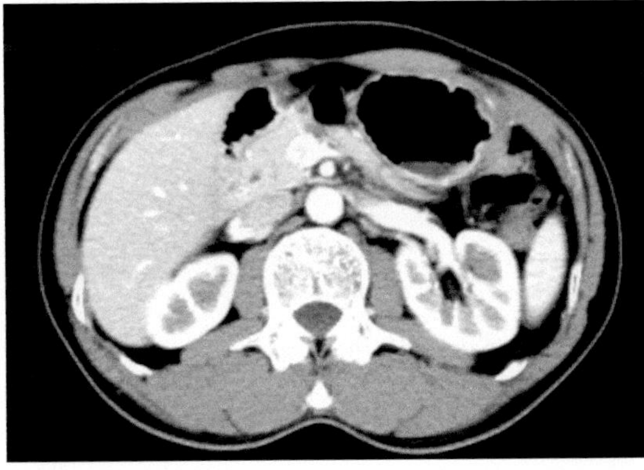

Fig. 4.7 Abdominal enhanced CT: The gastric wall along the greater curvature of the gastric body is thicken, measuring approximately 0.9 cm

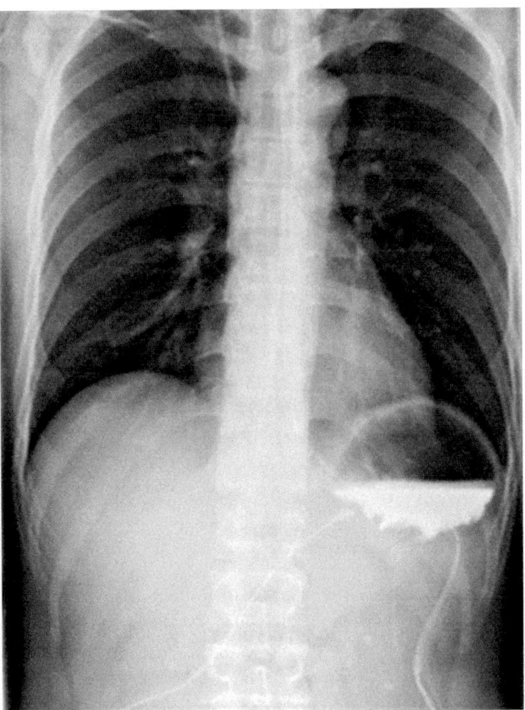

Fig. 4.8 Upper gastrointestinal contrast imaging conducted on the 12th day after surgery

was no tumor involvement of the pylorus, duodenal bulb, upper margin, lower margin, and greater omentum. Furthermore, no metastatic cancer was detected in the examined lymph nodes (0/37). TNM staging was pT2N0M0, stage I.

During the follow-up examination at the outpatient clinic, which took place 2 months after the surgery, the patient reported that oral intake had commenced approximately 2 weeks after discharge, approximately 40 days after the surgery. The patient's diet gradually transitioned to a semi-liquid consistency. Gastroscopy (Fig. 4.9) showed congestion and hematoma of the residual gastric mucosa with gastric and nutritional tubes. The gastrojejunal anastomosis was located approximately 46 cm from the incisors. The mucosa at the anastomotic site exhibited congestion and roughness, but no evident masses or ulcers were observed. The anastomotic site did not show significant narrowing, and the passage of the endoscope was smooth. Consequently, both the gastric and nutritional tubes were removed.

4.3.3 Case Analysis

Delayed gastric emptying (DGE) is a syndrome characterized by gastric motility disorders resulting in gastric dysmotility and delayed emptying, caused by non-mechanical obstruction factors after surgery, commonly observed after gastrectomy or pancreaticoduodenectomy. The reported incidence varies between 0.6% and 10% [23, 24]. Typically, DGE manifests between the sixth and 12th days following surgery and is characterized by persistent upper abdominal fullness, belching, acid reflux, and vomiting. Patients may also experience reduced appetite, weight loss, and continuous high-volume gastric drainage.

The pathogenesis of DGE remains unclear and is believed to be multifactorial. Potential contributing factors include:

1. Psychosocial factors: During the perioperative period, stress responses such as anxiety, tension, and insomnia can result in autonomic nervous system dysfunction. This can lead to

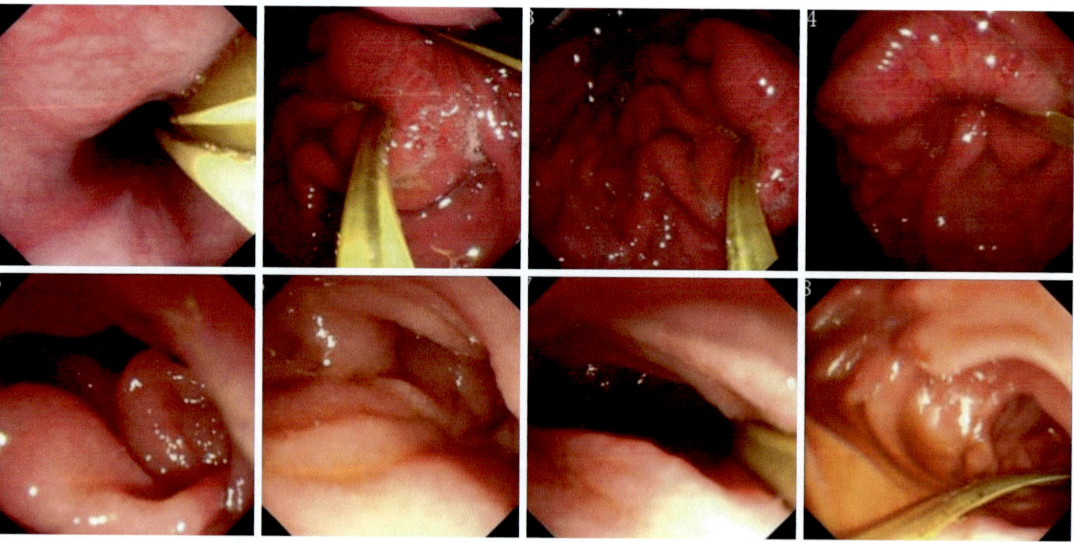

Fig. 4.9 Gastroscopy: The gastrojejunal anastomosis was located about 46 cm from the incisors, and the anastomotic site exhibits significant narrowing, allowing for smooth passage of the endoscope

increased sympathetic nervous system activity, inhibition of excitatory neurons in the enteric nervous system, and indirectly hinder smooth muscle contractions, ultimately causing delayed gastric emptying [25].

2. Surgical injury: The peristalsis and contraction of the stomach are regulated by the vagus nerve. Damage to the vagus nerve can result in prolonged gastric retention.
3. Digestive tract reconstruction: Currently, Billroth I and Billroth II procedures are commonly used for distal gastric surgery and digestive tract reconstruction. Billroth I closely resembles normal physiological conditions, but its indications are limited, leading to the more frequent use of Billroth II. Numerous studies have reported a higher incidence of DGE following Billroth II compared to Billroth I, highlighting it as a risk factor for DGE [26–28]. This may be attributed to the more complex anastomosis in Billroth II, which increases surgical and anesthesia duration and, consequently, surgical risks. Moreover, postoperative reflux of bile and pancreatic secretions into the residual stomach can cause gastric wall congestion and edema, impeding gastrointestinal function recovery [29].
4. Gastric pacemaker cells: Interstitial cells of Cajal (ICC) can generate electrical activity that triggers smooth muscle contraction in the stomach, acting as the pacemaker cells for gastric electrical activity. Gastric subtotal resection surgery removes the gastric pacemaker site on the greater curvature side of the stomach, resulting in the inability of the residual stomach to generate effective basic electrical rhythms and contraction waves, leading to disturbances in gastric rhythm [30].
5. Patient's general nutritional status and underlying diseases: Hyperglycemia can inhibit the secretion and release of gastric hormones. Blood glucose levels exceeding 10 mmol/L can induce gastric rhythm disturbances, decrease gastric pressure, and delay gastric emptying [31]. Postoperative hypoalbuminemia can cause local movement disorders due to edema at the surgical anastomosis site, prolonging the recovery time of gastrointestinal function.
6. Preoperative gastric outlet obstruction: Some studies have demonstrated that preoperative gastric outlet obstruction significantly increases the risk of DGE by 26 times [32]. This can be attributed to factors such as gastric wall edema, disruption of gastric smooth muscle, and impaired nerve conduction caused by the preexisting obstruction. Preoperative gastric decompression has been shown to effectively prevent the occurrence of DGE in these patients.

There is currently no internationally standardized diagnostic criterion for DGE. Some foreign scholars propose the use of a gastric emptying test with a 99mTc-labeled meal as the gold standard for diagnosis [33]. The International Study Group of Pancreatic Surgery (ISGPS) defines delayed gastric emptying as the requirement for continuous gastrointestinal decompression lasting more than 3 days after surgery, the inability to tolerate solid oral food by postoperative day 7, or radiographic evidence of weakened gastric motility [34]. Based on the impact on the clinical course and the degree of postoperative management, three different grades have been defined (Table 4.1). Currently, many hospitals in China follow the diagnostic criteria established by Zhongshan Hospital, affiliated with Fudan University. These criteria include: (1) confirmation of gastric outlet obstruction through examination such as electronic gastroscopy or X-ray gastrointestinal imaging, with evidence of gastric retention; (2) daily drainage of gastric and intestinal decompression exceeding 800 mL, lasting for more than 10 days; (3) absence of significant electrolyte or acid-base imbalances; (4) exclusion of underlying conditions that may cause gastric motility disorders, such as hypothyroidism; and (5) no history of perioperative administration of smooth muscle contraction-inhibiting drugs like morphine and atropine [35].

Table 4.1 Consensus definition of DGE after surgery

DGE grade	NGT required	Unable to tolerate solid oral intake by POD	Vomiting/gastric distension	Use of prokinetics
A	4–7 days or reinsertion > POD 3	7	No/yes	No/yes
B	8–14 days or reinsertion > POD 7	14	Yes	Yes
C	>14 days or reinsertion > POD 14	21	Yes	Yes

DGE delayed gastric emptying; *POD* postoperative day; *NGT* nasogastric tube

The treatment of DGE primarily involves conservative measures, and surgical intervention should be avoided unless there is a mechanical obstruction. The following treatment options can be considered:

1. General treatment: Strict restriction of oral fluid intake, continuous gastrointestinal decompression, and gastric lavage using warm saline through a gastric tube can help reduce anastomotic edema and promote early recovery of gastrointestinal function. Regular monitoring of blood parameters including complete blood count, liver and kidney function, and electrolyte levels is necessary to correct any disturbances in the internal environment.
2. Nutritional support: In the early postoperative period, complete parenteral nutrition is administered, followed by enteral nutrition once intestinal function is restored. The approach is to start with small amounts and gradually increase the volume. The infusion rate should be adjusted based on the patient's tolerance to avoid severe abdominal pain and bloating.
3. Drug therapy: Pharmacological agents that promote gastrointestinal motility are commonly employed and can be categorized based on their mechanisms of action. (1) Dopamine receptor blockers, such as metoclopramide (ganaton) and domperidone (motilium) act by blocking dopamine receptors either centrally or peripherally. (2) Benzamide derivatives, such as mosapride, are selective 5-hydroxytryptamine 4 receptor agonists that promote acetylcholine release and exert prokinetic effects. (3) Macrolide antibiotics, such as erythromycin and its derivatives, can bind to high-density gastrin receptors on the surface of gastric smooth muscle, promoting gastrointestinal motility. However, their routine use has diminished over time.
4. Psychological therapy: Psychological counseling is an essential aspect of the treatment for patients with delayed gastric emptying (DGE). The stress induced by surgery, prolonged placement of gastric tubes, and water restriction can contribute to increased levels of anxiety and depression in patients. Healthcare professionals should carefully observe the psychological status of patients, provide patient education, and address any concerns or questions they may have. By offering emotional support and increasing patients' confidence in their treatment, psychological therapy can help alleviate the psychological burden associated with DGE.
5. Traditional Chinese medicine treatment: Traditional Chinese medicine plays a vital role in the management of DGE and serves as a valuable complement to Western medical treatments. In the concept of traditional Chinese medicine, DGE belongs to postoperative damage to the spleen and stomach. This damage leads to spleen deficiency and dysfunction, impairment of qi descent in the stomach, and disruption of meridian pathways, ultimately resulting in qi stagnation and dampness obstruction, which contributes to an increase in gastric drainage volume [36]. Currently, traditional Chinese medicine treatment methods include the external

application of herbal medicine, enema using Chinese herbal formulations, acupuncture of the Zusanli acupoint, and moxibustion. These approaches have demonstrated notable therapeutic effects in the management of DGE [37].

4.3.4 Expert Comments

Delayed gastric emptying (DGE) is a common complication following gastric cancer surgery, resulting in challenges such as impaired oral intake, prolonged hospital stays, and increased medical expenses. This condition imposes substantial psychological pressure on both patients and healthcare providers. Fortunately, the majority of DGE cases can be effectively managed through conservative treatment, with resolution typically occurring within a period of 10–60 days. However, a small percentage of patients may experience symptoms for several months. Given the functional nature of DGE, it is crucial to incorporate psychological counseling into the treatment regimen to enhance patients' confidence in their recovery process.

Case provider: Chongyuan Sun, Xiaofeng Bai.

Commentary: Xiaofeng Bai.

4.4 Case 28: Anastomotic Strictures After Radical Gastrectomy

4.4.1 Brief History

The patient is a 71-year-old male admitted to the hospital with a chief complaint of "upper abdominal pain over a span of 1 month." Roughly a month ago, the patient commenced experiencing intermittent discomfort localized to the upper abdomen, accompanied by sporadic mild pain. Notably, there were no associated symptoms of nausea, vomiting, diarrhea, constipation, or melena. Upon conducting a physical examination of the abdomen, no positive indicators were detected. Pertaining to tumor markers, the following values were obtained: tissue polypeptide antigen (TPS) displayed an elevated level of 173.175 U/L, while CEA, AFP, CA724, CA199, and CA242 all exhibited values within the normal range. Gastroscopy revealed a superficial elevated lesion situated at the cardia, featuring congested, rough, and erosive mucosa, along with a slightly rigid gastric wall encompassing the junction, fundus, and body of the stomach (Fig. 4.10). Histopathological examination of the biopsy specimens confirmed the presence of mucosal adenocarcinoma. Abdominal enhanced

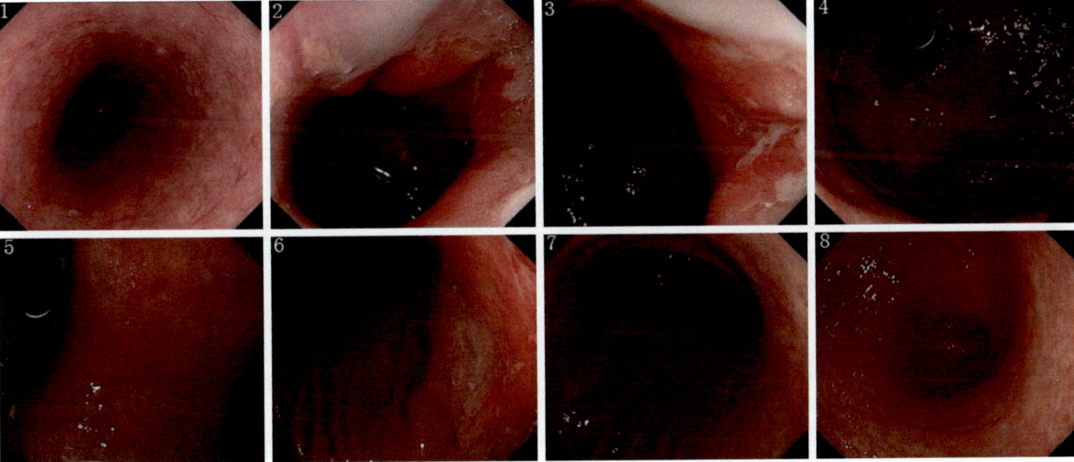

Fig. 4.10 Gastroduodenoscopy: A superficial elevated lesion located at the cardia, which extends to involve the junction, fundus, and body of the stomach

CT scan showed exhibited adequate gastric filling, devoid of discernible wall thickening or masses, and no anomalous enhancements upon contrast administration (Fig. 4.11). The patient's medical history encompasses a 3-year-long hypertension diagnosis, with a recorded highest blood pressure measurement of 160/90 mmHg, and a 4-year-long diabetes diagnosis, characterized by the highest blood glucose level reaching 18 mmol/L, which is ordinarily managed with insulin aspart administration.

Diagnosis: Gastric cancer (cT1N0M0), hypertension, diabetes.

4.4.2 Treatment

After completing the preoperative preparation, the patient underwent laparoscopic-assisted proximal gastrectomy. During the surgery procedure, a tumor measuring 4 cm × 2 cm was identified at the cardia, which did not infiltrate the serosa layer of the gastric wall. Subsequently, laparoscopic dissection was performed to remove the proximal stomach and adjacent lymph nodes. Following the dissection, a 10 cm auxiliary incision was made in the upper abdomen. The esophagus was transected 3 cm above the cardia, and a 25 mm anastomosis stapler was inserted. The stomach was transected 5 cm below the tumor, and the specimen was removed. A gastroesophageal anastomosis was performed. Postoperatively, the patient received symptomatic supportive treatment, including fluid replacement, acid suppression, pain management, antiemetics, and nebulization.

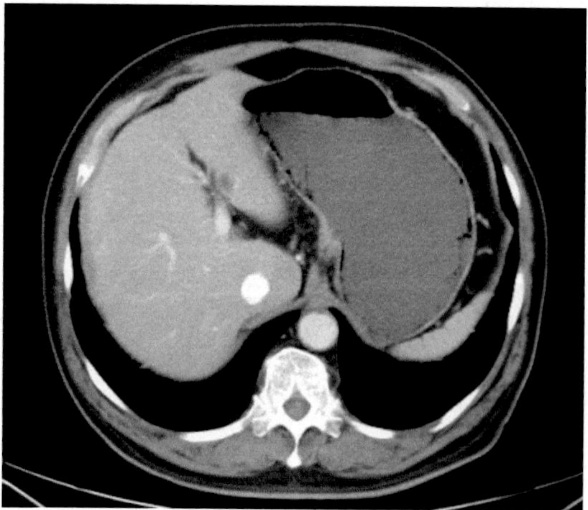

Fig. 4.11 Abdominal contrast-enhanced CT: No significant abnormal enhancement observed

On the ninth day after the surgery, the patient is presented with nausea and dysphagia after ingesting water. An upper gastrointestinal contrast study demonstrated stenosis of the anastomotic stoma, obstructing the passage of contrast agent (Fig. 4.12a). Gastroscopy revealed that the anastomotic stoma, located 37 cm from the incisors, exhibited rough and edematous mucosa. No definitive mass or ulceration was observed. The anastomotic stoma appeared twisted and narrowed, with only limited traversal possible using an ultra-thin endoscope. Subsequently, a gastrointestinal feeding tube was inserted under endoscopic guidance (Fig. 4.13). On the 13th day post-surgery, an upper gastrointestinal contrast study demonstrated persistent narrowing of the anastomotic stoma, resulting in contrast agent obstruction, as observed in previous imaging (Fig. 4.12b). By the 18th day, the patient continued to experience postprandial vomiting. Gastroscopy revealed twisting and narrowing of the anastomotic stoma. Although the ultra-thin endoscope could pass through with difficulty after dilation, the effect was unsatisfactory. Under X-ray monitoring, a 20 mm × 60 mm stent was endoscopically implanted (Fig. 4.14), resulting in successful stent expansion. Subsequently, the patient could consume small, frequent meals and was discharged on the 31st postoperative day.

The histopathological analysis confirmed the presence of a Siewert II-type, low-to-moderately differentiated adenocarcinoma at the gastroesophageal junction in the patient. The tumor exhibited invasion into the submucosal layer without evident nerve involvement or vascular tumor embolism. No signs of cancer were detected in the greater omentum or the resection margins. Furthermore, lymph node metastasis was absent, with all 36 examined lymph nodes showing no evidence of malignancy. The TNM staging was pT1bN0M0, stage I.

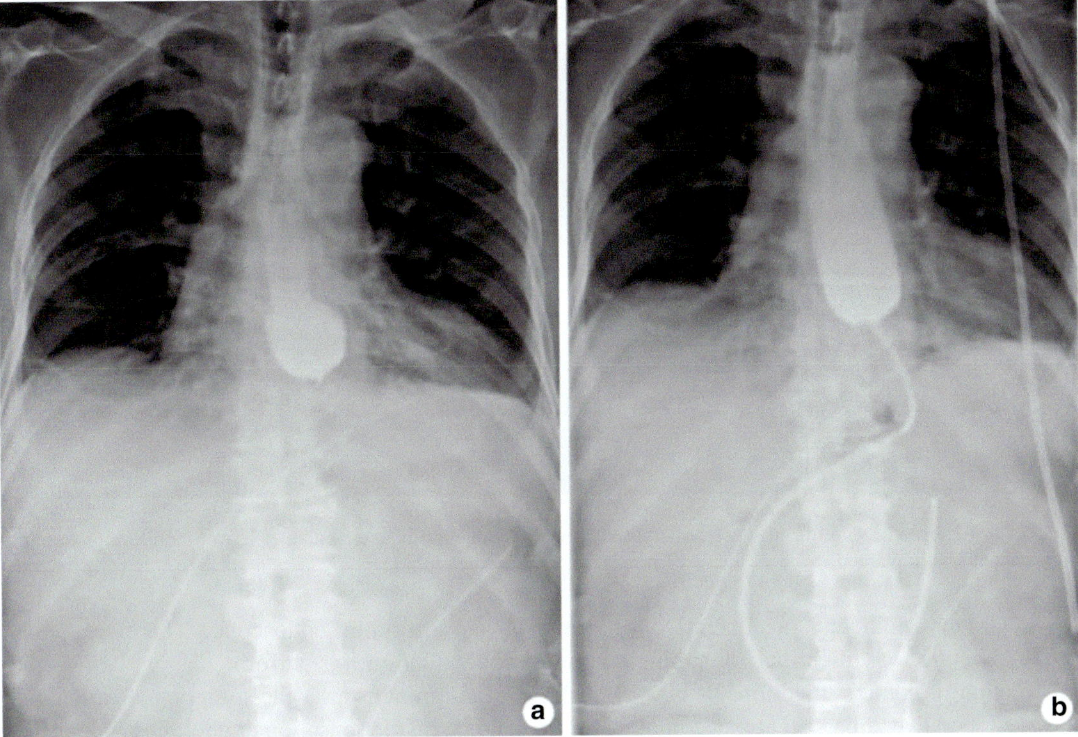

Fig. 4.12 Upper gastrointestinal contrast study (**a**) On POD 9, an anastomotic stricture was identified, leading to the blockage of contrast medium. (**b**) On POD 13, a persistent anastomotic stricture was observed, to the previous image

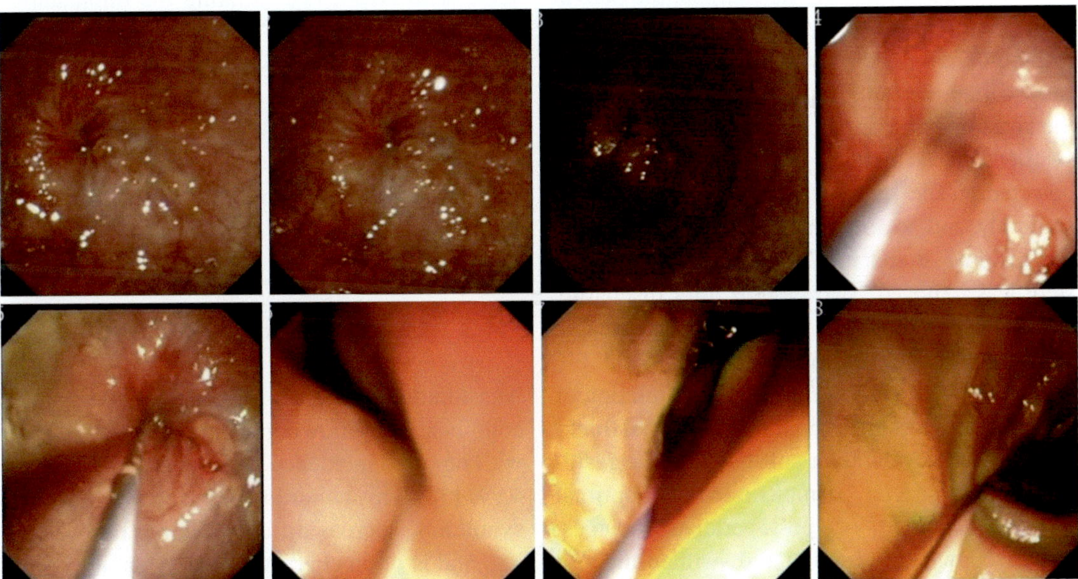

Fig. 4.13 Gastroscopy shows the anastomosis was twisted and narrowed, and the ultra-thin endoscope could pass through with difficulty. A nasointestinal feeding tube was inserted under endoscopy

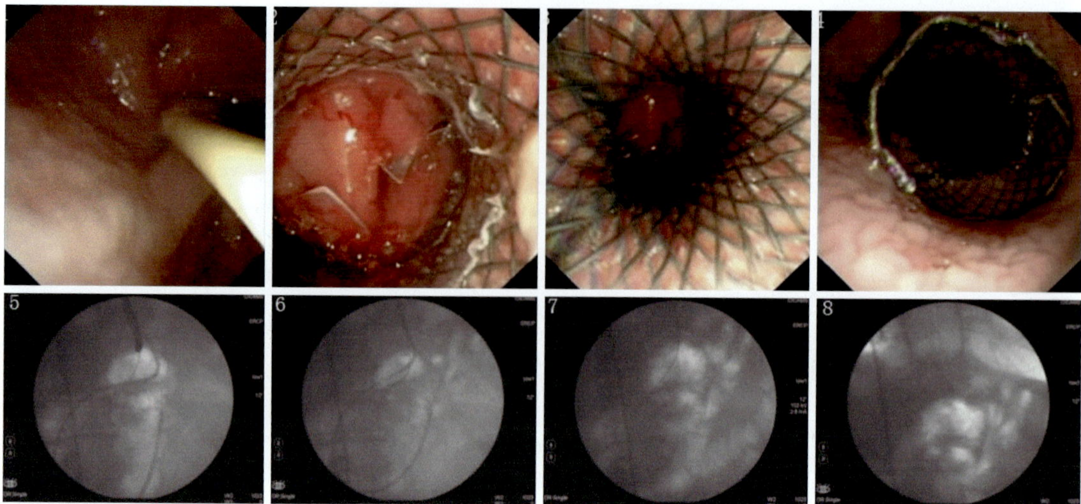

Fig. 4.14 Endoscopic dilation was performed, but the effect was unsatisfactory. Under X-ray monitoring, an endoscopic stent was implanted

A: On the ninth day postoperative, anastomotic stricture was identified, resulting in the obstruction of contrast medium. B: On the 13th day postoperative, a persistent anastomotic stricture was observed, with contrast medium blockage resembling the findings from the previous image.

One month after being discharged, the patient underwent a gastroscopy examination, revealing the presence of the previously implanted metal stent within the esophageal lumen. At the site of the anastomosis, the mucosa appeared rough and swollen, but no definite mass or ulceration was detected. The endoscope passed through smoothly, and no abnormalities were observed in the residual stomach. Consequently, the metal stent was removed. Two months after discharge, the patient experienced a recurrence of dysphagia and postprandial vomiting. An abdominal CT scan with contrast showed inadequate dilation of the anastomotic site, without any abnormal thickening of the surrounding soft tissues. The residual gastric cavity demonstrated suboptimal filling, indicative of postoperative changes. Gastroscopy showed rough and swollen mucosa at the anastomotic site, with no definitive mass or ulceration. The anastomotic stoma displayed twisting and narrowing, obstructing the passage of an ultra-thin endoscope. Therefore, endoscopic dilation was performed.

Four months after the surgery, the patient persisted with the sensation of choking while eating. Gastroscopy examination confirmed a twisted and narrow anastomotic stoma. Despite difficulty, the ultra-thin endoscope was able to traverse with effort, necessitating the implantation of a stent (Fig. 4.15). After 8 months since the operation, a subsequent gastroscopy examination (Fig. 4.16) revealed the presence of the appropriately expanded and well-positioned metal stent. Routine endoscopy was successfully conducted, and it was advised to continue with regular follow-up.

4.4.3 Case Analysis

Anastomotic stenosis is a frequently encountered complication following gastric cancer surgery, with reported incidence rates ranging from 1.2 to 4.9% [38]. This condition can lead to obstructive symptoms, such as difficulty eating or swallowing, and is often characterized by manifestations such as abdominal distension, abdominal pain, dysphagia, and vomiting. While some patients may exhibit mild stenosis without apparent signs,

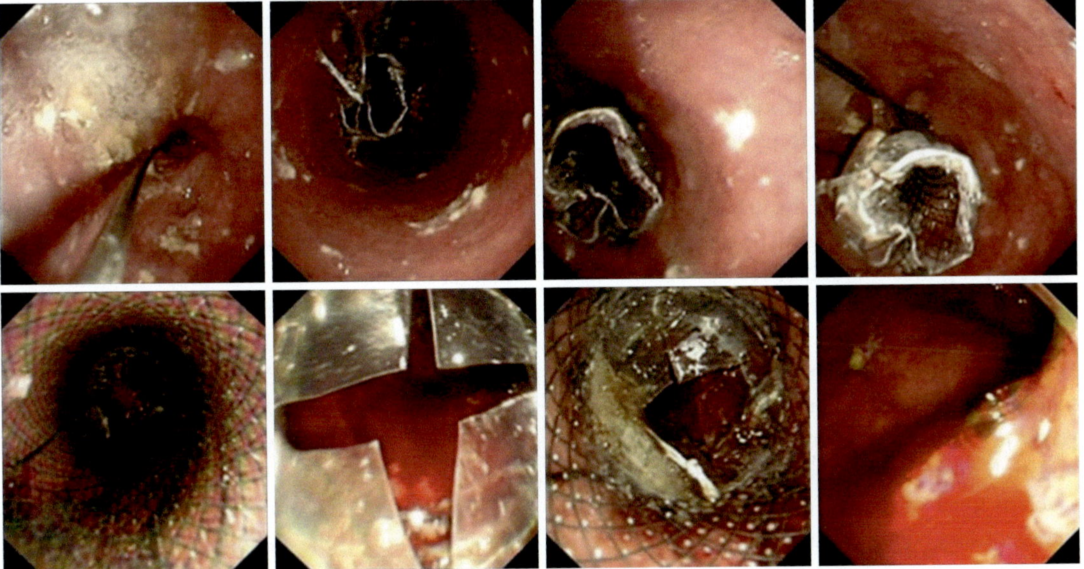

Fig. 4.15 Four months postoperative gastroscopy follow-up, with stent insertion performed

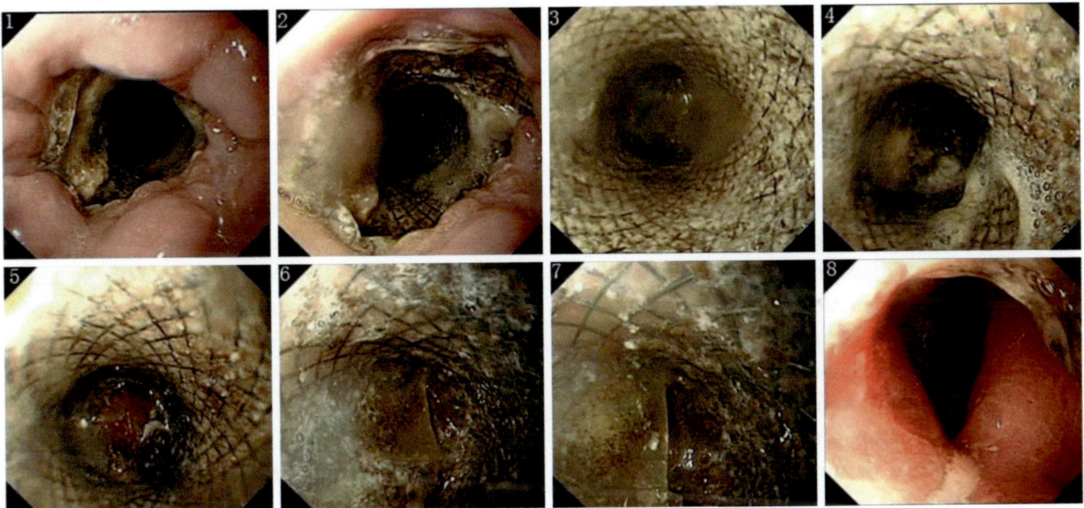

Fig. 4.16 Eight months postoperative gastroscopy follow-up, the position of the stent in the esophagus and residual gastric cavity is good

significant stenosis can result in noticeable symptoms and can be diagnosed and evaluated through upper gastrointestinal contrast studies or gastroscopy.

The common causes of anastomotic stenosis include [39]. (1) Inadequate selection of a small or inappropriate diameter circular stapler, or excessive tissue stapling leading to anastomotic stenosis or complete closure; (2) Use a linear stapler for closing a common opening, resulting in excessive tissue clamping and output loop stenosis; (3) Complications at the anastomotic site, such as ischemia, fistula, or ulcer, which can induce inflammatory reactions, scar tissue proliferation, and stenosis; (4) Excessive mucosal inversion during manual anastomosis or suturing on the opposite side of the mucosa during reinforcement suturing in surgery; (5) Some patients may experience postoperative anastomotic edema, which obstructs food passage. (6) In cases of proximal gastrectomy for gastric cancer, long-term reflux esophagitis can stimulate inflammatory stenosis of the anastomotic stoma.

According to the consensus among domestic experts [40], anastomotic strictures can be categorized into several levels based on the severity: Grade I: no specific intervention required; Grade II: medical intervention, reinsertion of the gastric tube or total parenteral nutrition >1 week after removal of the gastric tube; Grade IIIa: jejunal nutrition tube or other local anesthesia operation (such as local anesthesia endoscopy); Grade IIIb: intervention under general anesthesia; Grade IVa: at least one organ function failure; Grade IVb: sepsis or multiple organ dysfunction syndrome; Grade V: death.

As anastomotic stenosis is commonly associated with surgical procedures, it is essential to implement standardized intraoperative protocols to minimize the risk of postoperative strictures. The main measures include: (1) Selecting an appropriate anastomotic device based on the diameter of the anastomotic intestine. Generally, a 25 mm circular anastomotic device is suitable for intraoperative anastomosis; (2) Enhancing the condition of the gastrointestinal tract tissues before surgery to reduce edema; (3) Proper utilization of the anastomotic device to prevent misalignment of the mucosa at both ends of the anastomotic opening and avoid fixation issues with the intestinal tissue around the anastomotic site; (4) Proactive prevention and treatment of complications related to the anastomotic opening to ensure a tension-free and adequately vascularized anastomosis; (5) Avoiding excessive tightness in suture ligation of the anastomotic opening and preventing excessive inversion during the reinforcement of the muscular layer; (6) Post-anastomosis, conducting thorough inspections of the patency and potential weaknesses of the anastomotic opening; (7) Performing frozen pathological examinations during surgery to ensure negative margins, thereby reducing the recurrence rate of anastomotic tumors [41]·

The treatment of anastomotic stenosis follows a stepwise approach, beginning with conservative measures and progressing to surgical interventions, depending on the cause and severity of the stenosis. Conservative treatment is generally attempted first and is particularly effective for postoperative inflammatory edema compared to scar stenosis. This approach involves measures such as fasting, gastric tube placement, albumin supplementation, acid-inhibiting agents, mucosal protective agents, and high osmotic saline gastric lavage, which help reduce edema and provide rapid symptom relief. Mild to moderate scar stenosis can also be relieved by sufficient time of conservative treatment. For cases of severe stenosis, endoscopic balloon dilation [42] or endoscopic incision of the stenosis scar [43] should be considered, mostly performed 3–4 weeks after surgery. If the dilation effect is not satisfactory, the insertion of a stent should be considered. In instances where stenosis is caused by anastomotic tumor recurrence, the resection of the recurrent tumor and re-anastomosis may be considered if the patient's condition allows. If complete tumor removal is not possible, palliative treatments such as bypass surgery, stoma surgery, or endoscopic stent insertion can be considered to alleviate symptoms and improve the patient's quality of life [44]· For patients with systemic nutritional disorders, the placement of a nasointestinal nutrition tube under endoscopy is recommended to provide enteral nutrition support.

4.4.4 Expert Comments

Postoperative gastrointestinal reconstruction plays a critical role in gastric cancer surgery, and effectively managing anastomotic-related complications is a challenge faced by gastrointestinal surgeons. Given the frequent association between anastomotic stenosis and surgical procedures, adhering to standardized intraoperative protocols and selecting suitable anastomotic devices and gastrointestinal reconstruction methods are paramount for preventing stenosis. During the perioperative management phase, it is important to promptly identify anastomotic stenosis. Careful attention should be paid to distinguishing between gastrointestinal functional recovery disorders and mechanical obstruction, as distinct treatment approaches are warranted based on the underlying cause.

Case provider: Chongyuan Sun, Xiaofeng Bai.

Commentary: Yuemin Sun.

4.5 Case 29: Laparoscopic Surgery for the Internal Hernia After Gastrectomy

4.5.1 Brief History

The present case involves a 60-year-old male patient who was admitted to the hospital due to persistent upper abdominal discomfort spanning a period of 2 years, with a recent exacerbation lasting over 1 month. Previously, the patient experienced intermittent upper abdominal discomfort, for which he received pharmacological treatment for "gastritis" at an alternative medical facility. Unfortunately, the symptoms have progressively worsened within the past month, with no substantial relief observed from medication. Gastroscopy revealed gastric ulcerative-type gastric cancer, histologically characterized as adenocarcinoma, following the Lauren classification of the intestinal type. Notably, the patient has a significant history of tobacco and alcohol consumption, while abdominal examination did not reveal any positive signs. Pertaining to tumor markers, elevated levels of CA19–9 (54.7 U/mL) and CA24–2 (33.5 U/mL) were detected, while CEA, AFP, and CA72–4 levels remained within the normal range. Abdominal CT imaging displayed inadequate filling and expansion of the gastric cavity. Noteworthy findings included local irregular thickening and enhancement of the gastric wall adjacent to the gastric angle on the small curvature of the stomach. These features exhibited indistinct boundaries, with a diameter of approximately 3.1 cm and a maximum thickness of about 1.2 cm. Furthermore, the serosal surface appeared unclear. Additionally, multiple enlarged lymph nodes were identified in the left gastric region, exhibiting heterogeneous enhancement and measuring approximately 1.0 cm in their short diameter (refer to Fig. 4.17).

Diagnosis: Gastric cancer (cT4N + M0).

4.5.2 Treatment

Following a comprehensive evaluation upon admission, no contraindications for surgery were identified. Consequently, routine preoperative preparation was conducted, leading to the performance of a laparoscopic distal gastrectomy utilizing the Billroth II + Braun technique.

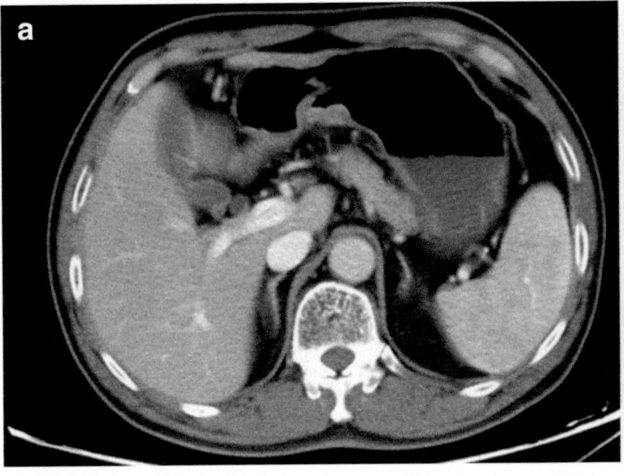

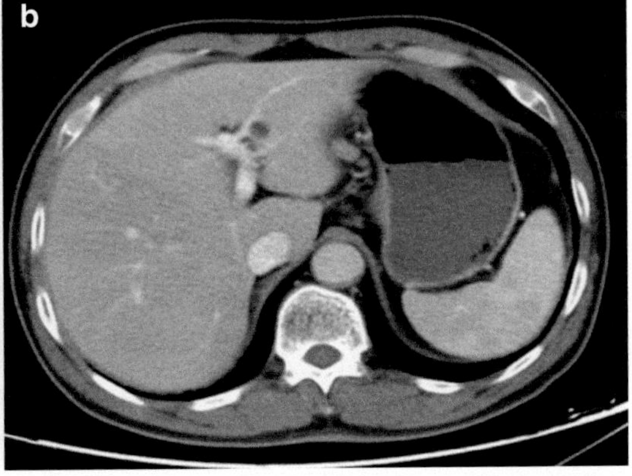

Fig. 4.17 Displays pertinent imaging findings. In (**a**). abdominal CT scan reveals conspicuous thickening of the gastric wall within the gastric antrum, a characteristic feature consistent with the appearance of gastric cancer. Moving on to (**b**), it showcases enlarged lymph nodes situated in the vicinity of the stomach

Postoperatively, the patient was encouraged to engage in early mobilization, and on the second day following the surgery, the gastric tube was removed. Subsequently, the abdominal drainage tube was removed on the fourth day, and the patient commenced a liquid diet on the sixth day. Ultimately, the patient was discharged on the seventh day.

Upon histopathological examination, the resected specimen exhibited localized ulcerative-type moderately to poorly differentiated adenocarcinoma of the stomach. According to the Lauren classification, the tumor predominantly displayed an intestinal type, with partly papillary structure comprising 30% and micro-papillary structure comprising 5% of the neoplastic architecture. Tumor foci infiltrating the serosa were observed, whereas the pylorus, duodenum, and greater omentum remained uninvolved. Noteworthy pathological features included evidence of neural invasion, vascular cancer embolus, and venous invasion. Importantly, no evidence of cancer involvement was detected at the upper and lower margins. Lymph node analysis revealed the presence of metastases in 5 out of 21 examined lymph nodes. According to the TNM staging system, the tumor was classified as pT4aN2M0, corresponding to stage III.

More than 10 days subsequent to the patient's discharge, he experienced a sudden onset of symptoms including abdominal distension, abdominal pain, vomiting, and cessation of gas and bowel movements. An emergent abdominal CT scan was conducted, revealing gastric fluid accumulation, proximal dilatation, and fluid accumulation at the site of intestinal anastomosis, indicative of intestinal obstruction (refer to Fig. 4.18a). To alleviate the obstruction, gastric and intestinal decompression was performed, with approximately 400 mL of gastric fluid being extracted daily. Subsequent gastroscopic examination demonstrated that the esophagogastric junction was located approximately 40 cm from the incisors. The residual gastric mucosa exhibited congestion and edema. Evaluation of the gastric-intestinal anastomosis, approximately 57 cm from the incisors, revealed mucosal congestion and edema, without discernible masses or ulcers and with no apparent stenosis. Importantly, successful passage of the endoscope was achieved. The intestinal anastomosis, located approximately 80 cm from the incisors, displayed

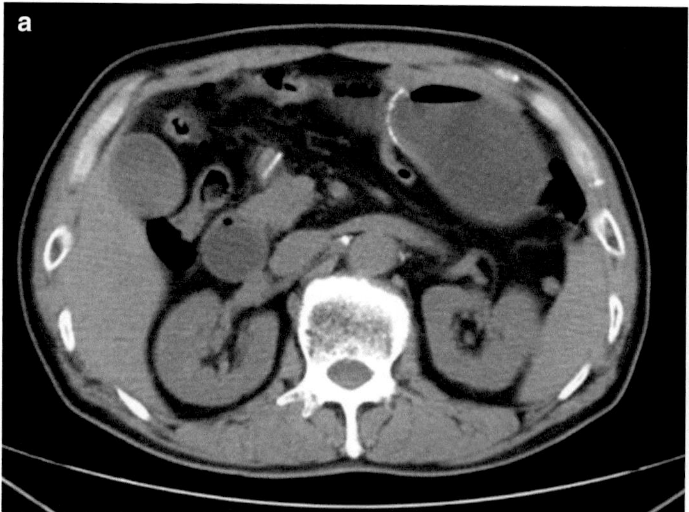

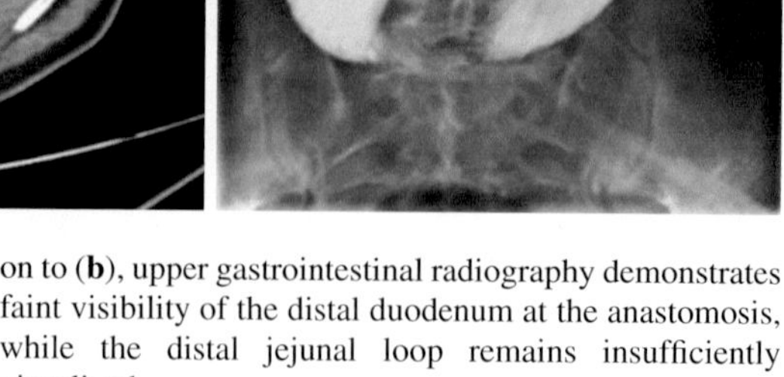

Fig. 4.18 displays relevant imaging findings pertaining to the patient's condition. In (**a**), a postoperative abdominal CT scan illustrates proximal dilatation and fluid accumulation at the site of the intestinal anastomosis. Moving on to (**b**), upper gastrointestinal radiography demonstrates faint visibility of the distal duodenum at the anastomosis, while the distal jejunal loop remains insufficiently visualized

local mucosal congestion and edema. In order to ensure enteral nutrition delivery, an enteral feeding tube was inserted under endoscopic guidance. However, subsequent administration of enteral nutrition resulted in the suctioning of the nutrition solution through the gastric tube, indicating a failure of the enteral nutrition tube to pass beyond the point of obstruction. Consequently, the tube was removed. Upper gastrointestinal radiography was repeated, revealing faint visualization of the distal duodenum at the anastomosis after oral administration of an iodine contrast agent for approximately 10 min. However, the distal jejunal loop remained inadequately visualized (see Fig. 4.18b). Despite 2 weeks of active conservative treatment, no improvement in the intestinal obstruction was observed, leading to the decision to proceed with laparoscopic surgical exploration. The subsequent surgical procedure is detailed as follows.

Under general anesthesia and in the modified lithotomy position, the patient underwent the surgical procedure. Following routine disinfection and draping, a 3-cm incision was made above the umbilicus, which was carefully opened layer by layer to access the abdominal cavity. Adequate visualization confirmed the absence of adhesions below the umbilicus, and pneumoperitoneum was established through an observation port. As the primary operative port, a 12 mm trocar was inserted at the midpoint between the umbilicus and the anterior superior iliac spine on the right lower abdomen, while a 5 mm trocar was placed at the initial puncture site on the right side of the navel.

Systematic exploration of the abdominal cavity revealed minor adhesions within the original surgical area. Specifically, adhesions were identified between the Braun anastomotic opening and the mesocolon in the lower abdomen, resulting in the formation of a hernia ring approximately 10 cm posterior to it. The anastomotic opening became twisted due to the herniation of the distal small intestine from the right to the left side. Additionally, scattered adhesion points were observed in the remaining distal small intestine and the pelvic cavity, limiting the mobility of the small intestine. To alleviate the pressure exerted on the adhered small intestine, the herniated small intestine on the left side was carefully repositioned to the right side. Subsequently, under direct visualization, the adherent points were released, and the pathogenic hernia ring was excised. Sequential examination was then performed to ensure the unobstructed flow of the small intestine from the Braun anastomotic opening to the ileocecal region, excluding any suspicious adhesions. Endoscopy confirmed the absence of obstruction at both the anastomotic opening and the Braun anastomotic opening. Suturing of the Petersen space and the interstitial space behind the Braun anastomotic opening was meticulously carried out, culminating in the completion of the surgical procedure.

The patient made a smooth recovery following the operation, and on the second day, a liquid diet was initiated. Ultimately, the patient was discharged on the seventh day, with no recurrence of intestinal obstruction observed post-discharge.

4.5.3 Case Analysis

Internal hernia refers to the displacement of organs or tissues within the abdominal cavity from their normal positions, entering specific anatomical gaps in the peritoneum or mesentery through either normal or abnormal openings or clefts. Following gastric cancer surgery, alterations in the anatomy can give rise to the formation of abnormal recesses, clefts, or defects, providing opportunities for abdominal organs and tissues to herniate. The entry of the intestinal tract into these gaps can lead to incarceration and torsion of the mesentery, resulting in intestinal obstruction and necrosis.

In a study conducted by Kang et al. [45], analysis of 6474 patients who underwent gastric cancer surgery revealed a postoperative internal hernia incidence of 1.7%. The incidence rates were found to be 0.9% for open surgery and 2% for laparoscopy. Other studies have reported the incidence of internal hernia after gastric cancer surgery to range from 0.19 to 5% [46, 47]. Various types of internal hernias can occur following gastric surgery, including mesenteric foramen hernia, Petersen hernia, diaphragmatic foramen hernia, adhesive hernia, and anastomotic hernia, with mesenteric foramen hernia being the most common.

4.5.3.1 Factors Influencing Internal Hernia After Gastric Cancer Surgery

Numerous factors influence the occurrence of internal hernia following gastric cancer surgery, including the surgical approach (open or laparoscopic), surgical technique (partial or total gastrectomy), anastomotic method, management of mesenteric defects (closure or non-closure of mesenteric gaps), and postoperative weight loss.

Laparoscopic gastrectomy has gained widespread use in gastric cancer treatment owing to its minimal surgical trauma, reduced risk of postoperative adhesions, early restoration of intestinal peristalsis, and shorter hospital stays. However, precisely because laparoscopic surgery minimizes tissue damage and adhesions, there is reduced adhesion formation between the small intestine and adjacent structures. This increased mobility of the small intestine predisposes it to herniate through mesenteric defects, leading to a higher incidence of internal hernia. Studies have demonstrated that the occurrence of internal hernia is significantly higher after laparoscopic gastrectomy compared to open gastrectomy. Furthermore, the incidence of internal hernia is higher after total laparoscopic gastrectomy compared to laparoscopic-assisted gastrectomy, and multi-port laparoscopy has a higher incidence than single-port laparoscopy [46, 48, 49].

The body mass index (BMI) index also exhibits a certain correlation with internal hernia. Patients with lower BMI tend to have less mesenteric fat, increasing the likelihood of mesenteric defects and subsequent internal hernia. Han et al. [50] identified low BMI (<23 kg/m^2), total gastrectomy, Roux-en-Y anastomosis, and laparoscopic surgery as associated factors for internal hernia. Multivariate analysis further revealed low BMI and laparoscopic surgery as independent risk factors for internal hernia.

The incidence of internal hernia varies among different reconstruction methods. Studies conducted abroad have reported a significantly higher incidence of internal hernia in patients with Roux-en-Y reconstruction and Uncut-Roux-en-Y reconstruction compared to those with Billroth-II reconstruction. This discrepancy may be attributed to the presence of two defects (mesenteric foramen and Petersen's defects) in Roux-en-Y reconstruction, whereas Billroth-II reconstruction only entails Petersen's defect [45, 46].

Internal hernia following gastric cancer surgery is also influenced by changes in intestinal function and disturbances in peristalsis. Factors such as overeating, vigorous physical activity after meals, and diarrhea can disrupt normal bowel movements, thereby facilitating the herniation of the intestinal tract into abdominal gaps and increasing the risk of internal hernia [51].

4.5.3.2 Diagnosis of Internal Hernia After Gastric Cancer Surgery

The clinical presentation of internal hernia is variable, with upper abdominal pain being a prominent symptom. Mild cases may exhibit intermittent abdominal pain that resolves spontaneously. Moderate cases are characterized by paroxysmal abdominal colic accompanied by nausea, vomiting, cessation of anal gas, and bowel movements. Severe cases manifest with symptoms such as chills, fever, shock, peritonitis, and signs of intestinal necrosis.

Diagnosing internal hernia can be challenging, as physical examination findings and laboratory test results alone are insufficient to confirm the diagnosis or determine the need for surgical intervention. Hence, immediate abdominal CT scan is recommended when there is suspicion of internal hernia. Abdominal CT typically reveals the aggregation of small bowel loops, small bowel obstruction, edema of mesenteric fat and vessels, and the presence of the characteristic "vortex sign." However, certain studies have reported the diagnostic challenges associated with CT scans, with specificity and sensitivity rates of 77% and 63%, respectively [52]. Consequently, only two-thirds of internal hernia cases are diagnosed preoperatively. Therefore, the diagnosis of internal hernia should not rely solely on specific symptoms or individual tests, but should integrate the patient's clinical presentation and various examinations, including CT imaging, endoscopic evaluation, and other relevant investigations, to promptly determine the appropriate treatment approach.

4.5.3.3 Treatment of Internal Hernia

Early intervention in cases of suspected internal hernia has been shown to yield better outcomes compared to late intervention. Although there may not be a statistically significant difference in the rate of intestinal resection, postoperative complications, and mortality between early and late intervention groups, the surgical outcomes of the late intervention group tend to be poorer. This finding suggests that early surgical treatment when internal hernia is suspected can help reduce surgical complications [53].

When choosing a surgical approach for treating internal hernia, a study comparing laparoscopic and open surgery for Petersen's hernia found no significant difference in operation time and the incidence of complications. However, laparoscopic surgery was associated with a shorter recovery time [9]. Therefore, laparoscopic surgery is considered safe for treating internal hernia, but the specific approach should be determined based on individual conditions. If there are severe intra-abdominal adhesions, open surgery may be safer. Laparoscopic exploration can also serve as a diagnostic tool to determine the appropriate surgical approach and method based on intraoperative findings and the severity of the hernia, such as reduction of the hernia, small bowel resection, and necessary intestinal ostomy.

Several measures can be taken during the operation to effectively prevent internal hernia: (1) Performing meticulous surgery to minimize surgical adhesions. (2) Routine closure of the mesenteric defect, as smaller defects are more prone to internal hernia. (3) Ensuring an appropriate length of the input loop, typically 8–12 cm in front of the colon and 4–8 cm behind the colon.

Internal hernia after gastric cancer surgery commonly occurs within months to years. According to Kang et al. [1], the median interval between gastric resection surgery and the occurrence of internal hernia was 450 days. However, in the case of the patient described, the internal hernia occurred more than 10 days after surgery, which represents a short-term complication with a relatively abrupt onset. This may be attributed to the patient's improper diet after surgery.

4.5.4 Expert Comments

Internal hernia following gastric cancer surgery is a grave complication, and its preoperative diagnosis poses a significant challenge. Failure to promptly diagnose and treat this condition can lead to severe consequences, potentially resulting in fatality. Hence, early surgical intervention is imperative when internal hernia is suspected. In the realm of gastric cancer surgery, employing non-absorbable sutures to meticulously close the mesenteric gap at the site of intestinal anastomosis, as well as addressing potential spaces like Petersen's defect and the defect in the transverse colon mesentery, is recommended to proactively prevent and diminish the incidence of internal hernia. This strategy aims to mitigate the occurrence of internal herniation, acknowledging its associated risks and the need for proactive measures during gastric cancer surgical procedures.

Case provider: Hong Zhou, Chunguang Guo.

Commentary: Dongbing Zhao.

References

1. Tanizawa Y, Bando E, Kawamura T, et al. Early postoperative anastomotic hemorrhage after gastrectomy for gastric cancer. Gastric Cancer. 2010;13(1):50–7.
2. Kim KH, Kim MC, Jung GJ, et al. Endoscopic treatment and risk factors of postoperative anastomotic bleeding after gastrectomy for gastric cancer. Int J Surg. 2012;10(10):593–7.
3. Park JY, Kim YW, Eom BW, et al. Unique patterns and proper management of postgastrectomy bleeding in patients with gastric cancer. Surgery. 2014;155(6):1023–9.
4. Yang J, Zhang XH, Huang YH, et al. Diagnosis and treatment of abdominal arterial bleeding after radical gastrectomy: a retrospective analysis of 1875 consecutive resections for gastric cancer. J Gastrointest Surg. 2016;20(3):510–20.

5. Li ZY, Wu ZQ. Prevention and management of postoperative bleeding in gastric cancer. Chin J Bases Clin General Surg. 2021;28(06):704–7. xx.
6. Zhu XF, Huang HP, Xiong WJ, et al. Clinical analysis of massive hemorrhage after radical gastrectomy with D2 lymph node dissection. J Digest Oncol (Electronic Version). 2020;12(01):26–30.
7. Song W, Yuan Y, Peng J, et al. The delayed massive hemorrhage after gastrectomy in patients with gastric cancer: characteristics, management opinions, and risk factors. Eur J Surg Oncol. 2014;40(10):1299–306.
8. Jeong O, Park YK, Ryu SY, et al. Predisposing factors and management of postoperative bleeding after radical gastrectomy for gastric carcinoma. Surg Today. 2011;41(3):363–8.
9. Li ZY, Li ZM, Li SX, et al. Causes and therapeutic strategies for postoperative bleeding after laparoscopic gastrectomy. Chin J Oper Proced General Surg (Electronic Edition). 2015;9(02):90–3.
10. Li ZY, Wu ZQ, Ji JF. Expert consensus on diagnostic registration standards for postoperative complications of gastrointestinal cancer surgery in China (2018 edition). Chin J Pract Surg. 2018;38(06):589–95.
11. Zhang YQ, Zhou PH. Value of endoscopy application in the management of complications after radical gastrectomy for gastric cancer. Chin J Gastrointest Surg. 2017;20(02):160–5.
12. Sung JJ, Tsoi KK, Lai LH, et al. Endoscopic clipping versus injection and thermo-coagulation in treating non-variceal upper gastrointestinal bleeding: a meta-analysis. Gut. 2007;56(10):1364–73.
13. Standop J, Schäfer N, Overhaus M, et al. Endoscopic management of anastomotic hemorrhage from pancreatogastrostomy. Surg Endosc. 2009;23(9):2005–10.
14. Blouhos K, Boulas KA, Konstantinidou A, et al. Early rupture of an ultralow duodenal stump after extended surgery for gastric cancer with duodenal invasion managed by tube duodenostomy and cholangiostomy. Case Reports Surg. 2013;2013:430295.
15. Cozzaglio L, Coladonato M, Biffi R, et al. Duodenal fistula after elective gastrectomy for malignant disease: an Italian retrospective multicenter study. J Gastrointest Surg. 2010;14(5):805–11.
16. Wu BY, Zhang JN. Reason, prevention, and treatment of gastrointestinal unplanned reoperation. Chin J Bases Clin General Surg. 2014;21(06):736–40.
17. Paik HJ, Lee SH, Choi CI, et al. Duodenal stump fistula after gastrectomy for gastric cancer: risk factors, prevention, and management. Ann Surg Treatment Res. 2016;90(3):157–63.
18. Suo J, Li W, Wang DG. Diagnosis and treatment of duodenal stump leakage after laparoscopic gastrectomy. Chin J Oper Proced General Surg (Electronic Edition). 2015;9(02):98–100.
19. Po Chu Patricia Y, Ka Fai Kevin W, Fong Yee L, et al. Duodenal stump leakage. Lessons to learn from a large-scale 15-year cohort study. Am J Surg. 2020;220(4):976–81.
20. Tang Y, Li R, Chen L, et al. Nutritional support of duodenal stump leakage after gastrectomy for gastric carcinoma. Chin J Gastrointest Surg. 2008;01:47–9.
21. Gong KM, Guo SK, Wang KH. Diagnosis and treatment of duodenal injury and fistula. Chin J Gastrointest Surg. 2017;20(03):266–9.
22. Aurello P, Sirimarco D, Magistri P, et al. Management of duodenal stump fistula after gastrectomy for gastric cancer: systematic review. World J Gastroenterol. 2015;21(24):7571–6.
23. Zhang HH, Wu BG, Du BL. Analysis of risk factors and their impact on prognosis for postoperative gastroparesis syndrome in radical resection of gastric cancer. Chin J Curr Adv Gen Surg. 2016;19(03):248–9.
24. Kim DH, Yun HY, Song YJ, et al. Clinical features of gastric emptying after distal gastrectomy. Ann Surg Treat Res. 2017;93(6):310–5.
25. Zárate N, Mearin F, Wang XY, et al. Severe idiopathic gastroparesis due to neuronal and interstitial cells of Cajal degeneration: pathological findings and management. Gut. 2003;52(7):966–70.
26. Meng H, Zhou D, Jiang X, et al. Incidence and risk factors for postsurgical gastroparesis syndrome after laparoscopic and open radical gastrectomy. World J Surg Oncol. 2013;11:144.
27. Zhang MJ, Zhang GL, Yuan WB, et al. Risk factors analysis of postsurgical gastroparesis syndrome and its impact on the survival of gastric cancer after subtotal gastrectomy. Zhonghua Wei Chang Wai Ke Za Zhi. 2013;16(2):163–5.
28. Chen XD, Mao CC, Zhang WT, et al. A quantified risk-scoring system and rating model for postsurgical gastroparesis syndrome in gastric cancer patients. J Surg Oncol. 2017;116(4):533–44.
29. Malagelada JR, Rees WD, Mazzotta LJ, et al. Gastric motor abnormalities in diabetic and postvagotomy gastroparesis: effect of metoclopramide and bethanechol. Gastroenterology. 1980;78(2):286–93.
30. Dong K, Yu XJ, Li B, et al. Advances in mechanisms of postsurgical gastroparesis syndrome and its diagnosis and treatment. Chin J Dig Dis. 2006;7(2):76–82.
31. Ishiguchi T, Tada H, Nakagawa K, et al. Hyperglycemia impairs antro-pyloric coordination and delays gastric emptying in conscious rats. Auton Neurosci. 2002;95(1–2, 112):–20.
32. Soenen S, Rayner CK, Horowitz M, et al. Gastric emptying in the elderly. Clin Geriatr Med. 2015;31(3):339–53.
33. Camilleri M, Parkman HP, Shafi MA, et al. Clinical guideline: management of gastroparesis. Am J Gastroenterol. 2013;108(1):18–37; quiz 8.
34. Wente MN, Bassi C, Dervenis C, et al. Delayed gastric emptying (DGE) after pancreatic surgery: a suggested definition by the international study Group of Pancreatic Surgery (ISGPS). Surgery. 2007;142(5):761–8.
35. Liu T, Fu WH. Postoperative gastric emptying dysfunction after laparoscopic radical gastrectomy: causes and management. Chinese J Oper Proc General Surg. 2015;9(02):94–7.

36. Dong WB, Qiao HP, Xi JW, et al. Acupuncture and Chinese herbal enema for the treatment of 26 patients with postoperative gastroparesis syndrome. Global Tradit Chinese Med. 2016;9(06):740–2.
37. Huang JF, Chen CY, Tan CF, et al. Effect of acupuncture at Zusanli (ST36) for gastroparesis syndrome after radical subtotal gastrectomy. Shanghai J Acupunct Moxibustion. 2020;39(11):1429–33.
38. Fetzner UK, Hölscher AH. A prospective randomized controlled trial of semi-mechanical versus handsewn or circular stapled esophagogastrostomy for prevention of anastomotic stricture. World J Surg. 2013;37(9):2246–7.
39. Huang CM, Zheng CH, Lin JX. Chinese expert consensus on the prevention and treatment of esophagojejunostomy complications after total gastrectomy for gastric cancer (2020 edition). Chinese J Pract Surg. 2021;41(02):121–4.
40. Li ZY, Wu ZQ, Ji JF. Chinese experts consensus on the diagnosis and registration criteria of postoperative complications in gastrointestinal surgery (2018 edition). Chinese J Pract Surg. 2018;38(06):589–95.
41. Hu JK, Yang K. Prevention and treatment of anastomosis-related complications after gastrectomy for gastric cancer. Chinese J Pract Surg. 2017;37(04):362–6.
42. Lee HJ, Park W, Lee H, et al. Endoscopy-guided balloon dilation of benign anastomotic strictures after radical gastrectomy for gastric cancer. Gut Liver. 2014;8(4):394–9.
43. Zhang YQ, Zhou PH. Value of endoscopy application in the management of complications after radical gastrectomy for gastric cancer. Chin J Gastrointes Surg. 2017;20(02):160–5.
44. Hu JK, Zhang WH. Prevention and treatment of anastomosis-related complications after gastric cancer surgery. Chinse J Dig Surg. 2020;19(09):946–50.
45. Kang KM, Cho YS, Min SH, et al. Internal hernia after gastrectomy for gastric cancer in minimally invasive surgery era. Gastric Cancer. 2019;22(5):1009–15.
46. Kelly KJ, Allen PJ, Brennan MF, et al. Internal hernia after gastrectomy for cancer with Roux-Y reconstruction. Surgery. 2013;154(2):305–11.
47. Miyagaki H, Takiguchi S, Kurokawa Y, et al. Recent trend of internal hernia occurrence after gastrectomy for gastric cancer. World J Surg. 2012;36(4):851–7.
48. Yoshikawa K, Shimada M, Kurita N, et al. Characteristics of internal hernia after gastrectomy with Roux-en-Y reconstruction for gastric cancer. Surg Endosc. 2014;28(6):1774–8.
49. Gunabushanam G, Shankar S, Czerniach DR, et al. Small-bowel obstruction after laparoscopic Roux-en-Y gastric bypass surgery. J Comput Assist Tomogr. 2009;33(3):369–75.
50. Han WH, Eom BW, Yoon HM, et al. Clinical characteristics and surgical outcomes of internal hernia after gastrectomy in gastric cancer patients: retrospective case control study. Surg Endosc. 2019;33(9):2873–9.
51. 魏法才，杨道贵，于俊秀，等. 手术后腹内疝27例. 中国现代普通外科进展. 2007;(01):92–3.
52. Blachar A, Federle MP, Brancatelli G, et al. Radiologist performance in the diagnosis of internal hernia by using specific CT findings with emphasis on transmesenteric hernia. Radiology. 2001;221(2):422–8.
53. Min JS, Seo KW, Jeong SH, et al. A comparison of postoperative outcomes after open and laparoscopic reduction of Petersen's hernia: a multicenter observational cohort study. BMC Surg. 2021;21(1):195.

The Comprehensive Treatment for Gastric Cancer

5

Tongbo Wang, Lulu Zhao, Zefeng Li, Chunguang Guo, Dongbing Zhao, Yingtai Chen, and Xiaofeng Bai

5.1 Case 30: Enhanced Recovery After Surgery in the Perioperative Management of Gastric Cancer

5.1.1 Brief History

The patient, a 26-year-old female, was admitted due to persistent dull upper abdominal pain lasting for 2 months, with exacerbation over the past week. Initially, she experienced intermittent epigastric dull pain accompanied by mild nausea and acid reflux, which did not exhibit a significant correlation with food intake. Seeking medical attention, she visited a local hospital where she received sporadic medication for a presumed "gastric ulcer." However, her symptoms continued to worsen despite the treatment. Five days prior, a follow-up gastroscopy revealed the presence of "gastric antrum carcinoma," with pathology confirming it to be signet ring cell carcinoma. Abdominal physical examination did not reveal any positive findings. The patient's tumor markers, including CEA, AFP, CA724, CA19–9, and CA242, all fell within the normal range. Gastroscopy findings indicated gastric cancer located at the stomach's corner, presenting as a superficial depressed + elevated type lesion measuring approximately 2.5 cm × 3.0 cm (Fig. 5.1). Abdominal enhanced CT imaging demonstrated slight thickening of the gastric wall at the gastric corner, reaching a maximum thickness of 0.8 cm. The mucosal surface displayed slight uneven enhancement, while the serous surface appeared smooth. Notably, no definitive enlarged lymph nodes were detected in the abdominal pelvic cavity, retroperitoneum, or bilateral inguinal area (Fig. 5.2).

Diagnosis: Gastric cancer (cT2N1M0, Stage II).

5.1.2 Treatment

Following admission, comprehensive examinations were conducted, revealing no contraindications for surgery. A rapid rehabilitation surgical approach was adopted during the perioperative period. Preoperative education was provided, emphasizing specific instructions such as unrestricted water intake, avoidance of skin preparation, and omission of intestinal preparation on the day prior to the operation. Gastric tube placement was not performed before surgery. A complete laparoscopic radical gastrectomy (triangular anastomosis) was performed at the designated time. Postoperatively, the patient was encouraged to drink water on the first day and to mobilize and

T. Wang · L. Zhao · Z. Li · C. Guo (✉) · D. Zhao
Y. Chen · X. Bai
Department of Pancreatic and Gastric Surgical Oncology, National Cancer Center/National Clinical Research for Cancer/Cancer Hospital, Chinese Academy of Medical Sciences and Peking Union Medical College, Beijing, China

J. Cai (ed.), *Interpretation of Gastric Cancer Cases*, Experts' Perspectives on Medical Advances,
https://doi.org/10.1007/978-981-99-5302-8_5

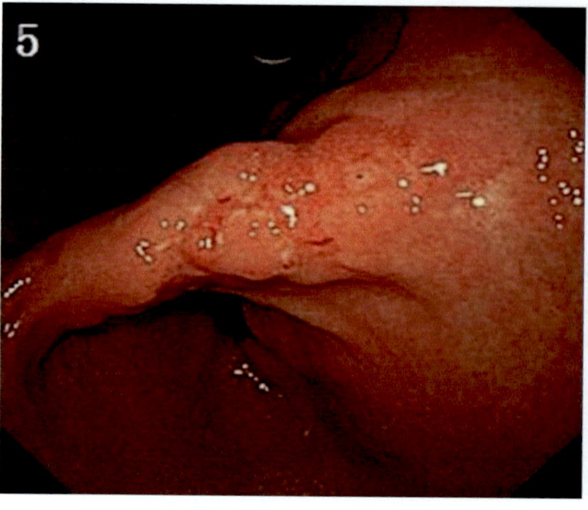

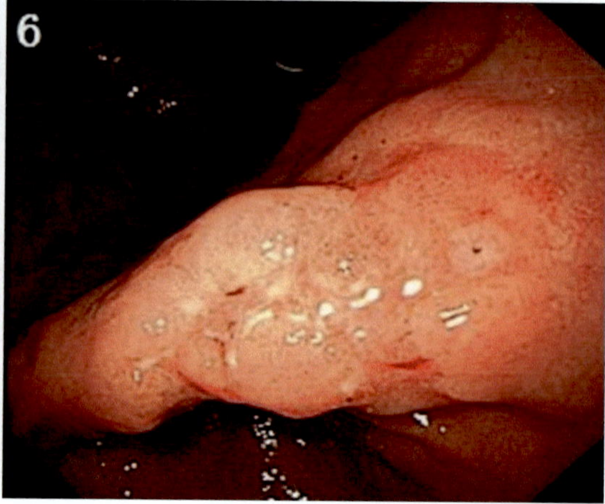

Fig. 5.1 Depicts the gastroscopic view of the patient's condition, revealing gastric cancer situated at the corner of the stomach. The lesion is characterized by a superficial depressed + elevated morphology and measures approximately 2.5 cm × 3.0 cm in size

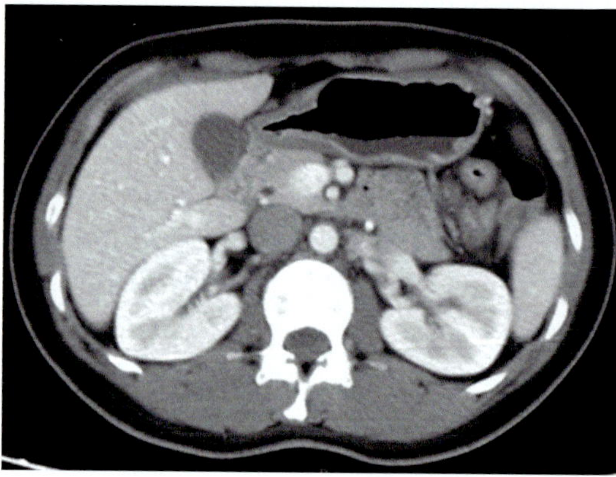

Fig. 5.2 The image illustrates a localized thickening of the gastric wall at the gastric angle, reaching a maximum thickness of approximately 0.8 cm. The mucosal surface displays slight uneven enhancement, while the serous surface appears smooth

ambulate. Clear fluids were introduced on the third day, followed by a liquid diet on the fourth day. The patient was discharged on the sixth day post-surgery.

Pathology examination of the resected gastric specimen (macroscopic) revealed a greater curvature length of 13 cm, a lesser curvature length of 8 cm, a duodenum measuring 0.6 cm in length and 5 cm in width, with the lesser curvature lateral margin located 2.5 cm away from the upper incisal margin. Notably, a superficial ulcerative mass measuring 3 × 1.5 × 0.2 cm was observed, while the pylorus remained uninvolved. Microscopic analysis identified the diagnosis as gastric limited ulcerative poorly differentiated adenocarcinoma, classified according to Lauren's classification as diffuse type, with some areas exhibiting signet ring cell carcinoma. The tumor invaded the muscularis propria with evidence of nerve invasion but no definitive vascular tumor thrombus. There was no involvement of the pylorus or duodenal wall. Furthermore, no metastatic lymph nodes were detected among the 20 examined (0/20), resulting in a TNM stage of pT2N0M0, corresponding to stage I.

5.1.3 Case Analysis

Enhanced Recovery After Surgery (ERAS) is a comprehensive treatment concept that focuses on minimizing surgical trauma and expediting postoperative recovery through a series of evidence-based perioperative interventions. The concept of ERAS was initially proposed by Kehlet in 1997 and encompasses various models aimed at optimizing perioperative care based on well-founded medical evidence. The overarching goal is to reduce stress responses, facilitate postoperative recovery, and ultimately improve patient outcomes [1].

The classic ERAS protocol comprises several key components, including preoperative education, preoperative nutritional support therapy, shortened fasting periods, avoidance of bowel preparation, optimized anesthesia regimens, reduced use of gastric tubes and abdominal drains, early mobilization, and prompt initiation of oral intake. Implementing these measures has been associated with notable benefits, such as decreased hospital stays, reduced rates of surgical complications, and improved postoperative recovery [1].

In accordance with the expert consensus on accelerated rehabilitation surgery for gastric cancer gastrectomy in China, perioperative management for gastric cancer is typically divided into three stages: preoperative preparation, intraoperative planning, and postoperative care. Multidisciplinary collaboration among surgical, nursing, anesthesia, and nutrition teams is crucial for promoting rapid postoperative recovery, serving as the foundation for the implementation of ERAS in gastric cancer surgery [2].

During the preoperative preparation stage, patients and their families are educated about the goals and components of the ERAS program to alleviate their concerns and enhance compliance. Preoperative nutritional support therapy, primarily enteral nutrition, is favored to address malnourished states and eliminate the need for preoperative bowel preparation, fasting, and fluid restrictions. In the intraoperative planning phase, laparoscopic or robotic minimally invasive surgery is recommended for patients with tumor infiltration depth less than T4a. Routine placement of nasogastric tubes and abdominal drainage tubes is avoided, but their utilization is considered on a case-by-case basis. Efforts are made to prevent intraoperative hypothermia. Postoperative management entails multimodal analgesia, early mobilization, prompt initiation of oral intake, and promotion of gastrointestinal motility [2].

The application of ERAS in gastric cancer surgery has gained increasing recognition. A recent meta-analysis incorporating 18 studies on rapid recovery from gastric cancer revealed that ERAS implementation significantly reduces hospital stay duration, hospitalization costs, and time to first vent, defecate, mobilize, and initiate oral intake [3]. It also demonstrated a reduction in postoperative lung infections. However, it should be noted that ERAS was associated with increased readmission rates among patients. Thus, while ERAS offers numerous advantages in postoperative rehabilitation, it also presents certain challenges for clinicians.

One pertinent concern revolves around the decision of whether to employ abdominal drainage tubes following surgery. A meta-analysis encompassing four randomized controlled trials, involving a total of 438 patients, examined this issue. The patients were divided into two groups: one with an indwelling drainage tube ($n = 220$) and the other without ($n = 218$). The results indicated no significant differences in perioperative mortality, secondary surgeries, time to resume feeding, and postoperative complications between the two groups. However, the presence of an abdominal drainage tube was associated with prolonged surgical duration, extended hospital stay, and an increased incidence of drainage-related complications [4]. Consequently, some scholars argue against routine placement of abdominal drainage tubes in patients undergoing radical gastrectomy for early or advanced gastric cancer [5]. Nonetheless, given the extensive lymph node dissection involved in gastric cancer surgery and the potential for significant postoperative wound exudation, complications related to gastric cancer surgery, albeit not frequent, should not be overlooked. Therefore, the guidelines recommend the use of abdominal drainage tubes based on individual circumstances [2]. Certain studies suggest that prophylactic indwelling of abdominal drainage tubes may benefit patients at high intraoperative risk, such as those experiencing substantial blood loss or prolonged operations [6]. Consequently, the decision regarding the retention of peritoneal drainage tubes in gastric cancer surgery within the ERAS framework should be guided by evidence-based medical data and specific clinical conditions. It should be gradually promoted, taking into account the practical medical environment.

5.1.4 Expert Comments

As laparoscopy has become increasingly established and widely adopted, the concept of ERAS has gained recognition and implementation in numerous medical centers. ERAS represents a multidisciplinary approach to diagnosis and treatment, employing a comprehensive array of accelerated rehabilitation techniques to minimize perioperative trauma and facilitate swift patient recovery. With the continuous advancement of minimally invasive surgical principles, ERAS is poised to further leverage the benefits of minimally invasive surgery, ultimately bestowing advantages upon individuals undergoing gastric cancer treatment.

Case provider: Tongbo Wang, Chunguang Guo.

Comment expert: Dongbing Zhao.

5.2 Case 31: Surgical Management of the Proximal Gastric Cancer

5.2.1 Brief History

The patient under consideration is a 60-year-old female who presented with a chronic history of upper abdominal pain spanning 6 months, with recent exacerbation over the past month. The initial onset of intermittent upper abdominal pain occurred 5 months prior to admission, independent of food consumption, and subsided following periods of rest. One month preceding hospitalization, the patient noticed a progression in the severity of the abdominal pain following meals, prompting her to seek medical evaluation at a local healthcare facility. Subsequent gastroscopy examination unveiled the presence of cardia-fundus cancer, with histopathological analysis confirming a poorly differentiated adenocarcinoma. Notably, the patient's levels of carcinoembryonic antigen (CEA), alpha-fetoprotein (AFP), cancer antigen 72-4 (CA72-4), cancer antigen 19-9 (CA19-9), and cancer antigen 24-2 (CA24-2) all fell within the normal range. The gastroscopy further revealed cardia cancer, located approximately 38–43 cm from the incisors, invading the lower esophagus and gastric fundus (as illustrated in Fig. 5.3). An enhanced computed tomography (CT) scan demonstrated the following findings: (1) Serosal invasion by the cardia cancer. The gastric wall adjacent to the cardia displayed irregular thickening, with a maximal thickness of approximately 1.8 cm, exhibiting moderate and heterogeneous enhancement on enhanced scanning, along with an indistinct outer membrane. (2) Multiple lymph nodes in the vicinity of the cardia and left side of the stomach were visualized, with the largest node measuring approximately 0.5 cm along its short axis (depicted in Fig. 5.4). The final diagnosis rendered was cardiac carcinoma (cT3N0M0).

5.2.2 Treatment

Upon admission, thorough examinations were conducted, and no indications for surgical contraindications were identified. Subsequently, the patient underwent fast-track surgery without preoperative water intake, skin preparation, intestinal preparation, or placement of a gastric tube. A laparoscopic proximal gastric cancer radical surgery (double-channel anastomosis) was per-

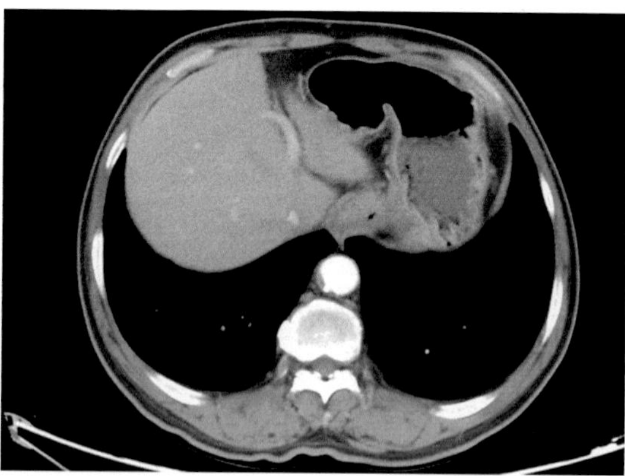

Fig. 5.3 Depicts a gastric endoscopy revealing the presence of cardia cancer, located approximately 38–43 cm from the incisors. This malignancy is observed to invade both the lower esophagus and gastric fundus

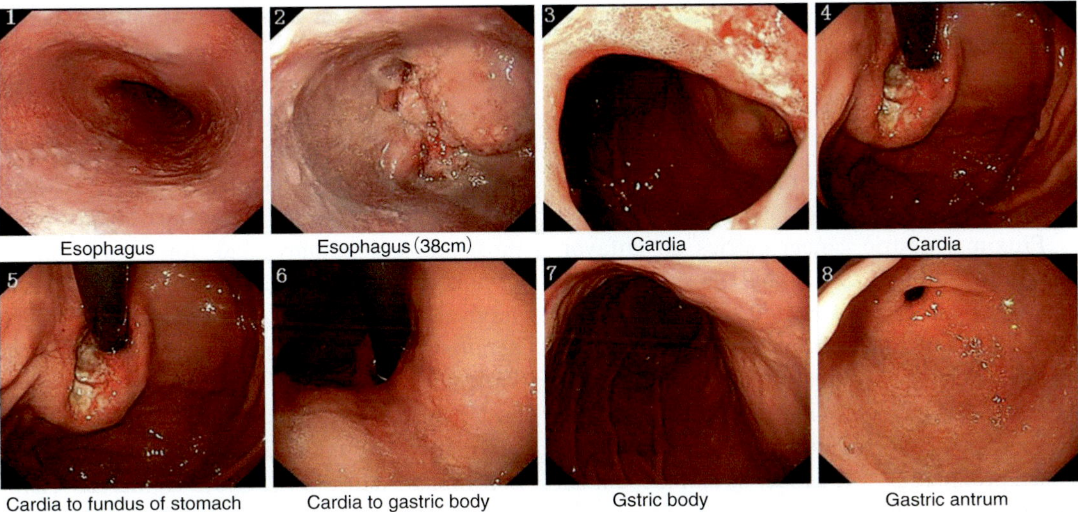

Fig. 5.4 We observe carcinoma originating from the cardia, demonstrating invasion into the adventitia. The gastric wall surrounding the cardia exhibits irregular thickening, with maximum thickness measuring approximately 1.8 cm

formed at a selected time. Postoperatively, on the first day, the gastric tube was removed, and the patient was encouraged to mobilize and ingest water. By the third day, a clear liquid diet was initiated, followed by a liquid diet on the fifth day. Upper gastrointestinal radiography revealed no abnormalities. On the sixth day, the abdominal drainage tube was removed, and ultimately, the patient was discharged on the ninth day.

Pathological examination of the resected specimen disclosed a poorly differentiated adenocarcinoma, classified according to the Lauren classification as intestinal type, exhibiting ulceration at the gastroesophageal junction. The tumor infiltrated the gastric wall, extending to the subserosal adipose tissue, while infiltration into the esophageal wall was observed at the fibrous layer. The interstitial tissue exhibited significant lymphocyte infiltration, and nerve invasion was noted, while no evidence of vascular tumor emboli was detected. The greater omentum and upper and lower margins exhibited absence of cancer involvement. Moreover, there were no metastatic lesions in the examined lymph nodes (0/33). Based on these findings, the final TNM staging was designated as pT3N0M0, corresponding to stage IIA. The precise pTNM staging confirmed pT3N0M0, stage IIA.

5.2.3 Case Analysis

Gastric cancer represents a prevalent malignancy worldwide and stands as the third leading cause of cancer-related mortality. While gastric cancer primarily manifests in the middle and distal regions of the stomach, the incidence of proximal gastric cancer (PGC) has been steadily rising in recent years [7–12]. Analysis of the US SEER (Surveillance, Epidemiology, and End Results) database revealed a significant increase in cardia cancer incidence, escalating from 1.22/100,000 to 1.94/100,000 between 1970 and 2010 [8]. The precise mechanisms driving this surge in PGC incidence remain elusive; however, evidence suggests plausible associations with widespread usage of anti-Hp drugs, gastroesophageal reflux disease, excessive obesity, and dietary factors [13].

Esophagogastric junction adenocarcinoma (AEG) denotes tumors located within 5 cm of the esophagogastric junction (EGJ) [14]. Presently, the widely adopted Siewert classification categorizes AEG [15]. Siewert type I tumors exhibit their epicenter 1–5 cm above the EGJ, Siewert type II tumors possess their epicenter between 1 cm above and 2 cm below the EGJ, and Siewert type III tumors have their epicenter 2–5 cm below the EGJ [16]. Currently, proximal gastric cancer encompasses tumors occurring in the upper one-third of the stomach, encompassing lesions within the region extending from 1 cm above to 5 cm below the EGJ (i.e., Siewert type II and III), as well as tumors within the upper one-third of the gastric body and the greater curvature.

Proximal gastric cancer carries an unfavorable prognosis [17–19]. In 2001, a study from a single Italian center reported a 5-year overall survival rate of 17.7% for patients with proximal gastric cancer, significantly lower than that observed for patients with distal gastric cancer (36.4%, $p < 0.01$). Multivariate analysis established proximal gastric cancer as an independent prognostic factor for poor outcomes [17]. However, certain subgroup analyses failed to demonstrate a statistically significant survival disparity between proximal and distal gastric cancer when matched for pathological stage [18]. Findings from our center indicated that the location of gastric cancer was not significantly correlated with prognosis (HR = 0.94, 95% CI: 0.88–1.00, $p = 0.058$) [20]. An analysis based on the American NCDB database revealed that proximal gastric cancer exhibited a worse prognosis than distal gastric cancer for early and locally advanced cases, whereas a more favorable prognosis was observed for proximal gastric cancer in late-stage cases [21]. Thus, we postulate that variations in survival prognosis for proximal gastric cancer may be intricately linked to geographical location, ethnicity, and distinct genetic factors, necessitating further validation through large-scale clinical trials.

The standard treatment options for proximal gastric cancer typically involve total gastrectomy or proximal gastrectomy. Total gastrectomy may result in vitamin B12 absorption disorders, postoperative weight loss, and nutritional anemia [22]. Proximal gastrectomy, on the other hand, preserves a portion of the gastric cavity and gastric hormone secretion function, effectively alleviating postoperative anemia symptoms and improving the patient's nutritional status. However, it does disrupt the anatomical structure of the esophagogastric junction, leading to potential complications such as reflux and anastomotic stenosis, which can significantly impact patients' quality of life [14].

The treatment strategies for early and advanced proximal gastric cancer differ slightly, considering the balance between nutritional status and curability of tumors. For early proximal gastric cancer, a wealth of evidence suggests that proximal gastrectomy and total gastrectomy exhibit no significant differences in long-term survival outcomes [23]. Consequently, the latest iteration of the "Japanese Gastric Cancer Treatment Guidelines" recommends proximal gastrectomy for select early proximal gastric cancer patients to maintain optimal postoperative nutritional status [24]. While numerous retrospective studies have demonstrated similar survival outcomes between proximal resection and total gastrectomy in the treatment of locally advanced proximal gastric cancer, total gastrectomy remains a commonly favored approach based on clinical guidelines and practice.

Several methods of digestive tract reconstruction are commonly employed following proximal gastrectomy, including esophagogastrostomy (EG) and double-tract reconstruction (DTR). Although esophagogastrostomy is a straightforward technique, it is associated with a higher incidence of anastomotic stricture and reflux esophagitis [25]. DTR is considered the most effective reconstruction method for mitigating postoperative reflux esophagitis after proximal gastrectomy [26]. The advantage of DTR lies in the insertion of the jejunum between the remnant stomach and the esophagus, increasing the distance for food reflux while preserving the remnant stomach and duodenal passage, thereby facilitating food storage. A meta-analysis revealed that the incidence of reflux symptoms, reflux esophagitis, and anastomotic stricture in patients undergoing DTR after proximal gastrectomy was comparable to those who underwent total gastrectomy [27]. However, this technique involves multiple anastomoses, increasing the risk of anastomotic leakage. The ongoing KLASS-05 study in Korea aims to compare the short-term and long-term outcomes of laparoscopic DTR and total gastrectomy, and its results are eagerly anticipated.

There have been reports suggesting that jejunal interposition (JI) reconstruction can serve as an alternative approach for managing reflux esophagitis, potentially yielding better outcomes compared to esophagogastrostomy (EG) [28]. In this method of digestive tract anastomosis, a segment of the jejunum is connected to both the esophagus and the residual stomach, creating a barrier against reflux and reducing the tension associated with direct gastroesophageal anastomosis, thereby ensuring safety. Some researchers advocate for the use of JI as a technique that preserves normal gastric digestive function [28]. However, following JI surgery, patients may occasionally experience discomfort in the stomach due to the folding of the jejunal segment, which may be attributed to compromised food movement.

5.2.4 Expert Comments

Epidemiological data indicates a rising incidence of proximal gastric tumors, which exhibit distinct clinical, pathological, and prognostic features compared to distal gastric cancer. However, there remains a considerable debate surrounding surgical approaches, the extent of resection, and reconstruction methods. Consequently, there is a pressing need for high-quality clinical research to generate robust evidence in this field. In response to advancements in surgical technology and the growing emphasis on enhancing quality of life, surgical procedures are shifting toward precision, minimally invasive, and personalized approaches.

Case provider:Lulu Zhao, Yingtai Chen.

Expert comments:Dongbing Zhao.

5.3 Case 32: Surgical Management of the Gastroesophageal Junction Adenocarcinoma

5.3.1 Brief History

A 72-year-old male patient was referred to our medical facility for management of gastric carcinoma. Approximately 1 month prior, he sought medical attention at a local clinic due to symptoms of hematemesis, nausea, and heartburn. Following intravenous fluid administration and acid-suppressive therapy at the aforementioned clinic, the patient ceased vomiting blood; however, he continued to experience upper abdominal discomfort in the absence of vomiting, dysphagia, abdominal pain, and abdominal distension. A comprehensive physical examination revealed no discernible abnormalities. Tumor marker levels, including CEA (carcinoembryonic antigen) at 32.35 ng/mL, CA242, CA199, CA724, and AFP (alpha-fetoprotein), remained within the normal range. Hematological assessment exhibited RBC (red blood cell) count at 3×10^{12}/L and hemoglobin level at 93 g/L. Subsequent gastroscope examination unveiled a protruding mass extending from the lower segment of the esophagus to the cardiac and fundic regions of the stomach (the proximal boundary being approximately 39 cm from the incisor tooth). The lesion exhibited an inactive base and displayed rough and erosive surface mucosa. Although the cardiac orifice appeared narrow, passage of the endoscope was feasible (Fig. 5.5). Pathological analysis confirmed the presence of moderately differentiated adenocarcinoma. Further evaluation through abdominal enhanced computed tomography (CT) demonstrated an irregular mass measuring 7.6 × 5.1 cm extending from the cardiac region to the fundus of the stomach. The local serosal surface displayed blurring, with involvement of the lower esophageal segment apparent (Fig. 5.6).

Diagnosis: Esophagogastric junction adenocarcinoma (cT4aN1M0).

5.3.2 Treatment

Following admission, the patient underwent relevant preoperative examinations prior to laparoscopic-assisted total gastrectomy. The postoperative recovery was uncomplicated. On the fourth day after the operation, the patient experienced flatus and initiated a liquid diet. The gastric tube was subsequently removed on the

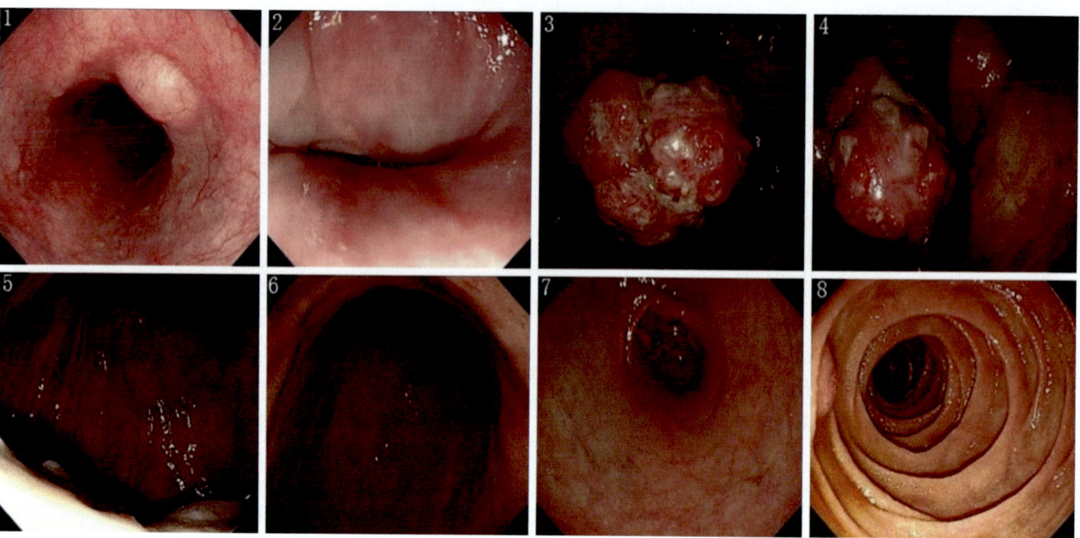

Fig. 5.5 Gastroscope examination reveals the presence of a prominent mass extending from the lower segment of the esophagus to the cardia and fundus of the stomach. The upper boundary of this mass was approximately 39 cm from the incisor tooth. The base of the lesion appeared inactive, while the surface mucosa exhibited a rough and erosive appearance

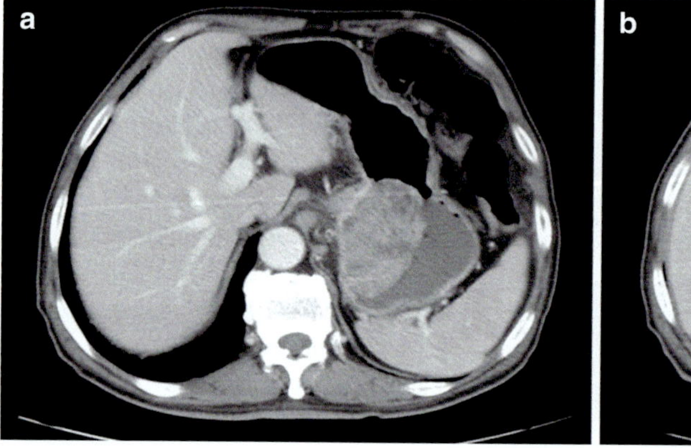

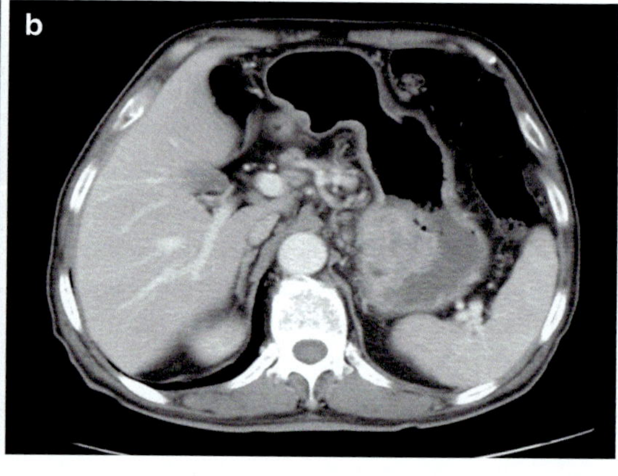

Fig. 5.6 The findings of CT was following. (**a**) CT reveals the presence of an irregular mass extending from the cardia to the fundus of the stomach, measuring 7.6 × 5.1 cm, with noticeable lobulation (**b**). The local serous surface appears blurred, indicating infiltration, and involvement of the lower esophageal segment is evident

sixth day, and the drainage tubes were removed on the ninth day. Subsequently, the patient was discharged on the eleventh day.

Pathological evaluation of the surgical specimen, consisting of a total gastrectomy specimen, revealed the following findings: The lesser curvature measured 17 cm in length, while the greater curvature measured 30 cm. The duodenum and esophagus measured 2 cm and 2.2 cm in length, and 6 cm and 3 cm in width, respectively. Notably, a protuberant tumor measuring 8 × 7.5 × 2.5 cm was observed near the cardia, specifically at the fundus of the stomach. The tumor exhibited proximity to the serosa, with its center located 4.5 cm away from the esophagogastric junction.

Microscopic analysis confirmed the diagnosis of medium to low differentiated adenocarcinoma of the stomach, classified as intestinal type

(Lauren type). The tumor displayed significant necrosis and had penetrated the muscular layer, reaching the gastric serosa and involving the esophagogastric junction. Nerve invasion and vascular tumor thrombus were observed. The tumor did not involve the duodenum, upper and lower incisional margins, or greater omentum. Additionally, no lymph node metastasis was identified among the examined 61 lymph nodes. The final TNM stage was determined as pT4aN0M0.

5.3.3 Case Analysis

Adenocarcinoma of the esophagogastric junction (AEG) commonly refers to adenocarcinoma occurring within a proximity of 5 cm above or below the esophagogastric junction (EGJ). It is important to highlight that the anatomical demarcation line differs from the dentate line, but rather corresponds to the proximal extent of the palisade vascular pattern in the lower esophageal segment or the gastric mucosal fold. The dentate line, on the other hand, represents the histological interface between the esophageal squamous and gastric columnar epithelium.

In recent years, the global incidence of AEG has exhibited a steady annual increase [8, 10]. Notably, the incidence of AEG in China has shown a significant rise, accounting for 26.7% of all gastric cancers [29]. This surge in incidence may be attributed to factors such as gastroesophageal reflux disease (GERD), which can be influenced by factors like obesity and alcohol consumption [30].

AEG classification and staging: Currently, the Siewert classification is widely utilized internationally to classify AEG tumors. According to this classification, the tumor first contacts or crosses the esophagogastric junction (EGJ) and is subsequently categorized into types I, II, or III based on the central position of the cancer. In type I AEG, the tumor center is located 1–5 cm above the EGJ. In type II AEG, the tumor center is situated 1 cm above to 2 cm below the EGJ. Type III AEG tumors have their center positioned 2–5 cm below the EGJ [31]. In Japan, the Nishi classification [32], proposed in 1973, is followed. According to this classification, the area 2 cm above or below the EGJ is considered the esophagogastric junction area. Based on the relationship between the tumor center and the EGJ, it is classified into five types: E type (mainly located on the esophageal side), EG type (partially on the esophageal side), E = G type (crossing the esophagogastric junction), GE type (partially on the gastric side), and G type (mainly located on the gastric side). In the past, staging AEG was a matter of controversy. After numerous revisions, the staging standards have been unified between Eastern and Western guidelines. In the eighth edition of the AJCC staging system, Siewert I and II AEG tumors are staged according to the esophageal cancer staging system, while Siewert III is staged according to the gastric cancer staging system [33].

Preoperative staging of AEG: As AEG is situated at the thoracoabdominal junction, the surgical approach depends on factors such as tumor stage, classification, tumor size, length of esophageal invasion, and other considerations. Preoperative imaging diagnosis is crucial, and in addition to conventional gastroscope and endoscopic ultrasound, gastrointestinal radiography can enhance the accuracy of determining the length of esophageal invasion and the location of tumor invasion. If necessary, three-dimensional CT reconstruction should be performed [34].

Selection of AEG surgical approach: The choice of surgical approach for Siewert I and III AEG is relatively straightforward. Siewert I, which is similar to esophageal cancer, is preferably approached through the right transthoracic approach. Siewert III, resembling gastric cancer, is managed via the abdominal esophageal hiatus approach. The optimal surgical approach for Siewert II AEG remains a subject of debate. A retrospective study conducted at West China Hospital demonstrated that the 3-year overall survival rate for Siewert II AEG was 78.1% with the abdominal approach and 46.3% with the thoracic approach (P = 0.001), favoring the abdominal approach [35]. Notable phase III clinical studies include the Dutch and Japanese JCOG 9502 studies, which were published in 2002. The Dutch study showed a high incidence of complications and poor short-term quality of life following the transthoracic approach, with no significant difference in the 5-year survival rates between the two approaches (36% and 34%, respectively). Subgroup analysis revealed that Siewert I type patients had better 5-year survival rates with the thoracic approach, particularly in stage N1 [36–38]. The Japanese JCOG 9502 study focused on advanced AEG (T2–4) with esophageal invasion less than 3 cm and compared the two surgical approaches. The results indicated that the transabdominal approach had superior long-term prognosis, with 5-year survival rates of 52.3% and 37.9% and 10-year survival rates of 37% and 24%, respectively [39, 40]. The choice of AEG surgical approach is also influenced by the extent of esophageal invasion. Nunobe et al. [41] found that when the length of esophageal involvement was less than 2 cm, the metastasis rate of lower mediastinal lymph nodes was 2%. When the esophagus was involved in 2–3 cm, the metastatic rate of lymph nodes in the lower mediastinum increased to 17.8%. Considering the lower complication rate of the transabdominal esophageal hiatus approach compared to the transthoracic or combined thoracoabdominal approach [40], a consensus has been reached recommending the transabdominal approach for esophageal invasion ≤2 cm and the transthoracic approach for esophageal invasion >2 cm [42, 43].

Lymph node dissection: In advanced-stage AEG (T2–4), the lymph node metastasis rate is 77.6%, with the majority of patients having abdominal lymph node metastasis. The mediastinal lymph node metastasis rates are 46.0%, 29.5%, and 9.3% for Siewert I, II, and III types, respectively [44]. Therefore, routine dissection of abdominal lymph nodes in groups 16–20 is recommended for Siewert type I AEG, along with mediastinal lymph node dissection for esophageal cancer. Siewert II AEG requires D1/D1+ or D2 lymph node dissection based on tumor size and resection range, while Siewert type III necessitates D2 lymph node dissection [45]. The JCOG 0110 study in Japan suggested that routine dissection of splenic hilar lymph nodes is not required for AEG without invasion of the greater curvature of the stomach [46]. However, for suspected splenic hilar lymph node metastasis, the decision to perform splenic hilar lymph node dissection can be based on intraoperative biopsy results of No.4 s lymph nodes, considering the correlation between the lymph drainage areas of No.10 and No.4 s [47].

Surgical margin: It is recommended to have a ≥ 5 cm upper esophageal margin for Siewert type I and II via the thoracic approach surgeries, and a ≥ 2 cm upper esophageal margin for Siewert type II AEG via the abdominal approach. The most important aspect is ensuring a negative frozen pathological margin during the operation [45]. Regarding the scope of resection, resection of the lower esophagus and proximal stomach is recommended for Siewert type I AEG, while total gastrectomy is recommended for Siewert type III. For Siewert type II AEG, the risk of distal perigastric lymph node metastasis and postoperative esophageal reflux should be considered when deciding to resect the whole stomach or the proximal stomach. Studies have shown a high rate of esophageal reflux and poor quality of life after proximal gastrectomy, hence total gastrectomy is generally recommended [48]. However, with improved digestive tract reconstruction techniques, the rate of esophageal reflux after proximal gastrectomy has decreased in recent years. Some researchers have suggested proximal gastrectomy for Siewert II AEG tumors ≤4 cm in length and total gastrectomy for tumors >4 cm [45].

5.3.4 Expert Comments

AEG is characterized by its unique anatomical location and has been increasingly recognized due to its rising incidence rate. The management of AEG often requires a multidisciplinary approach involving gastrointestinal surgery, thoracic surgery, endoscopy, medical oncology, and radiotherapy. Studies have shown that multidisciplinary management significantly improves the diagnosis and treatment outcomes for AEG. However, several aspects of AEG, such as tumor staging, surgical approaches, resection ranges, and the timing of radiotherapy and chemotherapy, remain areas of controversy and require further exploration in clinical practice.

In the future, efforts should be focused on enhancing the standardization and individualization of the diagnosis and treatment of AEG. This includes refining diagnostic criteria, improving surgical techniques, optimizing the selection of treatment modalities, and tailoring therapies to the specific needs of each patient. The ultimate goal is to improve the prognosis and quality of life for individuals with AEG. Continued research and advancements in the field will contribute to achieving these objectives and providing better outcomes for patients with AEG.

Case provider:Xiaofeng Bai, Zefeng Li.

Commentary:Xiaofeng Bai.

5.4 Case 33: Neoadjuvant Chemotherapy for Advanced Gastric Cancer

5.4.1 Brief History

The hospitalized patient, a 72-year-old male, presented with a chief complaint of chronic upper abdominal pain persisting for a duration of over 3 years. Initially, he experienced mild upper abdominal discomfort of unknown etiology and received treatment consisting of gastric motility and acid suppression therapy at a local medical facility, which resulted in symptomatic improvement. However, the patient subsequently reported recurring pain episodes accompanied by anorexia, reduced appetite, bloating, and acid reflux. Attempts at self-medication proved futile. Upon undergoing gastroscopy at a different medical institution, the patient was diagnosed with gastric antral cancer. Upon admission to our hospital, physical examination of the abdomen revealed no discernible positive findings. Notably, tumor markers, including CEA, AFP, CA72-4, CA19-9, and CA24-2, were all found to be within the normal range. Our gastroscopic examination revealed two significant findings: firstly, the presence of ulcerative lesions extending from the gastric antrum to the pylorus, and secondly, congestion and roughness observed in the cardiac mucosa approximately 41–43 cm from the incisors, indicative of either early-stage cardiac cancer or premalignant lesions (Fig. 5.7). Subsequent histopathological examination of biopsied tissue confirmed the presence of adenocarcinoma. Furthermore, an enhanced CT scan demonstrated thickening of the gastric wall within the gastric

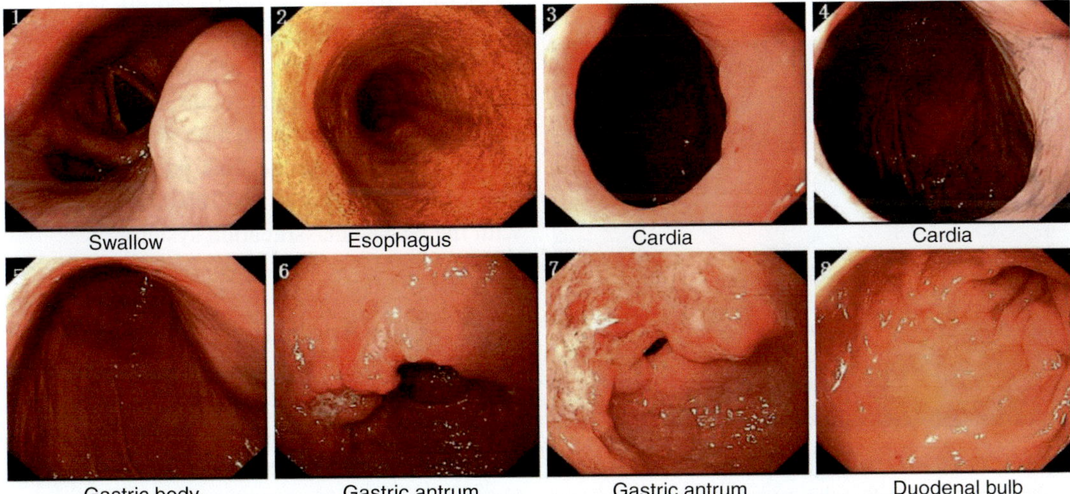

Fig. 5.7 Gastroscopic visualization exhibited ulcerative lesions extending from the gastric antrum to the pylorus, indicative of gastric cancer. Notably, congestion and roughness were observed in the cardiac mucosa located approximately 41–43 cm from the incisors, suggestive of early-stage cardiac cancer or premalignant lesions

antrum and pyloric regions, measuring approximately 2.0 cm × 1.9 cm, accompanied by a slightly irregular serosal surface and the discernible presence of multiple linear shadows, characteristic of malignant growth (Fig. 5.8). Based on the aforementioned clinical and imaging findings, a diagnosis of gastric cancer (cT4NxM0) was established.

5.4.2 Treatment

The patient underwent two cycles of neoadjuvant chemotherapy utilizing the DOS regimen, which consisted of intravenous administration of docetaxel (100 mg) on day 1, oxaliplatin (180 mg) on day 2, and oral S-1 (60 mg twice daily) from day 1 to day 14, repeated every 21 days. Following chemotherapy, the patient experienced grade I gastrointestinal reactions and grade III hand-foot syndrome, alongside achieving a stable disease (SD) response. Subsequently, the patient received a reduced dose of S-1 and continued with the third and fourth cycles of chemotherapy, consisting of intravenous docetaxel (100 mg) on day 1, oxaliplatin (180 mg) on day 2, and S-1 administered at a dose of 40 mg in the morning and 60 mg in the evening from day 7 to day 21, with each cycle lasting 28 days. The patient developed grade II hyperbilirubinemia, which was managed with hepatoprotective therapy at a local medical facility, resulting in a gradual return to normal bilirubin levels. Following the completion of four cycles of neoadjuvant chemotherapy, endoscopic examination revealed the following findings: (1) presence of ulcerative lesions from the gastric antrum to the pylorus, with suspicion of residual disease. However, compared to the initial endoscopy, there was localized improvement in the lesion; (2) congestion and roughness observed in the cardiac mucosa; (3) congestion, edema, and roughness of the posterior wall of the gastric body (Fig. 5.9). The patient exhibited an SD response. Subsequently, an open distal gastrectomy was scheduled and performed with curative intent.

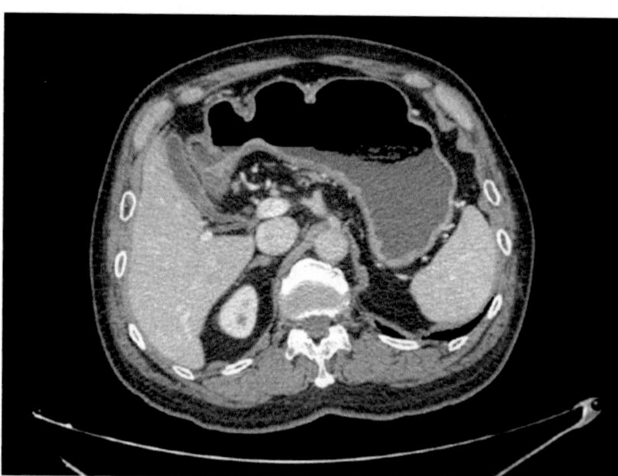

Fig. 5.8 Enhanced CT imaging demonstrated thickening of the gastric wall within the gastric antrum and pyloric regions, measuring approximately 2.0 cm × 1.9 cm, accompanied by a slightly irregular serosal surface. Furthermore, the presence of multiple linear shadows was observed, consistent with malignant growth

Pathological examination of the resected specimen revealed the presence of sufficient samples, with only a small amount of dysplastic glands observed in the mucosal lamina propria, indicating gastric remnant adenocarcinoma (Lauren classification: intestinal type). Tumor cells displayed severe degeneration, accompanied by mild fibrosis and a significant infiltration of inflammatory cells, consistent with substantial treatment-related changes (Mandard TRG grade: grade 2). The surrounding gastric mucosa exhibited intestinal metaplasia and mild to moderate dysplasia. Notably, the tumor did not invade the pylorus or duodenum, and both the proximal and distal margins were negative for cancer. Additionally, no lymph node metastasis was detected among the 22 lymph nodes examined (0/22). Accordingly, the final pathological staging was determined as ypT1aN0, in accordance with the pTNM classification system.

5.4.3 Case Analysis

5.4.3.1 The Concept of Neoadjuvant Chemotherapy for Gastric Cancer in Western Countries

Gastric cancer holds a prominent position among malignant tumors in China, ranking third in terms of both incidence and mortality. Radical surgery (R0 resection) serves as the primary treatment for

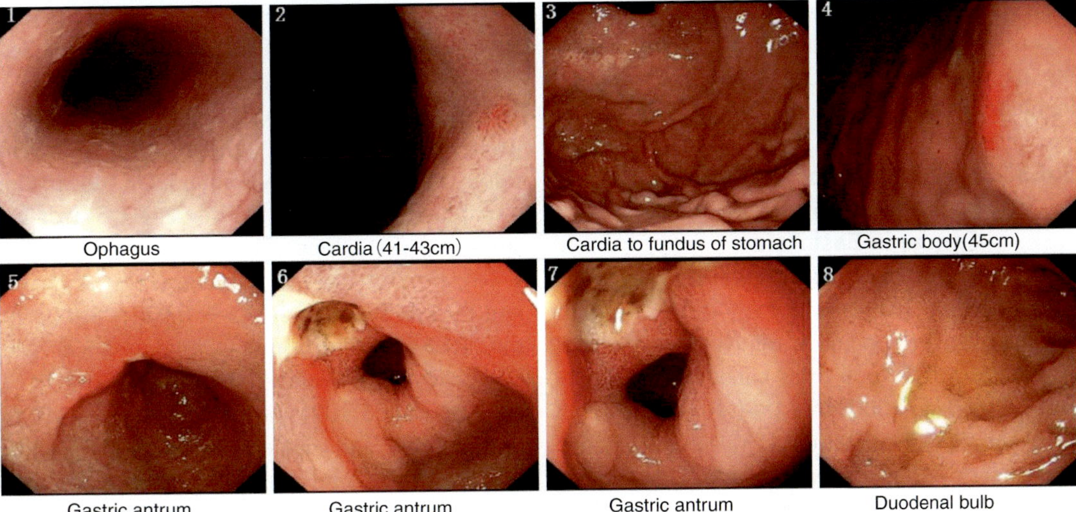

Fig. 5.9 Gastroscopic evaluation following four cycles of neoadjuvant chemotherapy demonstrated the presence of ulcerative lesions in the gastric antrum and pylorus, suggesting the possibility of residual disease. However, when compared to the initial gastroscopy, partial improvement in the lesions was observed

advanced gastric cancer. However, the effectiveness of simple surgical intervention and traditional surgery combined with postoperative adjuvant therapy has proven unsatisfactory [49, 50]. In recent years, a significant advancement in the management of advanced gastric cancer has emerged through the utilization of neoadjuvant therapy. This approach offers several advantages, including downstaging of tumors, reduction in primary tumor size, elimination of micrometastases, decreased intraoperative dissemination and tumor recurrence, and enhanced resectability of gastric cancer [49].

The concept of neoadjuvant chemotherapy, involving the administration of chemotherapy prior to surgery, was first proposed by Feri et al. in 1982 [51]. It has since become a crucial aspect of the comprehensive treatment of solid tumors. In 2006, the groundbreaking MAGIC study [52] became a milestone trial in neoadjuvant chemotherapy for gastric cancer. It demonstrated, for the first time, that perioperative chemotherapy with the ECF regimen (epirubicin, cisplatin, and fluorouracil) significantly improved the 5-year overall survival rate in gastric cancer patients when compared to surgery alone (36.3 months vs. 26.0 months). Subsequently, in 2007, the French FNCLCC-FFCD trial [53] reaffirmed the efficacy of perioperative chemotherapy. The CF regimen (cisplatin combined with fluorouracil) significantly increased the R0 resection rate (84% vs. 73%, $p = 0.04$), 5-year overall survival (38% vs. 24%, $p = 0.02$), and 5-year disease-free survival (34% vs. 19%, $p = 0.02$) in gastric cancer patients. Hence, these studies have firmly established the crucial role of neoadjuvant chemotherapy in the comprehensive treatment of gastric cancer.

In 2017, the results of the German FLOT4 trial [54] were published, revealing that the FLOT regimen (fluorouracil, leucovorin, oxaliplatin, and docetaxel) significantly improved the median overall survival of patients with locally advanced gastric cancer in comparison to the traditional ECX or ECF regimens (epirubicin, cisplatin, and fluorouracil/capecitabine). Consequently, the latest version of the National Comprehensive Cancer Network (NCCN) guidelines recommends neoadjuvant chemotherapy as the first-line treatment for patients with T2 + NxM0 stage or higher gastric cancer [55]. It is important to note, however, that the aforementioned trials primarily included European and American populations. Due to variations in tumor biology among different races, the application of these research regimens in Asian populations is limited, resulting in differences in dosage and an increased incidence of side effects.

5.4.3.2 The Concept of Neoadjuvant Chemotherapy for Gastric Cancer in East Asia

The exploration of neoadjuvant therapy for Asian gastric cancer has drawn upon the experience gained from postoperative adjuvant therapy for gastric cancer. Several trials conducted in Japan, such as the JCOG0002 trial [56], JCOG0210 trial [57], and JCOG0501 study [58], have evaluated the efficacy of neoadjuvant chemotherapy using irinotecan, S-1 monotherapy, and/or combined with cisplatin in locally advanced gastric cancer. Surprisingly, the long-term survival results of these trials were negative. Based on the analysis of the enrolled population, it was found that patients with larger tumors but earlier N staging (N0/N1) may not be the optimal population to benefit from neoadjuvant chemotherapy. As a result, neoadjuvant chemotherapy is not strongly recommended in Japan, as it has not been proven to be superior to the traditional surgical approach followed by postoperative adjuvant chemotherapy. However, it is worth noting that data from the Japanese JCOG0405 single-arm trial have identified a beneficiary population for neoadjuvant chemotherapy, which consists of locally advanced gastric cancer patients with bulky lymph node metastasis (Bulky N). This group received 2–3 cycles of S-1 combined with cisplatin before undergoing curative resection of gastric cancer, achieving an R0 resection rate of 82.35% and 5-year overall survival and recurrence-free survival rates (RFS) of 53% and 50%, respectively [59]. This has led to a basic consensus regarding the target population for neoadjuvant chemotherapy in locally advanced gastric cancer. The Chinese Society of Clinical Oncology (CSCO) gastric cancer guidelines recommend neoadjuvant chemotherapy for patients with clinical stage III gastric cancer and clinical stage II–III esophagogastric junction cancer [60].

In 2019, the 3-year follow-up data from the Korean PRODIGY trial [61] and the Chinese RESOLVE trial [62] were presented at the ESCO Annual Meeting. The PRODIGY trial included 530 patients with locally advanced (cT2, 3/N + M0, or cT4/NxM0) gastric or esophagogastric junction adenocarcinoma who were randomly assigned to receive either DOS (docetaxel, oxaliplatin, and S-1) + D2 surgery + S-1 or D2 surgery + S-1 alone. The trial demonstrated a 3-year progression-free survival (PFS) of 66.3% and 60.2%, respectively (p = 0.023). Similarly, the RESOLVE trial in China, which was launched concurrently with the PRODIGY study, enrolled 1094 patients (cT4a/N + M0 or cT4bNxM0) and randomized them into three groups: Group A received D2 surgery + XELOX, Group B received D2 surgery + SOX, and Group C received SOX + D2 surgery + SOX. The trial reported a 3-year recurrence-free survival (RFS) of 54.78%, 60.29%, and 62.02% for the respective groups (p = 0.045). A comparison of the two studies conducted in China and Korea revealed that despite differences in chemotherapy regimens, both studies demonstrated that neoadjuvant chemotherapy could achieve tumor reduction and improve survival. Furthermore, the 3-year disease-free survival (DFS) data from the two studies were similar, with rates of 6% and 7%, respectively. As the RESOLVE trial primarily enrolled Chinese patients, the perioperative SOX regimen is expected to become a new treatment model for locally advanced gastric cancer in China.

5.4.4 Expert Comments

The timing of neoadjuvant chemotherapy for gastric cancer and the selection of an effective regimen are currently significant areas of research. In clinical practice, it is crucial to adopt individualized treatment plans that consider various factors, including the patient's physical condition, surgical complexity, surgeon's expertise, HER-2 expression, and microsatellite instability. These plans should be continually modified based on the patient's evolving condition.

Case provider:Lulu Zhao, Yingtai Chen.

Expert comments:Dongbing Zhao.

5.5 Case 34: Pathological Complete Response After Concurrent Chemoradiotherapy for Gastric Cancer

5.5.1 Brief History

The patient, a 37-year-old female, was admitted to our facility presenting with a 2-week history of dysphagia. Additionally, she reported intermittent upper abdominal discomfort, although no symptoms of nausea or vomiting were reported. Prior to admission, a gastroscopy was performed at a local hospital, which revealed an elevated lesion located in the cardia region of the stomach. Subsequent pathological examination confirmed the presence of cardia adenocarcinoma. Laboratory analysis demonstrated a CA199 level of 149.20 U/mL, with no other abnormal tumor markers detected. A comprehensive gastroscopy performed at our hospital identified cardia cancer invading the lower esophagus and gastric fundus, as depicted in Fig. 5.10. To further evaluate the extent of the disease, a contrast-enhanced CT scan was conducted, revealing notable thickening of the gastric wall on the lesser curvature side of the cardia. The maximum thickness measured 2.6 cm, spanning a length of approximately 5.1 cm. Moreover, an internal ulcer and prominent heterogeneous enhancement were observed (Fig. 5.11). Consequently, a diagnosis of esophagogastric junction adenocarcinoma (cT4aN2M0) was established.

5.5.2 Treatment

Following thorough multidisciplinary consultation, a treatment plan was formulated involving neoadjuvant concurrent chemoradiotherapy. The regimen consisted of a radiation dose of 45 Gy delivered in fractions of 1.8 Gy over 25 sessions, targeting 95% of the planning target volume (PTV). Concurrently, the patient received oral administration of twice-daily 60 mg S-1. Subsequently, sequential chemotherapy was initiated, comprising three cycles of oxaliplatin in combination with S-1, followed by two cycles of single-agent S-1. Post-treatment evaluation through a follow-up CT scan revealed a reduction in thickening of the gastric wall on the lesser curvature side of the cardia, measuring approximately 1.1 cm compared to the pre-treatment assessment. Additionally, multiple lymph nodes with a short diameter of around 0.6 cm were

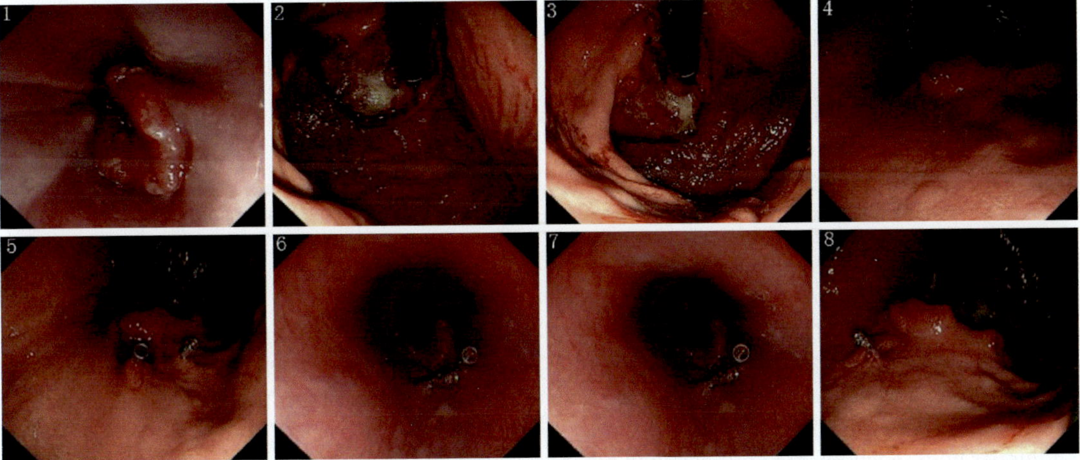

Fig. 5.10 Gastroscopic examination demonstrating the invasion of cardia cancer into the lower esophagus and gastric fundus

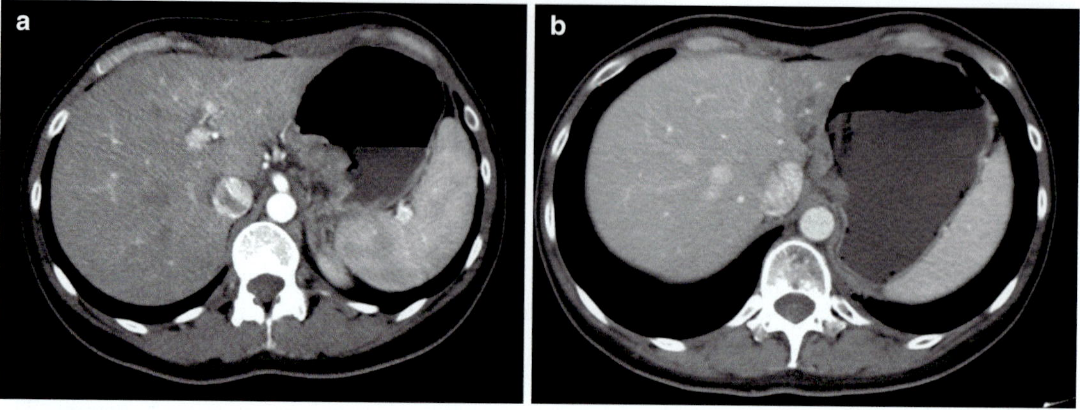

Fig. 5.11 (**a**) Contrast-enhanced CT scan illustrating thickening of the gastric wall on the lesser curvature side of the cardia, measuring up to 2.6 cm at its thickest point and involving a length of approximately 5.1 cm, with the presence of an internal ulcer during the pre-treatment evaluation. (**b**) Subsequent imaging after treatment displaying a reduction in the thickening of the gastric wall on the lesser curvature side of the cardia compared to the pre-treatment evaluation

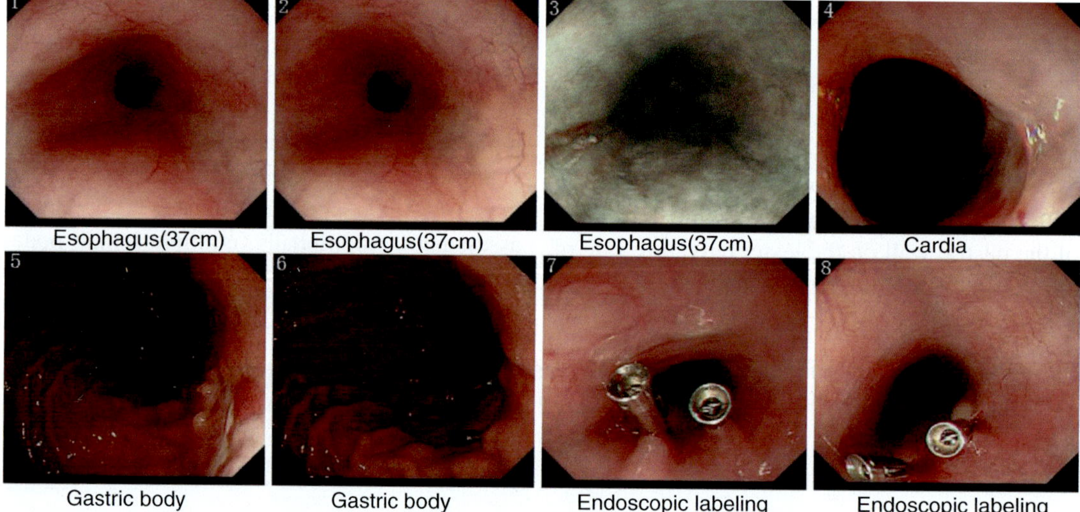

Fig. 5.12 Illustrates gastroscopy images displaying scar-like alterations in the mucosa of the cardia, lower esophagus, gastric fundus, and upper body, featuring localized ulcerative lesions approximately 40–43 cm from the incisors, suggestive of remaining lesions

identified on the lesser curvature side of the stomach (Fig. 5.10b). Gastroscopic examination further unveiled scar-like changes in the mucosa of the cardia, lower esophagus, gastric fundus, and upper body, accompanied by localized ulcerative lesions situated approximately 40–43 cm from the incisors, indicative of residual lesions (Fig. 5.12). Subsequent preoperative assessments were conducted, leading to the patient undergoing total gastrectomy with D2 lymphadenectomy under general anesthesia and laparoscopic guidance.

Pathological examination of the entire stomach, labeled as "Gastric cancer after neoadjuvant chemoradiotherapy," revealed the absence of residual tumor tissue in the esophagogastric junction or stomach wall. However, extensive infiltration of inflammatory cells was observed in the gastric tube and gastric wall tissues, alongside scattered calcifications, multinucleated giant cells, and interstitial fibrous tissue proliferation, consistent with a profound post-treatment response (Mandard TRG grade 1). The surrounding gastric mucosa exhibited chronic non-atrophic inflammation. No evidence of cancer was identified in the pylorus ring, duodenum, greater omentum, or margins (0/25), and lymph node metastases were absent (ypT0N0M0).

5.5.3 Case Analysis

5.5.3.1 Application of Radiation Therapy in Neoadjuvant Therapy for Gastric Cancer

Radiotherapy, also referred to as radiation therapy, employs high-energy radiation, including alpha, beta, gamma rays, X-rays, electron beams, proton beams, and other particle beams, generated by a radiation source, to irradiate and eliminate localized tumor tissue, thereby impeding tumor growth and metastasis. However, during the irradiation of cancerous tissues, radiation lacks the ability to differentiate between healthy and malignant cells, resulting in damage and adverse reactions to normal tissues, such as allergic reactions, ulcers, and even bone marrow suppression.

In 1998, the Cancer Hospital of the Chinese Academy of Medical Sciences conducted a clinical trial comparing neoadjuvant radiotherapy combined with surgery to surgery alone [63]. The study, which involved 370 patients with cardia cancer, demonstrated the potential of neoadjuvant radiotherapy in the management of locally advanced gastric cancer. The results indicated that neoadjuvant radiotherapy (40 Gy) increased the R0 resection rate (81.0% vs. 60.8%, $p < 0.001$) and the 10-year overall survival rate (20.3% vs. 13.3%, $p = 0.0094$). This investigation laid the foundation for the exploration of neoadjuvant radiotherapy, with subsequent studies focusing on the clinical effectiveness of combined radiotherapy and chemotherapy in patients with esophagogastric junction cancer.

The CROSS trial conducted in the Netherlands [64] established the crucial role of neoadjuvant radiochemotherapy in clinical practice for gastric cancer. In this trial, 366 patients with cT1N1M0 or cT2–3N0-1M0 esophageal or gastroesophageal junction cancer (including 275 adenocarcinomas and 84 squamous cell carcinomas) were randomly assigned to receive either neoadjuvant radiochemotherapy or surgery alone. Follow-up assessments revealed that neoadjuvant radiochemotherapy significantly improved median survival (49.4 months vs. 24.0 months, $p = 0.003$). However, the survival benefit observed in the trial may be primarily attributed to the squamous cell subtype, which exhibits sensitivity to radiation therapy. Further analysis indicated no survival benefit in the adenocarcinoma group.

In 2009, the results of the POET trial [65] were published. This trial involved 126 patients with locally advanced (T3-T4) gastroesophageal junction adenocarcinoma who were randomized to receive either neoadjuvant chemotherapy or radiochemotherapy before surgery. Although radiotherapy demonstrated a higher rate of pathologic complete response (pCR) (15.6% vs. 2.0%, $p = 0.03$) and increased the 3-year survival rate from 27.7 to 47.4%, the difference did not reach statistical significance ($p = 0.07$). A similar conclusion was drawn from a phase II clinical trial conducted in Australia [66]. Based on these studies, the NCCN and ESMO guidelines state that neoadjuvant chemotherapy and radiochemotherapy confer similar survival benefits for patients with gastroesophageal junction adenocarcinoma, and the addition of preoperative radiation therapy does not improve the prognosis of locally advanced gastric cancer [55, 67]. However, it is important to note that a limitation of these studies is that most enrolled patients did not undergo standard D2 lymph node dissection, which significantly impacts the surgical curative effect and patient prognosis.

5.5.3.2 Application of Targeted Therapy in Neoadjuvant Therapy for Gastric Cancer

Trastuzumab is a humanized monoclonal antibody that specifically targets cells with high expression of Her-2, inhibiting signal transduction. In 2010, the ToGA trial results were announced, establishing trastuzumab as the earliest targeted drug employed in the clinical management of gastric cancer. It was specifically indicated for patients with advanced gastric cancer who tested positive for Her-2 and were ineligible for surgery [68]. Subsequently, the NCCN guidelines emphasized that molecular typing of gastric cancer based on Her-2 expression status in tumor tissue serves as a critical basis for selecting anti-Her-2 targeted therapies. The combination of chemotherapy and trastuzumab has been recognized as an important approach in treating advanced gastric cancer.

Since the discovery in 1971 that tumor growth relies on angiogenesis, anti-angiogenic targeted drugs have remained at the forefront of targeted cancer therapies. In 2014, the NCCN guidelines recommended ramucirumab as a second-line treatment for advanced gastric cancer. The use of anti-angiogenic drugs in neoadjuvant therapy for gastric cancer has also been investigated. Ma et al. [69] examined the clinical efficacy of bevacizumab (a VEGF monoclonal antibody) in combination with DOF (docetaxel/oxaliplatin/5-FU) chemotherapy and chemotherapy alone in neoadjuvant therapy for gastric cancer. The study demonstrated a significant increase in the R0 resection rate (75% vs. 50%, $p = 0.0209$) and a significant prolongation of disease-free survival (15.2 months vs. 12.3 months, $p = 0.013$) in the experimental group, although there was no difference in overall survival ($p = 0.776$). Similarly, the ST03 trial [70] did not find that bevacizumab improved the survival outcomes in gastric cancer and raised concerns about delayed wound healing and increased incidence of anastomotic fistula. Based on these findings, bevacizumab did not receive approval for neoadjuvant therapy in gastric cancer.

Apatinib, the first small-molecule anti-angiogenic drug, has been demonstrated to be safe and effective in advanced gastric cancer globally. In 2020, Zheng et al. [71] reported the results of a trial investigating the use of apatinib in combination with SOX chemotherapy as neoadjuvant treatment for gastric cancer. The single-arm trial exhibited a high pathological response rate (pRR) of 89.7%. This study represented the initial exploration of apatinib in neoadjuvant treatment for locally advanced gastric cancer; however, further validation is required to ascertain whether it can enhance long-term patient survival.

5.5.3.3 Application of Immunotherapy in Neoadjuvant Therapy for Gastric Cancer

Diverging from conventional treatment approaches, immunotherapy has emerged as a crucial strategy in the fight against cancer by harnessing the patient's immune system and counteracting immune suppression. A phase III clinical trial (ATTRACTION-2) conducted in 2017 on patients with advanced gastric or gastroesophageal junction adenocarcinoma demonstrated that nivolumab, a PD-1 monoclonal antibody, yielded a significant improvement in median survival compared to placebo (5.26 months vs. 4.14 months, $p < 0.001$) [72]. Subsequent survival analysis revealed 1-year and 2-year overall survival rates of 27.3% vs. 11.6% and 10.6% vs. 3.2%, respectively, further affirming the therapeutic benefit of PD-1 blockade in patients with advanced gastric cancer [73]. Consequently, nivolumab received approval as a third-line treatment for advanced gastric cancer, marking the first immune-oncology drug approved for gastric cancer treatment. In contrast, the PD-L1 monoclonal antibody, vedolizumab, failed to achieve its intended study objectives, as no significant difference in median survival was observed [74].

Regrettably, the aforementioned trials exclusively focused on patients with advanced gastric cancer who were not suitable candidates for surgery. Recent studies have revealed that chemotherapy and radiation can impact the expression levels of molecular targets associated with gastric cancer [75]. Specifically, one study found that the overall expression of PD-1 and PD-L1 in gastric cancer was upregulated following neoadjuvant chemotherapy, implying that neoadjuvant treatment may enhance the response rate of gastric cancer patients to immunotherapy [76].

To date, no definitive clinical trial has established the benefits of immunotherapy in neoadjuvant treatment for gastric cancer. Nevertheless, the trend in neoadjuvant treatment for gastric cancer is to guide the use of immunotherapeutic agents based on genetic testing, such as in patients with MSI-H gastric cancer, those with a PD-1 CPS score ≥ 1, and individuals with TMB-H gastric cancer.

5.5.4 Expert Comments

The utilization of neoadjuvant therapy has emerged as a promising and advantageous approach in addressing the challenges posed by locally advanced gastric cancer. This treatment strategy offers several benefits, including tumor downstaging, reduction in tumor size, eradication of micrometastases, decreased risk of intraoperative dissemination and postoperative recurrence, and improved rates of achieving R0 resection. While radical surgery remains the mainstay treatment for advanced gastric cancer, the effectiveness of adjuvant therapy following surgery has been less than satisfactory. However, with the rapid advancements in targeted therapies and immune-based treatments, there is potential for further advancements in the management of locally advanced gastric cancer.

Case provider:Lulu Zhao, Yingtai Chen.

Expert comments:Dongbing Zhao.

5.6 Case 35: Hyperthermic Intraperitoneal Chemotherapy in Advanced Gastric Cancer

5.6.1 Brief History

The patient, a 62-year-old male, presented with a chief complaint of abdominal distension persisting over the past 2 months. Upon abdominal examination, no positive signs were observed. However, elevated tumor markers were detected (CEA: 8.26 ng/mL, CA199: 38.78 U/mL, CA724: 15.68 U/mL). Subsequent gastroscope examination revealed an irregular tumor located at the lesser curvature of the stomach. Histopathological analysis confirmed the presence of moderately and poorly differentiated adenocarcinoma. Abdominal computed tomography (CT) exhibited uneven thickening of the gastric wall along the greater curvature, lesser curvature, and cardia, accompanied by roughening of the local serous surface and blurred fat spaces in the vicinity, consistent with gastric cancer. Notably, multiple lymph nodes were detected in the vicinity of the cardia, abdominal trunk, and retroperitoneum, with the larger nodes measuring 1.2 cm in short diameter, indicative of a high likelihood of metastasis (Fig. 5.13).

Diagnosis: gastric cancer (cT4aN1M0).

5.6.2 Treatment

Complete preoperative examinations were conducted due to the advanced stage of the tumor. Neoadjuvant treatment was recommended. However, after thorough discussion, the patient

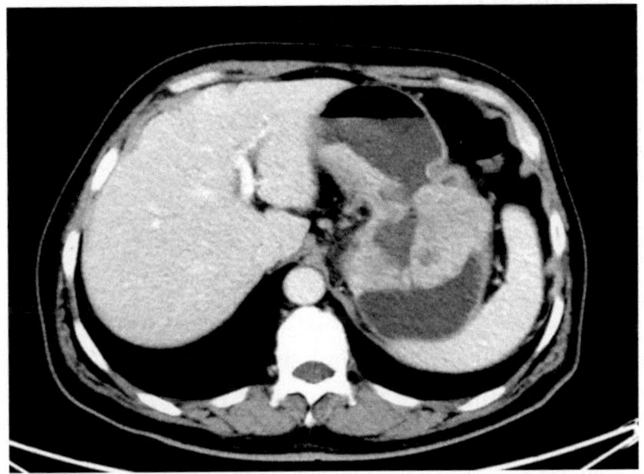

Fig. 5.13 CT demonstrated uneven thickening of the gastric wall along the greater curvature and lesser curvature of the cardia, as well as the stomach body. The local serous surface exhibited roughness, accompanied by blurred fat spaces in the surrounding area, consistent with findings indicative of gastric cancer. Notably, multiple lymph nodes were visualized adjacent to the cardia, along the abdominal trunk, and within the retroperitoneum. Among them, the larger lymph nodes displayed a short diameter of 1.2 cm, suggesting a substantial likelihood of metastatic involvement

and his family declined and strongly insisted on surgical intervention to remove the lesion. Laparoscopic exploration during the operation revealed minor adhesions in the upper abdomen, minimal ascites in the abdominal and pelvic cavities, and no evidence of implant metastasis. The tumor, measuring approximately 12 × 10 cm, was situated in the stomach. It had invaded the body and tail of the pancreas, with multiple enlarged lymph nodes surrounding the stomach, some of which displayed partial fusion. The largest lymph node, measuring approximately 3 × 3 cm, had encroached upon the splenic hilum. Subsequently, an open abdominal approach was employed, and a total gastrectomy was performed, along with distal pancreatectomy and splenectomy (left upper abdominal combined visceral resection). Following the procedure, two hyperthermic intraperitoneal chemotherapy tubes were inserted into the abdominal cavity, while one intraperitoneal drainage tube was placed in the left abdominal wall. After the abdomen was meticulously closed in layers, hyperthermic intraperitoneal chemotherapy was administered for 60 min, with the infusion of chemotherapy drugs consisting of 5% glucose injection (250 mL) and 90 mg of lobaplatin injection. The perfusion process proceeded uneventfully.

On the second and fifth postoperative days, hyperthermic intraperitoneal chemotherapy was repeated, utilizing the same chemotherapy regimen as before. On the sixth day after the operation, the patient experienced flatus and commenced a liquid diet. The drainage tube was removed on the 12th day postoperatively, and all tumor markers returned to within normal ranges. Subsequently, the patient was discharged on the 14th day following the surgical procedure.

Pathological examination revealed a 14 cm long lesser curvature, and a 20 cm long greater curvature of the stomach. The specimen of the pancreatic body and tail measured 8 × 4 × 3 cm. A large ulcerative mass measuring 13 × 10 × 5 cm was observed at the lesser curvature of the gastric fundus and posterior wall. The cross-section displayed a grayish-white appearance with medium hardness. The tumor exhibited adhesion to the pancreatic body and tail at the small curvature of the stomach, with a grayish-yellow appearance upon sectioning. The spleen weighed 600 g and measured 13 × 11 × 7 cm, displaying a gray-red and soft appearance. The greater omental area measured 42 × 20 cm, with no palpable nodules. Microscopic examination revealed a poorly differentiated adenocarcinoma of the gastric ulcer type, with focal signet ring cell carcinoma. Extensive nerve invasion, vascular invasion, and lymphatic invasion were observed. The tumor had penetrated the serosa and invaded the pancreatic tissue and dentate line. No cancer cells were detected in the omentum, spleen, esophageal stump, duodenal stump, pancreatic stump, or upper incisal margin. Lymph node metastases were present in 20 out of 60 lymph nodes examined. Immunohistochemical analysis showed negative staining for CgA, Syn, CD56, SALL4, Glypican3, AFP, and HER2. Positive staining was observed for DNA mismatch repair proteins MSH2, MSH6, MLH1, PMS2, and CK. The TNM stage was classified as pT4bN3M0.

5.6.3 Case Analysis

Hyperthermic intraperitoneal chemotherapy (HIPEC) is a therapeutic approach that involves heating the chemotherapy solution to an appropriate temperature, infusing it into the abdominal cavity of cancer patients, and maintaining it for a specific duration to prevent and treat peritoneal cancer and malignant ascites [77]. In 1980, Spratt et al. [78] pioneered the application of this technique in the treatment of pseudomyxoma peritonei, demonstrating no apparent adverse reactions associated with HIPEC postoperatively. Subsequent studies have shown the effectiveness of HIPEC in various abdominal malignancies, including advanced gastric cancer [79]. The advancement of HIPEC equipment has led to precise temperature control, accurate positioning, and enhanced clearance, substantially mitigating concerns related to equivocal efficacy and a high incidence of perfusion-related complications [80].

The principles underlying the efficacy of HIPEC are as follows: (1) Malignant tumor cells and normal cells exhibit differential temperature tolerances. Malignant tumor cells experience irreversible damage when exposed to a temperature of 43 °C for 1 h, while normal tissue cells can withstand temperatures of 47 °C for the same duration [77]. By leveraging precise temperature control, HIPEC can selectively target and eliminate tumor cells without causing harm to normal tissues [81]. (2) HIPEC enables enhanced drug concentration in the abdominal cavity. Due to the presence of the peritoneum-plasma barrier and the adhesive and isolative properties of the peritoneum, traditional systemic chemotherapy drugs often fail to achieve adequate concentration in peritoneal tumors. HIPEC, on the other hand, can elevate the concentration of intraperitoneal chemotherapy drugs to levels 20–1000 times higher than plasma levels, effectively exerting their therapeutic effects on tumor cells [82]. (3) Mechanical lavage facilitates the removal of residual cancer cells. In contrast to early-stage approaches that involved draining perfusion fluid from the abdominal cavity, current high-precision continuous circulation thermal perfusion methods employ cyclic lavage of the abdominal cavity at a fixed flow rate. This process effectively filters out free cancer cells larger than 40 μm, thereby eliminating them from the abdominal cavity.

Currently, the widely used method for assessing the extent of peritoneal involvement is the Sugarbaker Peritoneal Cancer Index (PCI) zoning counting method [83], as depicted in Fig. 5.14. This approach, developed by Sugarbaker, divides the abdomen into 13 regions, and the largest visible nodules are used as representative scoring objects. Lesions that are not detected are assigned 0 points, lesions with a diameter of ≤0.5 cm receive 1 point, lesions with a diameter of 0.5–5 cm receive 2 points, and lesions with a diameter > 5 cm or those exhibiting fusion with other lesions receive 3 points. The total score ranges from 0 to 39 points. It is important to evaluate the PCI index both before and after surgery, excluding primary or resectable metastatic cancers. The PCI index can serve as a prognostic indicator for patients. However, further research is needed to establish specific thresholds for risk stratification.

Peritoneal metastasis is a common type of recurrence in gastric cancer patients after surgery and is associated with poor prognosis [84]. Traditionally, peritoneal metastasis in gastric cancer has been considered an advanced stage of the disease, limiting the value of surgical intervention. However, in recent years, a growing body of evidence suggests that selected cases of peritoneal metastasis can be treated as a form of localized metastasis, with the potential for

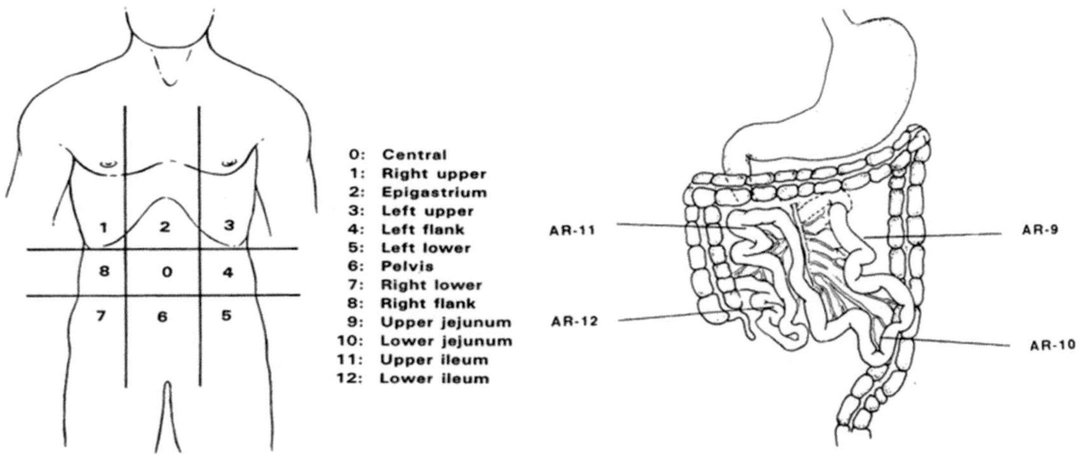

Fig. 5.14 Sugarbaker Peritoneal Cancer Index (PCI) zoning counting method

achieving long-term survival through active treatment. Numerous studies have demonstrated that prophylactic hyperthermic intraperitoneal chemotherapy (HIPEC) following surgery for advanced gastric cancer can effectively reduce the recurrence of gastric cancer and prolong patient survival [85–88]. Commonly used chemotherapy agents for HIPEC in gastric cancer include paclitaxel, docetaxel, oxaliplatin, cisplatin, 5-fluorouracil, and epirubicin, which are also utilized in systemic chemotherapy. However, the characteristics of systemic chemotherapy and HIPEC differ. In theory, chemotherapy agents with higher molecular weight, superior tumor tissue penetration, and synergy with hyperthermia may yield better outcomes [89]. According to the consensus among Chinese experts [77], HIPEC can be employed for the following purposes: (1) prevention of peritoneal implantation metastasis in gastric cancer; (2) postoperative treatment of peritoneal implantation metastasis in gastric cancer; (3) conversion or palliative therapy. Experience has shown that repeated laparoscopic HIPEC treatments allow for continuous monitoring and assessment of gastric cancer progression, treatment response, and metastasis. HIPEC can also improve the quality of life for patients who are not candidates for surgery due to ascites [90].

5.6.4 Expert Comments

Peritoneal metastasis represents an advanced stage of gastric cancer and is often challenging to manage with traditional cytotoxic chemotherapy due to the presence of the peritoneum-plasma barrier, which limits drug penetration. However, the emergence of HIPEC as an effective treatment for pseudomyxoma peritonei has sparked increased interest in its potential application for gastric cancer. Although HIPEC is not currently recommended as a first-line treatment for gastric cancer, the completion of several high-quality clinical studies will hold promise for its broader utilization in the future, leading to improved outcomes for patients with advanced gastric cancer.

Case provider:Xiaofeng Bai, Zefeng Li.

Commentary:Xiaofeng Bai.

5.7 Case 36: The Management of Ovarian Metastases from Primary Gastric Cancer

5.7.1 Brief History

The patient, a 33-year-old female, presented with a chief complaint of persistent upper abdominal pain lasting for a duration exceeding 2 months. Notably, the pain exhibited a temporal association with hunger and was alleviated upon consumption of food. A prior gastroscopic examination conducted at a different medical facility revealed the presence of poorly differentiated adenocarcinoma localized to the gastric antrum. Subsequent imaging via a computed tomography (CT) scan performed at our institution revealed notable thickening of the gastric wall within the antrum, reaching a maximum thickness of approximately 1.5 cm. Additionally, deep ulcers were visualized, and the serosal surface exhibited a roughened appearance. Intriguingly, multiple linear shadows were discernible within the surrounding adipose interstitial spaces. Furthermore, bilateral adnexal regions appeared enlarged with indistinct boundaries, displaying significant localized enhancement characterized by ring enhancement, as illustrated in Fig. 5.15. Gastroscopic assessment unveiled the lesion's location spanning from the lower segment of the gastric body to the antrum, involving the lesser curvature of the gastric antrum, as depicted in Fig. 5.16. The final diagnosis rendered was gastric cancer classified as cT4NxMx, indicating advanced disease staging.

5.7.2 Treatment

Under the administration of general anesthesia, an exploratory laparotomy was conducted, revealing extensive metastatic lesions within the abdominal and pelvic cavities. Consequently, the revised diagnosis was established as gastric cancer classified as cT4NxM1, prompting a recommendation for internal medicine treatment.

The patient underwent an initial course of 8 cycles of PD-1100 mg immunotherapy, fol-

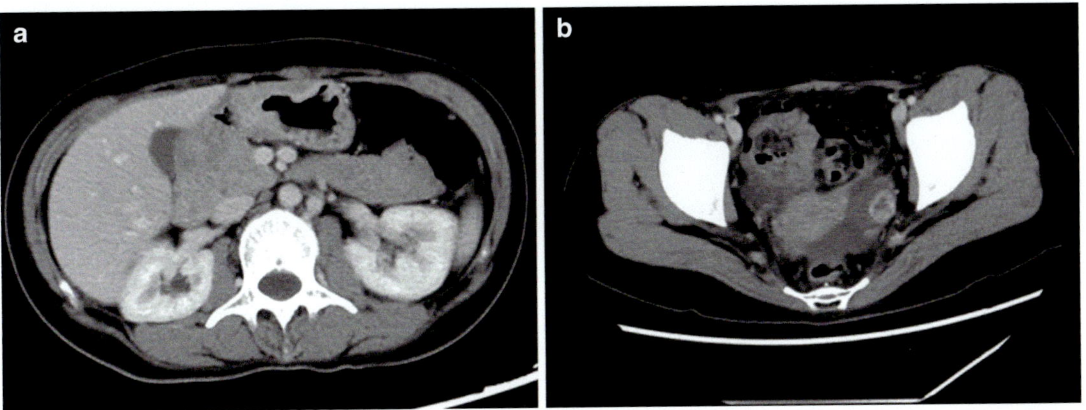

Fig. 5.15 Illustrates the following findings: (**a**) Thickening of the gastric wall in the gastric angle, and (**b**) bilateral adnexal fullness characterized by indistinct borders and notable local enhancement, presenting as ring enhancement

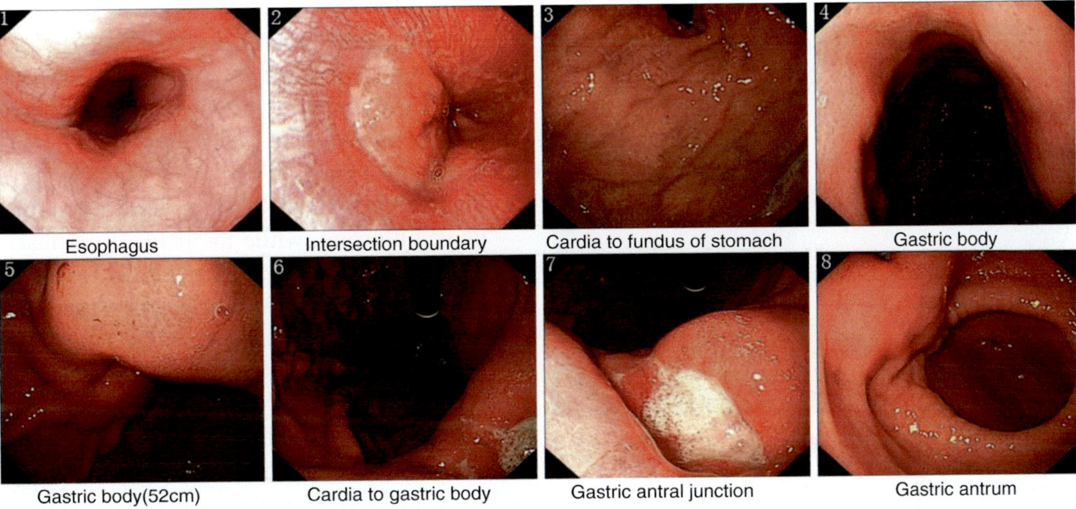

Fig. 5.16 Showcases a gastroscopic view revealing the presence of gastric cancer situated at the junction between the lower body and antrum of the stomach, as well as involving the lesser curvature of the stomach

lowed by 5 cycles of SOX chemotherapy. Subsequent evaluation via a follow-up CT scan demonstrated the gastric cavity to be replete, accompanied by slight thickening of the walls in the gastric antrum and lesser curvature, which displayed indistinct borders akin to the previous scan. Furthermore, the left adnexal mass exhibited a reduction in size relative to its previous dimensions, measuring approximately 3.8 × 2.5 cm in maximum cross-sectional area. Conversely, the right adnexal area appeared to be filled, lacking clear demarcation on the plain scan and exhibiting ambiguous separation from the uterus and intestinal tract, as depicted in Fig. 5.17.

Following thorough multidisciplinary discussions, given the inadequate control of ovarian metastasis, palliative debulking surgery was recommended. Consequently, an open bilateral salpingo-oophorectomy was performed, as illustrated in Fig. 5.18. Subsequent pathological examination confirmed the presence of infiltrating poorly differentiated adenocarcinoma within both the left and right ovaries, consistent with gastric adenocarcinoma metastasis, as supported by the patient's medical history and immunohistochemistry results. Notably, no evidence of cancer was observed in the left and right fallopian tubes. Immunohistochemical staining revealed

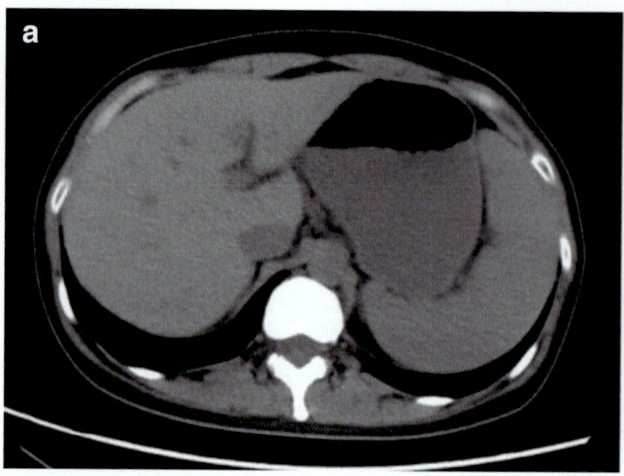

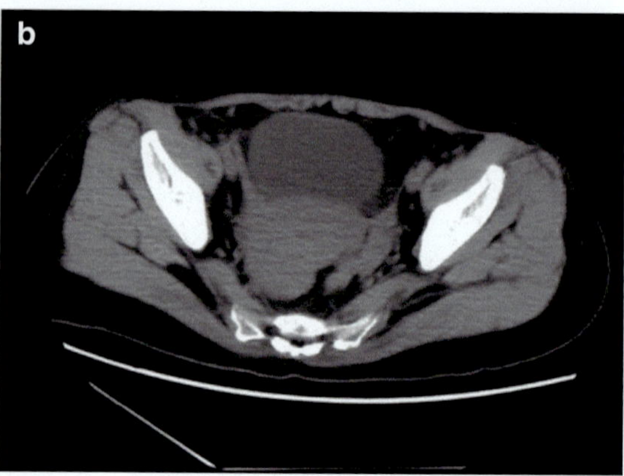

Fig. 5.17 Post-treatment CT scan findings include (**a**) slightly thickened walls of the gastric antrum and lesser curvature with indistinct borders on the plain scan, akin to the previous scan; (**b**) reduced size of the left adnexal mass compared to the previous scan and persistent fullness of the right adnexal area

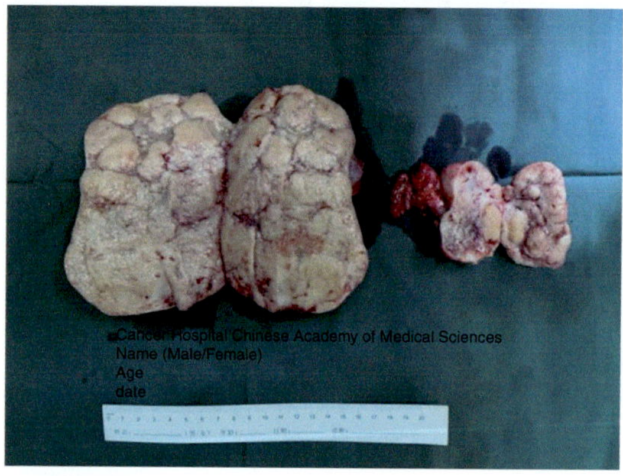

Fig. 5.18 Bilateral ovaries displaying metastatic tumors

AE1/AE3 (3+), CK7 (−), CK20 (+), CDX-2 (3+), CEA (3+), PAX8 (−), ER (−), WT-1 (−), and HER2 (1+). Additionally, in situ hybridization for Epstein-Barr virus-encoded RNA (EBER) yielded a negative result.

Following the completion of 6 cycles of PD-1 combined with toripalimab, the patient's response was evaluated as stable disease (SD). A CT scan performed 8 months after the bilateral salpingo-oophorectomy yielded the following observations:

1. The gastric cavity remained discernible, and the thickening of the gastric antrum and lesser curvature appeared comparable to the previous scan.
2. The fat planes within the abdominal cavity exhibited indistinct boundaries, accompanied by the identification of multiple small lymph nodes in the mesentery and retroperitoneum.
3. Post-pelvic surgery, the edge of the uterus displayed blurring, while the pelvic floor fascia exhibited thickening, characterized by visible cord-like shadows. These changes were attributed to postoperative effects, as depicted in Fig. 5.19.

Following the administration of PD-1, albumin-bound paclitaxel, and apatinib for 6 cycles, the patient achieved a partial response. Subsequent monitoring via a CT scan conducted 16 months after the bilateral salpingo-oophorectomy yielded the following findings:

1. The thickening of the gastric antrum and lesser curvature remained similar to previous scans.
2. The fat planes within the abdominal cavity exhibited blurred demarcations, and there was evidence of omental thickening and nodular changes in both the abdominal and pelvic cavities. Some regions showed signs of improvement, while others remained unchanged. The largest measurable nodule had a longitudinal diameter of approximately 1.4 cm, suggesting metastatic involvement.

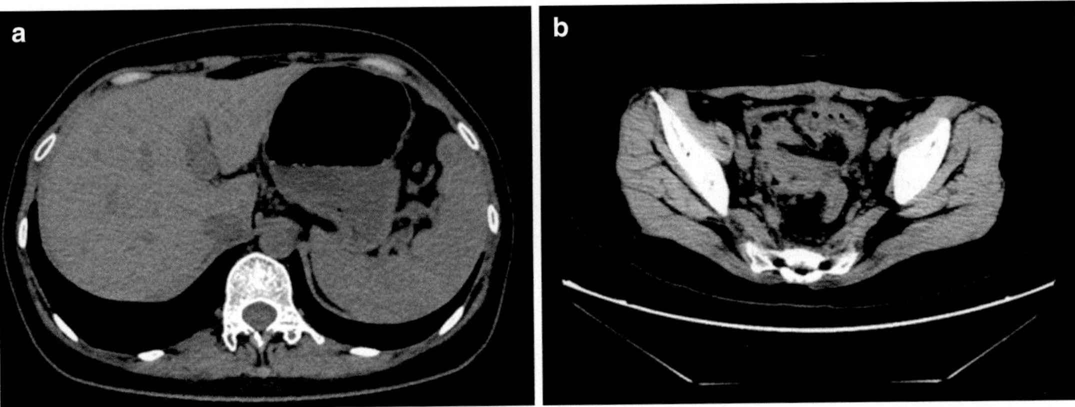

Fig. 5.19 (**a**) Persistence of thickening in the gastric antrum and lesser curvature 8 months post bilateral salpingo-oophorectomy; (**b**) Postoperative alterations in the pelvic region

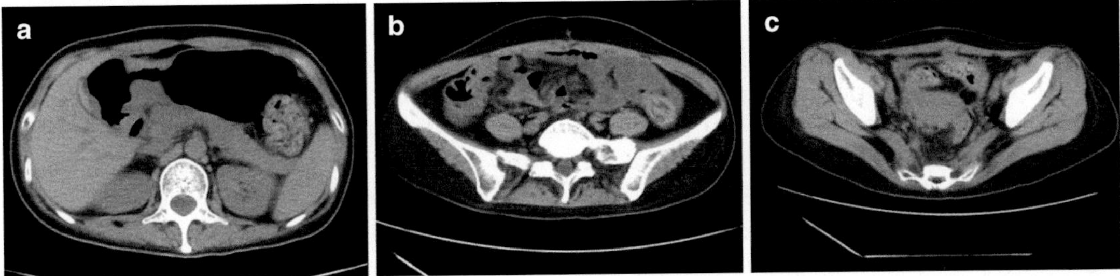

Fig. 5.20 (**a**) Persistence of thickening in the lesser curvature and antrum of the stomach 16 months after bilateral salpingo-oophorectomy. (**b**) Thickening of the peritoneum within the abdominal and pelvic cavities, displaying both nodular and fibrous changes. Partial improvement observed in certain regions, while others exhibited findings similar to previous scans. The largest nodular lesion measured approximately 1.4 cm in its longest dimension, indicative of metastasis. (**c**) Identification of a low-density nodule with indistinct margins on the left side of the uterus

3. A low-density nodule with indistinct margins was identified on the left side of the uterus, necessitating further follow-up, as illustrated in Fig. 5.20. The diagnosis of peritoneal metastasis is being considered.

5.7.3 Case Analysis

5.7.3.1 Gastric Cancer with Ovarian Metastasis

Ovaries serve as prominent target organs for distant metastasis in female patients with gastric cancer. The seminal report by German pathologist and gynecologist Krukenberg in 1896 documented six distinctive cases of ovarian metastases originating from gastric cancer, subsequently leading to the coining of the term "Krukenberg tumor" [91]. In 1973, the World Health Organization introduced a revised histological definition for Krukenberg tumor, characterizing it as the presence of tumorous proliferation consisting of mucin-secreting signet ring cells within the ovary, accompanied by stromal sarcoma-like infiltration [92]. The incidence of ovarian metastasis in gastric cancer patients varies from 0.3 to 6.7%, while postmortem studies reveal a much higher rate of 30–40% compared to clinical statistics. Such a discrepancy may suggest potential challenges in timely and accurate diagnosis of Krukenberg tumor [93, 94].

5.7.3.2 The Mechanism of Ovarian Metastasis

The mechanism underlying ovarian metastasis in gastric cancer has remained a subject of controversy and significant scientific discourse. The implantation theory was initially proposed, positing that gastric cancer cells infiltrate the serosal layer and subsequently detach into the peritoneal cavity. Utilizing intestinal peristalsis, these cells ultimately implant and proliferate on the ovarian capsule [95]. Nevertheless, this theory has been met with skepticism, as certain primary gastric lesions do not invade the serosal layer, and metastatic lesions often manifest within the ovarian stroma while the ovarian capsule remains intact [96]. Currently, lymphatic metastasis is considered the most plausible route of dissemination [97]. Gastric cancer cells have the ability to migrate to the perigastric lymph nodes, forming cancer emboli that obstruct normal lymphatic flow. Consequently, these cells reflux into the peritoneal and pelvic lymph nodes through lymphatic vessels. Given the abundance of lymphatic networks in the pelvic cavity, the retrograde lymphatic pathway provides a means for gastric cancer cells to metastasize to the ovaries [97–99]. There exists a discernible association between blood metastasis and Krukenberg tumors. Notably, Krukenberg tumors primarily affect premenopausal women, and the rich vascularization of the ovaries in young individuals, along with the observed tendency for tumors to invade the ovarian stroma, substantiate the notion of hematogenous spread [100]. Currently, several studies propose that the occurrence of Krukenberg tumors may be attributed to the combined influence of the aforementioned pathways [101].

5.7.3.3 Treatment of Ovarian Metastasis in Gastric Cancer

Comprehensive treatment for gastric cancer with ovarian metastases primarily revolves around a surgical approach; however, there is currently a lack of clinical trial evidence supporting this practice.

The indication for surgery in cases of gastric cancer with ovarian metastases has been a topic of debate, particularly regarding the optimal management of the primary lesion and metastases. The 2020 Chinese Society of Clinical Oncology (CSCO) gastric cancer guidelines suggest that systemic chemotherapy remains the mainstay treatment for patients with gastric cancer and a solitary ovarian metastasis [102]. Nevertheless, retrospective studies have demonstrated potential benefits of aggressive surgery combined with systemic chemotherapy, resulting in extended median survival periods from 6–9 months to 19–23.7 months [103]. However, a consensus regarding the specific patient population suitable for surgical treatment, optimal timing of surgery, and appropriate surgical methods has yet to be reached. Consequently, the CSCO guidelines classify these recommendations as Class 2B evidence. The American National Comprehensive Cancer Network (NCCN) guidelines [104] and the Japanese gastric cancer guidelines [105] have not provided surgical recommendations for gastric cancer with ovarian metastases at present.

Systemic chemotherapy serves as the standard treatment for advanced-stage gastric cancer with recurrence or metastasis. Additionally, the investigation of intraperitoneal hyperthermic chemotherapy and cytoreductive surgery for gastric cancer with ovarian metastasis has garnered significant attention. However, the benefit of cytoreductive surgery in such cases remains a subject of controversy. While maximal cytoreductive surgery is widely acknowledged as beneficial for primary ovarian cancer, Bozzetti et al. [106] argue that most cases of gastric cancer with ovarian metastasis involve signet ring cell carcinoma, which is relatively insensitive to chemotherapy. Consequently, cytoreductive surgery is unlikely to confer significant survival benefits and is primarily employed for symptom relief. Wu et al. [107] demonstrated that patients with peritoneal dissemination undergoing simple cytoreductive surgery exhibited a median survival time of only 10.4 months. However, when combined with intraperitoneal hyperthermic chemotherapy, the median survival time increased to 15.5 months. These findings underscore the need for well-designed clinical trials to definitively establish the therapeutic value of cytoreductive surgery and intraperitoneal hyperthermic chemotherapy in the management of gastric cancer with ovarian metastasis.

5.7.4 Expert Comments

Gastric cancer with ovarian metastasis is associated with a dismal prognosis, and early diagnosis and comprehensive therapy are crucial for effective management. However, standardized diagnostic and treatment approaches for this condition are still under investigation. The implementation of a multidisciplinary collaborative system and the adoption of comprehensive treatment strategies, primarily involving surgical resection of metastatic lesions in conjunction with systemic chemotherapy, have shown potential for improving patient outcomes to some extent.

Case provider:Lulu Zhao, Chunguang Guo.

Expert comments:Dongbing Zhao.

5.8 Case 37: The Surgical Resection for Advanced Gastric Cancer After Translational Therapy

5.8.1 Brief History

The patient, a 62-year-old male, presented with episodic upper abdominal discomfort and nausea unaccompanied by vomiting or acid reflux. These symptoms emerged approximately 2 months ago, without any discernible triggering factors. Initial treatment for "gastric ulcer" at a local hospital yielded unsatisfactory outcomes, prompting the patient to seek medical care at our institution.

Laboratory assessments conducted at our hospital revealed normal levels of carcinoembryonic antigen (CEA), alpha-fetoprotein (AFP), cancer antigen 72–4 (CA72–4), cancer antigen 19–9 (CA19–9), and cancer antigen 24–2 (CA24–2). Gastroscopy examination unveiled an ulcerative lesion located at the junction between the gastric body and antrum, raising suspicions of its malignant nature (refer to Fig. 5.21). Subsequent pathological evaluation confirmed the presence of poorly differentiated cancer.

Enhanced computed tomography (CT) scan depicted thickening of the gastric wall at the gastric angle, indicative of gastric cancer. Additionally, mild thickening of the gastric wall at the gastric antrum was observed during the imaging (as demonstrated in the endoscopy findings). Noteworthy, numerous scattered small lymph nodes were identified in the vicinity of the pylorus, necessitating caution for potential metastasis. Further lymph nodes were also detected in the mesentery and retroperitoneum, warranting a follow-up investigation. Additionally, a lesion was detected in the left lobe of the liver, raising suspicion of metastatic involvement (refer to Fig. 5.22).

Positron emission tomography-CT (PET-CT) examination revealed heightened metabolic activity in the thickened gastric wall at the gastric angle, consistent with the presence of gastric cancer. Increased metabolic activity was also detected in the lymph nodes surrounding the pylorus, multiple retroperitoneal lymph nodes, and a small lymph node in the left supraclavicular area, suggesting possible metastasis. For further confirmation, ultrasound examination and biopsy are recommended.

Final diagnosis: Gastric cancer (cT4aN3M1, H1, No.16+), indicating advanced disease with infiltration into adjacent structures and extensive lymph node involvement.

5.8.2 Treatment

Following thorough multidisciplinary consultation, it was determined that the patient should undergo the DOS chemotherapy regimen. This protocol involves the administration of paclitaxel at a dose of 150 mg intravenously on day 1, oxaliplatin at a dose of 150 mg intravenously on day 2, and tegafur gimeracil oteracil potassium capsules at a dose of 60 mg twice daily from day 1 to day 10. After completing four cycles of treatment, a CT evaluation revealed the following changes:

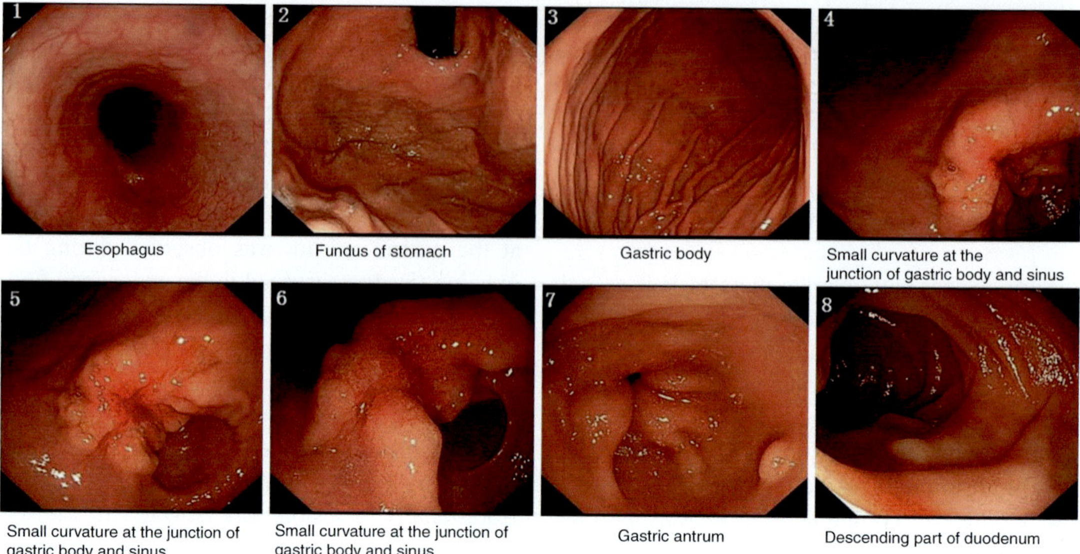

Fig. 5.21 Gastroscopy image displaying an ulcerative lesion located at the junction of the gastric body and antrum, indicative of carcinoma

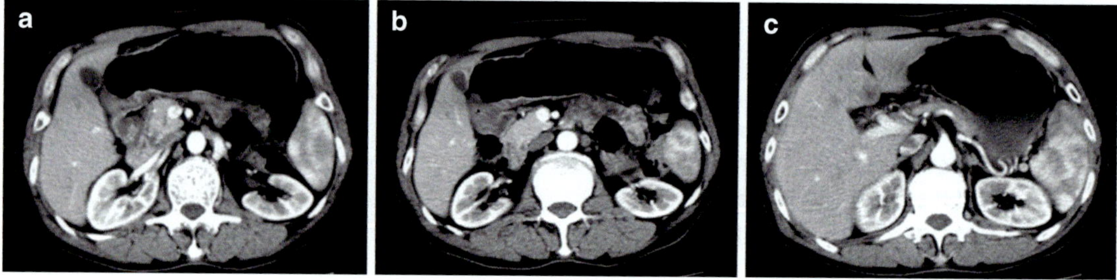

Fig. 5.22 (Before Treatment): (**a**) Gastric cancer; (**b**) peritoneal lymph node metastasis; (**c**) liver metastasis

1. The thickening of the gastric wall in the area of the gastric angle demonstrated a reduction, with the thickest part measuring approximately 0.8 cm and displaying mild enhancement. The thickening of the gastric wall in the antrum remained slightly increased, consistent with the findings observed during endoscopy.
2. Scattered small lymph nodes were observed around the gastric antrum and pylorus. Multiple lymph nodes in the mesentery and retroperitoneum exhibited a decrease in size, with the largest measuring approximately 0.4 cm in short diameter, necessitating further follow-up observation.
3. The size of the metastatic tumor in the left hepatic lobe decreased compared to the initial assessment and now measures approximately 0.7 cm x 0.7 cm with fuzzy edges (refer to Fig. 5.23).

Following the multidisciplinary consensus, the patient underwent radiofrequency ablation for hepatic metastasis. The original chemotherapy regimen was continued for the fifth cycle, and subsequent to treatment, a follow-up CT was conducted, revealing the following changes [108]: The degree of thickening of the gastric wall at the angle of the stomach displayed a reduction compared to the previous assessment,

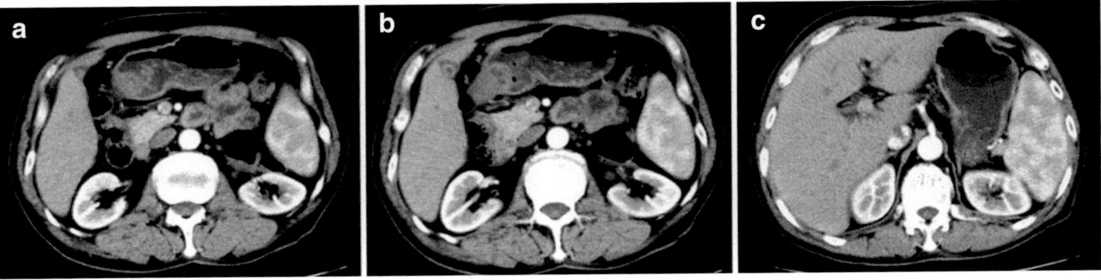

Fig. 5.23 (**a**) Illustrates gastric cancer after four cycles of chemotherapy; (**b**) depicts peritoneal lymph node metastasis; and (**c**) displays liver metastasis

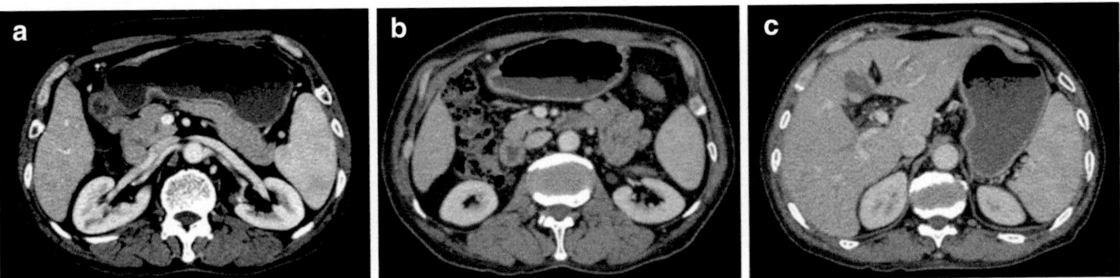

Fig. 5.24 (**a**) Depicts gastric cancer after five cycles of chemotherapy and liver radiofrequency ablation; (**b**) illustrates peritoneal lymph node metastasis; and (**c**) displays liver metastasis

with the thickest part measuring approximately 0.6 cm. The thickening of the gastric wall in the pyloric antrum remained similar to the previous findings [109]. The scattered small lymph nodes around the gastric antrum and pylorus exhibited a slight decrease in size compared to the previous evaluation. Multiple lymph nodes in the mesentery and retroperitoneum also displayed slight reductions in size, while some remained unchanged. The largest lymph node had a short diameter of approximately 0.6 cm. Further follow-up was recommended [55]. A low-density lesion with clear borders was identified in the left lobe of the liver, which was considered a post-radiofrequency ablation change. The size of the lesion was approximately 3.1 × 1.5 cm. Please consider the clinical significance (refer to Fig. 5.24). The evaluation indicated a partial response (PR).

Following the notable improvement in the patient's condition post-chemotherapy, a comprehensive multidisciplinary consultation was conducted. After thorough communication with the family, it was decided to proceed with a distal gastrectomy utilizing the Billroth II + Braun technique, accompanied by D3 lymph node dissection (refer to Fig. 5.25).

The patient experienced a smooth postoperative recovery, characterized by the following milestones: limited water intake on postoperative day 2 (POD2), a gradual introduction of rice soup on POD3, removal of the gastric tube and urinary catheter on POD4, transition to a semi-liquid diet on POD4, removal of bilateral abdominal drainage tube and pelvic drainage tube on POD7, and subsequent discharge on POD12.

Pathology: Macroscopic examination of the obtained distal gastrectomy specimen revealed measurements of 12 cm in length for the small curvature and 16 cm in length for the greater curvature. The distance from the pyloric ring was 3.8 cm, while the distance from the upper margin was 6.2 cm. An observed scar area in the lesser curvature of the stomach measured 1.5 × 1.5 × 0.3 cm and appeared to invade the muscular layer.

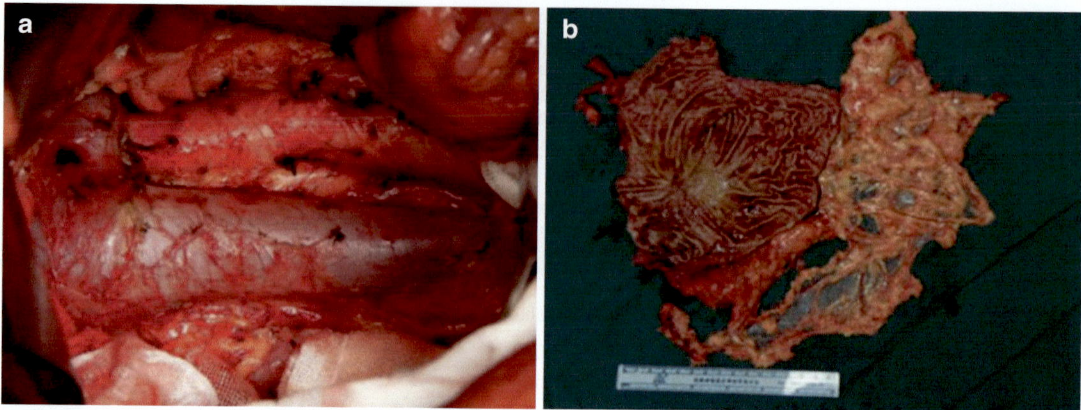

Fig. 5.25 (**a**) Illustrates the surgical field following the dissection of retroperitoneal lymph node No. 16, and (**b**) depicts the excised specimen

Microscopic examination of the lesion confirmed the diagnosis of a locally advanced ulcerative, moderately to poorly differentiated adenocarcinoma of the stomach with an intestinal type Lauren classification. The tumor exhibited invasion of the superficial muscular layer and showed evidence of vascular invasion. Resected margins were negative for malignancy. Following mild treatment, the tumor regression grade was determined to be 4 according to the Mandard tumor regression grading system. Lymph node involvement was confirmed, with metastatic cancer present in 11 out of 51 examined lymph nodes. The metastases were observed in the following lymph nodes: No.1 (1/5), No.3 (1/10), No.4sb (0/1), No.4d (4/8), No.5 (0/1), No.6 (1/1), No.7 (0/4), No.8a (0/5), No.9 (0), No.11p (1/8), No.12a (0), No.13 (0), No.14v (1/1), No.16b1 left (2/2), and No.16b1 right (0/5).

Following the surgery, a postoperative CT scan conducted at 4 months revealed the presence of multiple lymph nodes in the left subclavian region, left supraclavicular region, and mediastinal 1L, 3A, 4L, and 6 zones, some of which were newly identified, indicating the likelihood of metastasis. Subsequently, the patient underwent three cycles of trastuzumab plus irinotecan treatment, resulting in a progressive disease response. The treatment regimen was then switched to oral apatinib hydrochloride in combination with capecitabine for one cycle. During the 12-month follow-up period after surgery, the patient was found to have survived with residual tumor.

5.8.3 Case Analysis

5.8.3.1 Surgical Treatment of Liver Metastasis from Gastric Cancer

Gastric cancer metastasis can be classified into three main types: lymph node metastasis, liver metastasis, and peritoneal metastasis. Among these, liver metastasis is the most common type of distant metastasis for gastric cancer, and it often presents with multiple lesions involving multiple liver lobes, sometimes accompanied by other distant metastases. Surgical treatment for liver metastasis should be approached cautiously.

Systemic treatment is the primary approach for managing gastric cancer liver metastasis, and there is no consensus on the optimal surgical treatment strategies for liver metastases. The results of the 2016 REGATTA trial showed that palliative resection of the primary tumor does not extend the survival of advanced gastric cancer patients. Therefore, palliative surgical treatment is generally recommended only for patients with severe complications such as obstruction or bleeding in metastatic gastric cancer, according to the American NCCN guidelines.

Considering the diverse biological behavior and significant prognostic differences in stage IV gastric cancer, treatment approaches should be tailored based on the specific characteristics of the disease. For example, surgical resection may be considered for isolated liver metastases or a small number of lymph node metastases located adjacent to the abdominal aorta, as suggested by Yoshida et al. Neoadjuvant chemotherapy is recommended for potentially resectable metastases, such as multiple liver metastases with a diameter greater than 5 cm or those located near the hepatic or portal veins, to reduce tumor burden and increase the likelihood of achieving R0 resection.

The 2019 Chinese expert consensus on gastric cancer liver metastasis proposed a new classification system called C-GCLM (Chinese Type for Gastric Cancer Liver Metastasis) to aid in clinical decision-making [110]. This classification system categorizes cases into different types based on resectability and comprehensive assessment by a multidisciplinary team. Type I cases are considered resectable, where both the gastric primary tumor and liver metastases can be surgically removed. For Type I cases, direct surgical resection or neoadjuvant systemic treatment, combined with chemotherapy and targeted therapy for HER-2-positive cases, is recommended. R0 resection of both the primary tumor and liver metastases should be attempted, followed by systemic treatment consisting of 4–8 cycles.

Similar recommendations can be found in the Chinese Society of Clinical Oncology Gastric Cancer Diagnosis [111] and Treatment Guidelines, as well as the fifth edition of the Japanese Gastric Cancer Diagnosis and Treatment Guidelines [112]. The Japanese guidelines provide a treatment roadmap for M1 cases, with mild recommendations for surgical resection when there are few liver metastases and no other factors precluding a curative approach.

It is important to note that treatment decisions should be made in consultation with a multidisciplinary team of healthcare professionals who can assess the individual patient's condition and make personalized recommendations based on the specific characteristics of the disease.

5.8.3.2 The Significance of No.16 Lymph Node Dissection

The role of para-aortic lymph node dissection (PAND) in the management of locally advanced gastric cancer has been a topic of debate within the surgical community. Traditionally, the Japanese surgical community has advocated for PAND in patients with advanced gastric cancer, including those with para-aortic lymph node metastasis. Retrospective studies have shown that patients who underwent PAND for advanced gastric cancer with para-aortic lymph node metastasis had higher 5-year survival rates of 16–21% compared to other stage IV gastric cancer patients [113].

However, the Japanese JCOG9501 study did not confirm the clinical value of prophylactic PAND [114]. This study did not find a significant survival benefit in patients who underwent PAND compared to those who received standard D2 lymphadenectomy. Additionally, the REGATTA trial, which investigated the effectiveness of palliative resection of the primary tumor in stage IV gastric cancer, including cases with para-aortic lymph node metastasis, did not recommend surgical treatment for these patients.

In recent years, the effectiveness of neoadjuvant chemotherapy has improved, leading to increased success in conversion therapy for advanced gastric cancer. Conversion therapy refers to the use of neoadjuvant chemotherapy to downstage tumors and convert unresectable or borderline resectable tumors into resectable ones. Some studies have suggested that patients with isolated No.16 lymph node metastasis who respond well to conversion therapy may benefit from subsequent surgery [115–118]. These findings have brought hope to patients with isolated No.16 lymph node metastasis and have prompted the need for future trials to further investigate the role of surgery in these cases.

5.8.4 Expert Comments

With the progression of surgical techniques, the introduction of novel pharmaceutical agents, and the swift evolution of multidisciplinary diagnosis and treatment (MDT) frameworks, the management of advanced gastric cancer through surgical interventions has undergone continuous conceptual revisions and expanded indications. Moving forward, as the treatment paradigm for advanced gastric cancer is further optimized, the precise identification of suitable patient cohorts and the accurate determination of surgical indications, it is anticipated that conversion therapy will find broader application and foster significant advancements.

Case provider:Lulu Zhao, Tongbo Wang, Chunguang Guo.

Expert comments:Dongbing Zhao.

References

1. Wilmore DW, Kehlet H. Management of patients in fast track surgery. BMJ. 2001;322(7284):473–6.
2. Anon. Expert consensus of accelerated rehabilitation surgery after gastrectomy for gastric cancer (2016 edition). Chin J Gastrosurg. 2017;16(001):14–7.
3. Lee Y, Yu J, Doumouras AG, et al. Enhanced recovery after surgery (ERAS) versus standard recovery for elective gastric cancer surgery: a meta-analysis of randomized controlled trials. Surg Oncol. 2020;32:75–87.
4. Wang Z, Chen J, Su K, et al. Abdominal drainage versus no drainage post gastrectomy for gastric cancer. Cochrane Database Syst Rev. 2011;8:CD008788.
5. Ma Y, Jixiang C. Accelerate the application progress of rehabilitation surgery concept in gastric cancer patients. Chin J Surg Oncol. 2020;12(3):276–80.
6. Hirahara N, Matsubara T, Hayashi H, et al. Significance of prophylactic intra-abdominal drain placement after laparoscopic distal gastrectomy for gastric cancer. World J Surg Oncol. 2015;13:181.
7. Ahn HS, Lee HJ, Yoo MW, et al. Changes in clinicopathological features and survival after gastrectomy for gastric cancer over a 20-year period. Br J Surg. 2011;98(2):255–60.
8. Buas MF, Vaughan TL. Epidemiology and risk factors for gastroesophageal junction tumors: understanding the rising incidence of this disease. Semin Radiat Oncol. 2013;23(1):3–9.
9. Kusano C, Gotoda T, Khor CJ, et al. Changing trends in the proportion of adenocarcinoma of the esophagogastric junction in a large tertiary referral center in Japan. J Gastroenterol Hepatol. 2008;23(11):1662–5.
10. Liu K, Yang K, Zhang W, et al. Changes of Esophagogastric junctional adenocarcinoma and gastroesophageal reflux disease among surgical patients during 1988-2012: a single-institution, high-volume experience in China. Ann Surg. 2016;263(1):88–95.
11. Sano T. Gastric cancer: Asia and the world. Gastric Cancer. 2017;20(Suppl 1):1–2.
12. Zhao L, Niu P, Zhao D, et al. Regional and racial disparity in proximal gastric cancer survival outcomes 1996-2016: results from SEER and China National Cancer Center database. Cancer Med. 2021a;10(14):4923–38.
13. Mukaisho K, Nakayama T, Hagiwara T, et al. Two distinct etiologies of gastric cardia adenocarcinoma: interactions among pH, helicobacter pylori, and bile acids. Front Microbiol. 2015;6:412.
14. Jiafu J, Ke J. Przgress in surgical treatment of esophagogastric junction adenocarcinoma. Chin J Basic Clin Gen Surg. 2019;9:1021–4.
15. Fenglin L, Xinyu Q. Looking back at 2019—focusing on research progress in gastric tumors. Chin J Gastrointes Surg. 2020;023(001):10–4.
16. Siewert JR, Hölscher AH, Becker K, et al. Cardia cancer: attempt at a therapeutically relevant classification. Der Chirurg; Zeitschrift fur alle Gebiete der operativen Medizen. 1987;58(1):25–32.
17. Pacelli F, Papa V, Caprino P, et al. Proximal compared with distal gastric cancer: multivariate analysis of prognostic factors. Am Surg. 2001;67(7):697–703.
18. Park JC, Lee YC, Kim JH, et al. Clinicopathological features and prognostic factors of proximal gastric carcinoma in a population with high helicobacter pylori prevalence: a single-center, large-volume study in Korea. Ann Surg Oncol. 2010;17(3):829–37.
19. Piso P, Werner U, Lang H, et al. Proximal versus distal gastric carcinoma--what are the differences? Ann Surg Oncol. 2000;7(7):520–5.
20. Zhao L, Huang H, Zhao D, et al. Clinicopathological characteristics and prognosis of proximal and distal gastric cancer during 1997-2017 in China National Cancer Center. J Oncol. 2019:9784039.
21. Wang X, Liu F, Li Y, et al. Comparison on Clinicopathological features, treatments and prognosis between proximal gastric cancer and distal gastric cancer: a National Cancer Data Base Analysis. J Cancer. 2019;10(14):3145–53.
22. Yura M, Yoshikawa T, Otsuki S, et al. Oncological safety of proximal gastrectomy for T2/T3 proximal gastric cancer. Gastric Cancer. 2019;22(5):1029–35.
23. Zhao L, Ling R, Ma F, et al. Clinical outcomes of proximal gastrectomy versus total gastrectomy for locally advanced proximal gastric cancer: a propensity score matching analysis. Translat Cancer Res. 2020;9(4):2769–79.
24. Youth Committee of the Gastric Cancer Professional Committee of the Chinese Anti-Cancer Association. Interpretation of clinical issues in the 5th edition of the Japanese. Gastric Cancer Treatment Guidelines. 2019;1(1):1.
25. Rosa F, Quero G, Fiorillo C, et al. Total vs proximal gastrectomy for adenocarcinoma of the upper third of the stomach: a propensity-score-matched analysis of a multicenter western experience (on behalf of the Italian research Group for Gastric Cancer-GIRCG). Gastric Cancer. 2018;21(5):845–52.
26. Sun KK, Wu YY. Current status of laparoscopic proximal gastrectomy in proximal gastric cancer: technical details and oncologic outcomes. Asian J Surg. 2021;44(1):54–8.
27. Zhao L, Ling R, Chen J, et al. Clinical outcomes of proximal gastrectomy versus Total gastrectomy for

proximal gastric cancer: a systematic review and meta-analysis. Dig Surg. 2021b;38(1):1–13.
28. Du N, Wu P, Wang P, et al. Reconstruction methods and complications of Esophagogastrostomy and Jejunal interposition in proximal gastrectomy for gastric cancer: a meta-analysis. Gastroenterol Res Pract. 2020:8179254.
29. Wang W, Sun Z, Deng JY, et al. Integration and analysis of associated data in surgical treatment of gastric cancer based on multicenter, high volume databases Chinese. J Gastrointest Surg. 2016;19(2):179–85.
30. Chen ZF. Adenocarcinoma of the esophagogastric junction: epidemic trends, causes, prevention and therapy. Chinese J Pract Surg. 2012;32(4):267–70.
31. Rüdiger Siewert J, Feith M, Werner M, et al. Adenocarcinoma of the esophagogastric junction: results of surgical therapy based on anatomical/topographic classification in 1,002 consecutive patients. Ann Surg. 2000;232(3):353–61.
32. Anon. Japanese classification of gastric carcinoma: 3rd English edition. Gastric Cancer. 2011;14(2):101–12.
33. Amin MB, Edge S, Green FL, et al. AJCC cancer staging manual. 8th ed. New York: Springer; 2017.
34. Tang L, Li JZ. Radiological evaluation on invasive extent of adenocarcinoma of esophagogastric junction. Chin J Gastrointes Surg. 2019;22(2):119–25.
35. Yang SJ, Yuan Y, Hu HY, et al. Survival comparison of Siewert II adenocarcinoma of esophagogastric junction between transthoracic and transabdominal approaches: a joint data analysis of thoracic and gastrointestinal surgery. Chin J Gastrointes Surg. 2019;22(2):132–42.
36. De Boer AG, Van Lanschot JJ, Van Sandick JW, et al. Quality of life after transhiatal compared with extended transthoracic resection for adenocarcinoma of the esophagus. J Clin Oncol. 2004;22(20):4202–8.
37. Hulscher J, Van Sandick J, De Boer A, et al. Extended transthoracic resection compared with limited transhiatal resection for adenocarcinoma of the esophagus. N Engl J Med. 2002;347(21):1662–9.
38. Omloo J, Lagarde S, Hulscher J, et al. Extended transthoracic resection compared with limited transhiatal resection for adenocarcinoma of the mid/distal esophagus: five-year survival of a randomised clinical trial. N Engl J Med. 2007;246(6):992–1000; discussion 1000–1001.
39. Kurokawa Y, Sasako M, Sano T, et al. Ten-year follow-up results of a randomised clinical trial comparing left thoracoabdominal and abdominal transhiatal approaches to total gastrectomy for adenocarcinoma of the oesophagogastric junction or gastric cardia. Br J Surg. 2015;102(4):341–8.
40. Sasako M, Sano T, Yamamoto S, et al. Left thoracoabdominal approach versus abdominal-transhiatal approach for gastric cancer of the cardia or subcardia: a randomised controlled trial. Lancet Oncol. 2006a;7(8):644–51.
41. Nunobe S, Ohyama S, Sonoo H, et al. Benefit of mediastinal and Para-aortic lymph-node dissection for advanced gastric cancer with esophageal invasion. J Surg Oncol. 2008;97(5):392–5.
42. Guo CG, Tian YT. Controversy of surgical management for adenocarcinoma of esophagogastric junction. Chinese J Front Med Sci (Electronic Version). 2017;9(5):1–5.
43. Wang YK, Li ZY. Abdominal surgery for adenocarcinoma of esophagogastric junction. Int J Surg. 2020;47(8):510–3.
44. Pedrazzani C, De Manzoni G, Marrelli D, et al. Lymph node involvement in advanced gastroesophageal junction adenocarcinoma. J Thorac Cardiovascu Surg. 2007;134(2):378–85.
45. Multidisciplinary Union for Esophagogastric Junction Diseases of Chinese Society for Diseases of the Esophagus(CSDE; Laparoscopic Surgery Committee of the Endoscopist Branch in the Chinese Medical Doctor Association(CMDA; Upper Digestive Tract Surgeons Committee of the Surgeon Branch in the Chinese Medical Doctor Association(CMDA; Gastrointestinal Oncology Group of the Oncology Branch in the Chinese Medical Association(CM). Chinese expert consensus on the surgical treatment for adenocarcinoma of esophagogastric junction (2018 edition). Chin J Gastrointes Surg. 2018;21(9):961–75.
46. Sano T, Sasako M, Mizusawa J, et al. Randomised controlled trial to evaluate splenectomy in total gastrectomy for proximal gastric carcinoma. Ann Surg. 2017;265(2):277–83.
47. Chen L, Bian SB. Splenic hilar lymph node dissection should be performed selectively and individually. Chin J Gastrointes Surg, 2016, 19 (2): 172–173.
48. Tokunaga M, Ohyama S, Hiki N, et al. Endoscopic evaluation of reflux esophagitis after proximal gastrectomy: comparison between esophagogastric anastomosis and jejunal interposition. World J Surg. 2008;32(7):1473–7.
49. Das M. Neoadjuvant chemotherapy: survival benefit in gastric cancer. Lancet Oncol. 2017;18(6):e307.
50. Lulu Z, Dongbing Z, Yingtai C. Neoadjuvant therapy for locally advanced gastric cancer. Chin J Oncol. 2020;42(11):907–11.
51. Cats A, Jansen EPM, Van Grieken NCT, et al. Chemotherapy versus chemoradiotherapy after surgery and preoperative chemotherapy for resectable gastric cancer (CRITICS): an international, open-label, randomised phase 3 trial. Lancet Oncol. 2018;19(5):616–28.
52. Smyth EC, Wotherspoon A, Peckitt C, et al. Mismatch repair deficiency, microsatellite instability, and survival: an exploratory analysis of the Medical Research Council adjuvant gastric Infusional chemotherapy (MAGIC) trial. JAMA Oncol. 2017;3(9):1197–203.
53. Ychou M, Boige V, Pignon JP, et al. Perioperative chemotherapy compared with surgery alone for resectable gastroesophageal adenocarcinoma: an FNCLCC and FFCD multicenter phase III trial. J Clin Oncol. 2011;29(13):1715–21.

54. Al-Batran S-E, Homann N, Pauligk C, et al. Perioperative chemotherapy with fluorouracil plus leucovorin, oxaliplatin, and docetaxel versus fluorouracil or capecitabine plus cisplatin and epirubicin for locally advanced, resectable gastric or gastro-oesophageal junction adenocarcinoma (FLOT4): a randomised, phase 2/3 trial. Lancet. 2019;393(10184):1948–57.
55. National comprehensive cancer network. NCCN clinical practice guidelines in oncology (NCCN guidelines *): gastric cancer (version 1. 2020). 2020.
56. Kinoshita T, Sasako M, Sano T, et al. Phase II trial of S-1 for neoadjuvant chemotherapy against scirrhous gastric cancer (JCOG 0002). Gastric Cancer. 2009;12(1):37–42.
57. Iwasaki Y, Sasako M, Yamamoto S, et al. Phase II study of preoperative chemotherapy with S-1 and cisplatin followed by gastrectomy for clinically resectable type 4 and large type 3 gastric cancers (JCOG0210). J Surg Oncol. 2013;107(7):741–5.
58. Terashima M, Iwasaki Y, Mizusawa J, et al. Randomized phase III trial of gastrectomy with or without neoadjuvant S-1 plus cisplatin for type 4 or large type 3 gastric cancer, the short-term safety and surgical results: Japan clinical oncology group study (JCOG0501). Gastric Cancer. 2019;22(5):1044–52.
59. Yoshikawa T, Sasako M, Yamamoto S, et al. Phase II study of neoadjuvant chemotherapy and extended surgery for locally advanced gastric cancer. Br J Surg. 2009;96(9):1015–22.
60. Chinese Society of Clinical Oncology Guidelines Working Committee. Chinese Society of Clinical Oncology (CSCO) gastric cancer diagnosis and treatment guidelines (2020). Beijing People's Health Publishing House. 2020;3:1–175.
61. Endo S, Imano M, Furukawa H, et al. Phase II study of preoperative radiotherapy combined with S-1 plus cisplatin in clinically resectable type 4 or large type 3 gastric cancer: OGSG1205. Ann Oncol. 2019:30.
62. Zhang X, Liang H, Li Z, et al. Perioperative or postoperative adjuvant oxaliplatin with S-1 versus adjuvant oxaliplatin with capecitabine in patients with locally advanced gastric or gastro-oesophageal junction adenocarcinoma undergoing D2 gastrectomy (RESOLVE): an open-label, superiority and non-inferiority, phase 3 randomised controlled trial. Lancet Oncol. 2021;22(8):1081–92.
63. Zhang ZX, Gu XZ, Yin WB, et al. Randomized clinical trial on the combination of preoperative irradiation and surgery in the treatment of adenocarcinoma of gastric cardia (AGC)—report on 370 patients. Int J Radiat Oncol Biol Phys. 1998;42(5):929–34.
64. Van Hagen P, Hulshof MC, Van Lanschot JJ, et al. Preoperative chemoradiotherapy for esophageal or junctional cancer. N Engl J Med. 2012;366(22):2074–84.
65. Stahl M, Walz MK, Stuschke M, et al. Phase III comparison of preoperative chemotherapy compared with Chemoradiotherapy in patients with locally advanced adenocarcinoma of the Esophagogastric junction. J Clin Oncol. 2009;27(6):851–6.
66. Burmeister BH, Thomas JM, Burmeister EA, et al. Is concurrent radiation therapy required in patients receiving preoperative chemotherapy for adenocarcinoma of the oesophagus? A randomised phase II trial. Eur J Cancer. 2011;47(3):354–60.
67. Pentheroudakis G. Recent eUpdates to the ESMO clinical practice guidelines on hepatocellular carcinoma, cancer of the pancreas, soft tissue and visceral sarcomas, cancer of the prostate and gastric cancer. Ann Oncol. 2019;30(8):1395–7.
68. Bang YJ, Van Cutsem E, Feyereislova A, et al. Trastuzumab in combination with chemotherapy versus chemotherapy alone for treatment of HER2-positive advanced gastric or gastro-oesophageal junction cancer (ToGA): a phase 3, open-label, randomised controlled trial. Lancet. 2010;376(9742):687–97.
69. Ma J, Yao S, Li XS, et al. Neoadjuvant therapy of DOF regimen plus bevacizumab can increase surgical resection rate in locally advanced gastric cancer: a randomized, controlled study. Medicine (Baltimore). 2015;94(42):e1489.
70. Cunningham D, Stenning SP, Smyth EC, et al. Peri-operative chemotherapy with or without bevacizumab in operable oesophagogastric adenocarcinoma (UK medical research council ST03): primary analysis results of a multicentre, open-label, randomised phase 2-3 trial. Lancet Oncol. 2017;18(3):357–70.
71. Zheng Y, Yang X, Yan C, et al. Effect of apatinib plus neoadjuvant chemotherapy followed by resection on pathologic response in patients with locally advanced gastric adenocarcinoma: a single-arm, open-label, phase II trial. Eur J Cancer. 2020;130:12–9.
72. Kang YK, Boku N, Satoh T, et al. Nivolumab in patients with advanced gastric or gastro-oesophageal junction cancer refractory to, or intolerant of, at least two previous chemotherapy regimens (ONO-4538-12, ATTRACTION-2): a randomised, double-blind, placebo-controlled, phase 3 trial. Lancet. 2017;390(10111):2461–71.
73. Chen LT, Satoh T, Ryu MH, et al. A phase 3 study of nivolumab in previously treated advanced gastric or gastroesophageal junction cancer (ATTRACTION-2): 2-year update data. Gastric Cancer. 2020;23(3):510–9.
74. Bang YJ, Ruiz EY, Van Cutsem E, et al. Phase III, randomised trial of avelumab versus physician's choice of chemotherapy as third-line treatment of patients with advanced gastric or gastro-oesophageal junction cancer: primary analysis of JAVELIN gastric 300. Ann Oncol. 2018;29(10):2052–60.
75. Vrána D, Matzenauer M, Neoral Č, et al. From tumor immunology to immunotherapy in gastric and esophageal cancer. Int J Mol Sci. 2018;20(1).
76. Yu Y, Ma X, Zhang Y, et al. Changes in expression of multiple checkpoint molecules and infiltration of

tumor immune cells after Neoadjuvant chemotherapy in gastric cancer. J Cancer. 2019;10(12):2754–63.

77. Peritoneal Tumor Professional Committee of Chinese Anti-Cancer Association, Professional Committee of Tumor Hyperthermia of Guangdong provincial Anticancer Association. Expert consensus on clinical application of intraperitoneal perfusion chemotherapy technology in China (2019 version). National Med J China. 2020;100(2):89–96.
78. Spratt J, Adcock R, Muskovin M, et al. Clinical delivery system for intraperitoneal hyperthermic chemotherapy. Cancer Res. 1980;40(2):256–60.
79. He JM, Pu YD, Cao ZY, et al. Clinical study of detectable rate of intra-abdominal free cancer cells and Hyperthermic peritoneal perfusion chemotherapy of patients with gastric cancer. Chin J Base Clin Gen Surg. 2002;9(3):156–8.
80. Cui SZ, Ba MC, Tang HS. Changes and prospects of intraperitoneal hyperthermic perfusion chemotherapy. Chin J Clin. 2011;05(7):2039–42.
81. Cui SZ, Ba MC, Huang DW, et al. Animal experiment on the safety evaluation of BR-TRG-I body cavity thermal perfusion therapy system. Chin J Comp Med. 2009;19(10):27–31.
82. Lu Z, Wang J, Wientjes M, et al. Intraperitoneal therapy for peritoneal cancer. Future Oncol. 2010;6(10):1625–41.
83. Jacquet P, Sugarbaker P. Clinical research methodologies in diagnosis and staging of patients with peritoneal carcinomatosis. Cancer Treat Res. 1996;82:359–74.
84. Yoo C, Noh S, Shin D, et al. Recurrence following curative resection for gastric carcinoma. Br J Surg. 2000;87(2):236–42.
85. Bonnot P, Piessen G, Kepenekian V, et al. Cytoreductive surgery with or without Hyperthermic intraperitoneal chemotherapy for gastric cancer with peritoneal metastases (CYTO-CHIP study): a propensity score analysis. J Clin Oncol. 2019;37(23):2028–40.
86. Chen RY, Zhang L, Liu W. Effect of intraperitoneal hyperthermic perfusion chemotherapy on postoperative gastrointestinal function recovery in patients with gastric cancer. Chin J Curr Adv Gen Surg. 2017;20(6):458–9.
87. Hong YN, Pang HX, Zhu JF, et al. Clinical effect of hyperthermic intraperitoneal chemotherapy combined with intravenous chemotherapy in elderly gastric carcinoma patients complicated with malignant ascites. Jilin Med J. 2016;37(11):2645–7.
88. Wang QC, Qu ZY, Zhang H, et al. Clinical effect of intraperitoneal hyperthermic perfusion combined with systemic chemotherapy after radical resection of gastric cancer. Chongqing Medicine. 2017;46(15):2134–7.
89. Lemoine L, Sugarbaker P, Van Der Speeten K. Drugs, doses, and durations of intraperitoneal chemotherapy: standardising HIPEC and EPIC for colorectal, appendiceal, gastric, ovarian peritoneal surface malignancies and peritoneal mesothelioma. IntJ Hyperthermia. 2017;33(5):582–92.
90. Liao GQ, Qu YM, Wang HM, et al. Clinical research on continuous Hyperthermic perfusion in the treatment of peritoneal effusion induced by gastric carcinoma. Chin J Clin Oncol. 2012;39(8):452–4.
91. Aziz M, Kasi A. Krukenberg tumor. In: StatPearls. Treasure Island, FL: StatPearls Publishing; 2021.
92. Sobin LH. The international histological classification of tumours. Bull World Health Organ. 1981;59(6):813–9.
93. Wang J, Shi YK, Wu LY, et al. Prognostic factors for ovarian metastases from primary gastric cancer. Int J Gynecol Cancer. 2008;18(4):825–32.
94. Lionetti R, De Luca M, Travaglino A, et al. Treatments and overall survival in patients with Krukenberg tumor. Arch Gynecol Obstet. 2019;300(1):15–23.
95. Sodek KL, Murphy KJ, Brown TJ, et al. Cell-cell and cell-matrix dynamics in intraperitoneal cancer metastasis. Cancer Metastasis Rev. 2012;31(1–2):397–414.
96. Yoshida M, Sugino T, Kusafuka K, et al. Peritoneal dissemination in early gastric cancer: importance of the lymphatic route. Virchows Arch. 2016;469(2):155–61.
97. Al-Agha OM, Nicastri AD. An in-depth look at Krukenberg tumor: an overview. Arch Pathol Lab Med. 2006;130(11):1725–30.
98. Young RH. From krukenberg to today: the ever present problems posed by metastatic tumors in the ovary: part I. Historical perspective, general principles, mucinous tumors including the krukenberg tumor. Adv Anat Pathol. 2006;13(5):205–27.
99. Agnes A, Biondi A, Ricci R, et al. Krukenberg tumors: seed, route and soil. Surg Oncol. 2017;26(4):438–45.
100. Yook JH, Oh ST, Kim BS. Clinical prognostic factors for ovarian metastasis in women with gastric cancer. Hepato-Gastroenterology. 2007;54(75):955–9.
101. Yamanishi Y, Koshiyama M, Ohnaka M, et al. Pathways of metastases from primary organs to the ovaries. Obstet Gynecol Int. 2011;2011:612817.
102. Chinese Society of Clinical Oncology Guidelines Working Committee. Chinese Society of Clinical Oncology (CSCO) gastric cancer diagnosis and treatment guidelines (2018.V1). Beijing People's Medical Publishing House; 2018. p. 1–129.
103. Brieau B, Auzolle C, Pozet A, et al. Efficacy of modern chemotherapy and prognostic factors in patients with ovarian metastases from gastric cancer: a retrospective AGEO multicentre study. Dig Liver Dis. 2016;48(4):441–5.
104. National Comprehensive Cancer Network. NCCN clinical practice guidelines in oncology (nccnguidelines *): gastric cancer (version 1. 2020). 2020.
105. Japanese gastric cancer treatment guidelines 2018 (5th edition). Gastric Cancer. 2021;24(1):1–21.
106. Bozzetti F, Yu W, Baratti D, et al. Locoregional treatment of peritoneal carcinomatosis from gastric cancer. J Surg Oncol. 2008;98(4):273–6.

107. Wu XJ, Yuan P, Li ZY, et al. Cytoreductive surgery and hyperthermic intraperitoneal chemotherapy improves the survival of gastric cancer patients with ovarian metastasis and peritoneal dissemination. Tumour Biol. 2013;34(1):463–9.
108. Kodera Y, Fujitani K, Fukushima N, et al. Surgical resection of hepatic metastasis from gastric cancer: a review and new recommendation in the Japanese gastric cancer treatment guidelines. Gastric Cancer. 2014;17(2):206–12.
109. Fujitani K, Yang HK, Mizusawa J, et al. Gastrectomy plus chemotherapy versus chemotherapy alone for advanced gastric cancer with a single non-curable factor (REGATTA): a phase 3, randomised controlled trial. Lancet Oncol. 2016;17(3):309–18.
110. Jiyang L, Kecheng Z, Yunhe G, et al. Stomach cancer Chinese expert consensus on diagnosis and comprehensive treatment of liver metastases (2019 edition). Chin J Pract Surg. 2019;39(05):405–11.
111. Chinese Society of Clinical Oncology Guidelines Working Committee. Chinese Society of Clinical Oncology (CSCO) gastric cancer diagnosis and treatment guidelines (2020). Beijing People's Health Publishing House; 2020. p. 1–175.
112. Japanese Gastric Cancer Association. Japanese gastric cancer treatment Guidelines 2018 (5th edition). Gastric Cancer. 2021;24(1):1–21.
113. Morita S, Fukagawa T, Fujiwara H, et al. The clinical significance of Para-aortic nodal dissection for advanced gastric cancer. Eur J Surg Oncol. 2016;42(9):1448–54.
114. Sasako M, Sano T, Yamamoto S, et al. D2 lymphadenectomy alone or with Para-aortic nodal dissection for gastric cancer. N Engl J Med. 2008;359(5):453–62.
115. Katayama H, Ito S, Sano T, et al. A phase II study of systemic chemotherapy with docetaxel, cisplatin, and S-1 (DCS) followed by surgery in gastric cancer patients with extensive lymph node metastasis: Japan clinical oncology group study JCOG1002. Jpn J Clin Oncol. 2012;42(6):556–9.
116. Tsuburaya A, Mizusawa J, Tanaka Y, et al. Neoadjuvant chemotherapy with S-1 and cisplatin followed by D2 gastrectomy with Para-aortic lymph node dissection for gastric cancer with extensive lymph node metastasis. Br J Surg. 2014;101(6):653–60.
117. Wang Y, Yu YY, Li W, et al. A phase II trial of Xeloda and oxaliplatin (XELOX) neo-adjuvant chemotherapy followed by surgery for advanced gastric cancer patients with para-aortic lymph node metastasis. Cancer Chemother Pharmacol. 2014;73(6):1155–61.
118. Yoshida K, Yamaguchi K, Okumura N, et al. Is conversion therapy possible in stage IV gastric cancer: the proposal of new biological categories of classification. Gastric Cancer. 2016;19(2):329–38.

MIX
Papier aus verantwortungsvollen Quellen
Paper from responsible sources
FSC® C105338

If you have any concerns about our products, you can contact us on
ProductSafety@springernature.com

In case Publisher is established outside the EU, the EU authorized representative is:
Springer Nature Customer Service Center GmbH
Europaplatz 3, 69115 Heidelberg, Germany

Printed by Libri Plureos GmbH
in Hamburg, Germany